# Minimally Invasive Approaches to Pediatric Urology

To Anne, Katherine, William, Madeline and Danny

# Minimally Invasive Approaches to Pediatric Urology

**Edited by**

**Steven G Docimo MD**
*Division of Pediatric Urology*
*The Children's Hospital of Pittsburgh*
*The University of Pittsburgh Medical Center*
*Pittsburgh, PA 15213*
*USA*

**informa**
healthcare

New York  London

First published in 2005 by Taylor & Francis, an imprint of the Taylor & Francis Group.
This edition published in 2011 by Informa Healthcare, Telephone House, 69-77 Paul Street, London EC2A 4LQ, UK.

Simultaneously published in the USA by Informa Healthcare, 52 Vanderbilt Avenue, 7th Floor, New York, NY 10017, USA.

Informa Healthcare is a trading division of Informa UK Ltd. Registered Office: 37–41 Mortimer Street, London W1T 3JH, UK. Registered in England and Wales number 1072954.

A CIP record for this book is available from the British Library.

ISBN-13: 9781841845395

Orders may be sent to: Informa Healthcare, Sheepen Place, Colchester, Essex CO3 3LP, UK
Telephone: +44 (0)20 7017 5540
Email: CSDhealthcarebooks@informa.com
Website: http://informahealthcarebooks.com/

For corporate sales please contact: CorporateBooksIHC@informa.com
For foreign rights please contact: RightsIHC@informa.com
For reprint permissions please contact: PermissionsIHC@informa.com

Typeset by J&L Composition, Filey, North Yorkshire

Printed and bound by CPI Group (UK) Ltd, Croydon, CR0 4YY
Transferred to Digital Print 2012

# Contents

# Contributors

**David M Albala** MD
Professor of Urology
Head, Section of Minimally Invasive Urological Surgery
Duke University Medical Center
Durham, North Carolina
USA

**Brian K Auge** MD
Lieutenant Commander, Medical Corps
United States Navy Assistant
Professor of Surgery (Urology)
Naval Medical Center San Diego
San Diego, California
USA

**Linda A Baker** MD
Associate Professor of Urology
Director of Pediatric Urology Research
University of Texas Southwestern Medical Center at
Dallas
Department of Urology
5323 Harry Hines Boulevard
Dallas, TX 75390–9110
USA

**Jay T Bishoff** MD
Wilford Hall Medical Center
Department of Urology/MCSU
Lackland AFB, TX 78236
USA

**Victor Braren** MD FACS FAAP
Mid-South Pediatric Urology PC
Meharry & Vanderbilt Medical Schools
329 Twenty-first Av N
Nashville, TN 37203
USA

**Paolo Caione**
Head, Division of Pediatric Urology
'Bambino Gesù' Children's Hospital
Piazza S. Onofrio 4
00165 Rome
Italy

**Patrick C Cartwright** MD
Professor of Surgery and Pediatrics
University of Utah
Primary Children's Medical Center
Salt Lake City, Utah
USA

**Lars Cisek** MD
Texas Children's Hospital
Assistant Professor of Urology
Baylor College of Medicine
Scott Department of Urology
6560 Fannin, Suite 2100
Houston, Texas 77030
USA

**Michael J Conlin** MD FACS
Division of Urology
Oregon Health & Science University
3181 SW Sam Jackson Park Road L588
Portland
Oregon 97239
USA

**David Cuellar** MD
Department of Urology
The University of Pittsburgh School of Medicine
Pittsburgh, PA 15213
USA

**Steven G Docimo** MD
Professor and Director
Division of Pediatric Urology
The Children's Hospital of Pittsburgh
The University of Pittsburgh Medical Center
Pittsburgh, PA 15213
USA

**Alaa El-Ghoneimi** MD PhD
Professor of Pediatric Surgery
Consultant in Uro-Genital Pediatric Surgery
Department of Pediatric Surgery and Urology
Hôpital Robert Debré
48 Boulvard Sérurier
75019 Paris
France

**Michael J Erhard** MD
Nemours Children's Clinic
807 Children's Way
Jacksonville
FL 32207
USA

**Stephen V Jackman** MD
Associate Professor of Urology
University of Pittsburgh Medical Center
Pittsburgh, PA 15213
USA

**Gerald H Jordan** MD
University of Texas Southwestern Medical Center at Dallas
Children's Medical Center of Dallas
Dallas, TX 75390–9110
USA

**Thomas F Kolon** MD FAAP
The Children's Hospital of Philadelphia
Pediatric Urology
34ᵗʰ Street & Civic Center Boulevard
Robert Wood Johnson Center, 3ʳᵈ Floor
Philadelphia, PA 19104
USA

**Jaime Landman** MD
Assistant Professor
Division of Urology
Washington University
St. Louis, MO
USA

**Armando Lorenzo** MD
University of Texas Southwestern Medical Center at Dallas
Children's Medical Center of Dallas
Dallas, TX 75390–9110
USA

**Salvatore Micali** MD
Assistant Professor
Department of Urology
University of Modena and Reggio
Emilia
Italy

**John G Pattaras** MD
Assistant Professor
Department of Urology
Emory University
Atlanta, GA
USA

**Craig A Peters** MD FACS FAAP
Department of Urology
Children's Hospital
300 Longwood Avenue
Boston, MA 02115
USA

**Todd Renschler** MD
University of Utah
Salt Lake City, Utah
USA

**William Roberts** MD
The Johns Hopkins University School of Medicine
Brady Urological Institute
USA

**Brent W Snow** MD
Professor of Surgery and Pediatrics
University of Utah
Primary Children's Medical Center
Salt Lake City, Utah
USA

**J Stuart Wolf Jr** MD
University of Michigan, Department of Urology
1500 East Medical Center Drive
Ann Arbor
MI 48109
USA

# Preface

Pediatric urology has been at the forefront of endoscopic surgery since the advent of ureteroscopy and valve ablation. Despite this, complex minimally invasive procedures have been relatively slow to permeate our field. This is natural, since we tend to be protective of the child and the procedural outcome. If this tendency slows our progress, it enhances the thoughtfulness and elegance of the procedures we eventually adopt. The authors who contributed to this volume represent that thoughtfulness. All are pioneers and early adapters, but with an eye toward minimizing risk to their young patients. The applications and techniques represented here are a snapshot in time; the evolution of this field is rapid. This volume will be useful to both trainees and seasoned practitioners as a guide to established approaches, but will hopefully also serve as inspiration to those who have the creativity to envision tomorrow's techniques. Understanding that we did not get to this point in a vacuum, we have invited colleagues at the forefront of adult endourology to supply background material related to the anatomy, physiology and instrumentation of minimally invasive surgery.

I would like to acknowledge the efforts of Robert Moore, Stefan Loening and Jay Bishoff, without whose work and encouragement this volume would not exist. I would also like to thank my publisher Alan Burgess for the opportunity and technical expertise to succeed.

*Steven G Docimo MD*
*Pittsburgh PA*
*January 2005*

# 1

# Endourology surgical anatomy*

Brian K Auge and David M Albala

## Introduction

Endourology has come to the forefront of urologic surgery for the management of various stone and noncalculous conditions. With this, an increasing number of urologists are performing routine and complex endourologic procedures, all of which have the potential for significant patient morbidity. Understanding the anatomy and anatomic relationships of the urinary tract is, therefore, vital to minimizing complications and maximizing success rates. This chapter describes the basic anatomy of the male and female urinary systems and the relationships of urologic organs to surrounding structures. In addition, common congenital anomalies are discussed, with a focus on implications during endourologic procedures.

## Urethra

The urethra serves as a conduit for emptying of the urinary bladder and spans a distance from the bladder neck to the urethral meatus. Both male and female urethras are divided into sections with distinct landmarks. Due to the length of the urethra and the presence of the prostate gland, these landmarks are more prominent in men.

The male urethra can be divided into two distinct areas: the anterior and posterior portions. These areas are separated by the external striated sphincter or urogenital diaphragm (Figure 1.1), through which the membranous urethra traverses. The anterior urethra begins at the urethral meatus and is lined by squamous epithelium at its most distal extent, with transitional epithelium lining most of the remainder of the urethra. The fossa navicularis is a landmark within the glans penis, a point at which urethral strictures commonly occur. The penile, or pendulous, urethra is located within the shaft of the penis and contains the anteriorly located openings to

the ducts of Littre (Figure 1.2). These ducts drain the small periurethral mucous glands. The bulbar urethra is a dilated portion of the anterior urethra, beginning approximately at the level of the suspensory ligament of the penis. The bulbar urethra lies within the bulb of the penis, surrounded by bulbocavernosus muscle, and ends at the distal portion of the external sphincter. The most common location for a traumatic urethral stricture is the bulbar urethra, as seen in the retrograde urethrogram shown in Figure 1.3.

The posterior urethra progresses from this location proximally to the bladder neck and is covered with transitional epithelium that is similar to that in the remainder of the collecting system. Frequently, during endoscopic procedures using local anesthesia, the sphincter may take on a diaphragm-like appearance. The prostatic urethra will vary in length and appearance depending on patient age and degree of benign prostatic hyperplasia. The verumontanum defines the apical aspect of the prostatic urethra (see Figure 1.3), with the ejaculatory ducts situated on the lateral surface of the verumontanum. As patients age, the lateral lobes of the prostate will encroach upon the urethral lumen, potentially contributing to bladder outlet obstruction. Occasionally, a median lobe or median bar will be encountered, distorting the location of the ureteral orifices and causing J-hooking of the distal ureter. This J-hooking can result in significant difficulty in catheterizing the ureteral orifice when retrograde procedures are performed, and can make visualization of the ureteral orifices difficult when transurethral resections of the prostate are performed.

The female urethra is located within the anterior vaginal wall and is significantly shorter than the male urethra, a characteristic possibly contributing to the higher incidence of stress urinary incontinence and infections in women. Inspection of the female urethra begins at the introitus. Placement of the endoscope into the urethra must be

* The views expressed in this chapter are those of the authors and do not reflect the official policy of the United States Navy, Department of Defense, or U.S. Government.

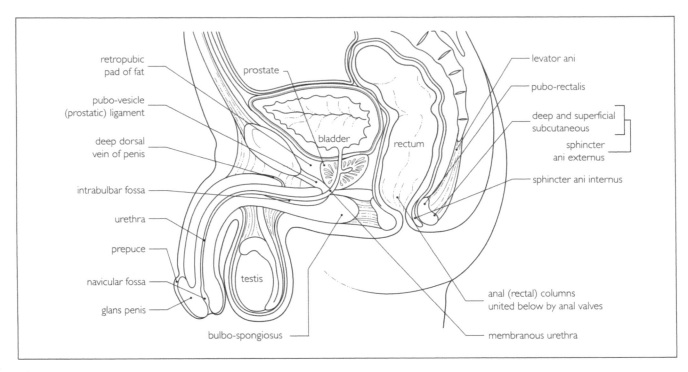

**Figure 1.1**
Sketch of the male pelvis, in median section. The external urinary sphincter separates the anterior urethra (distally) from the posterior urethra (proximally). The membranous urethra traverses the external sphincter.

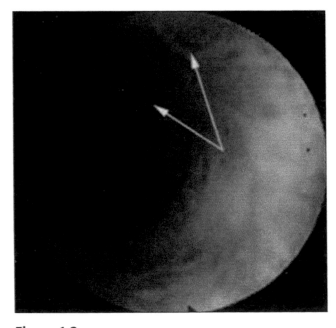

**Figure 1.2**
Endoscopic view of the anterior urethra, depicting the ducts of Littre, indicated by the arrows.

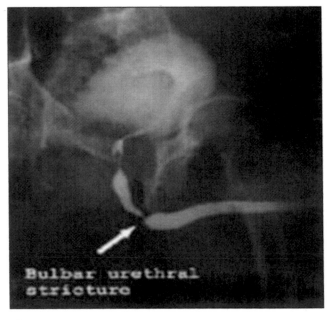

**Figure 1.3**
Retrograde urethrogram demonstrating a bulbar urethral stricture (arrow) secondary to a straddle injury to the perineum. Notice the narrowing of the striated sphincter proximal to the stricture, and the filling defect of the verumontanum.

accurate to avoid inadvertent vaginal endoscopy. The pink coapted appearance of the urethral mucosa and pale squamous appearance of the vagina enable the endoscopist to readily recognize proper positioning. The anterior and posterior components of the female urethra are distinct entities, yet less well defined. Again, these are separated by the urogenital diaphragm as in the male counterpart (Figure 1.4). Coaptation of the folded urethra mucosa gives the female urethra a diaphragm-like appearance from the meatus to the bladder neck (Figure 1.5). Urethral diverticula develop, occasionally, most commonly in a posterior or posterolateral orientation. Calculi can occasionally be seen if the orifice is open to endoscopic inspection (Figure 1.6).

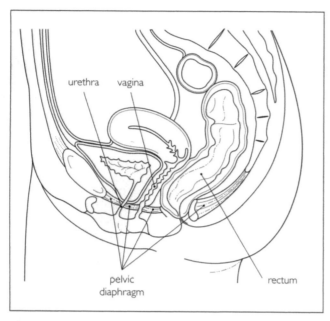

**Figure 1.4**
Anatomic relationships of the lower female urinary tract to surrounding structures.

# Urinary bladder

The urinary bladder is a hollow organ with two basic functions: to store urine at low pressures and to empty urine completely on demand once capacity is reached. The bladder is composed of several smooth muscle layers: an outer serosal membrane and an inner 'mucosa', or lining of transitional epithelium. It is located extraperitoneally within the pelvis, with the uterus causing an extrinsic compression on the dome due to the cephalad position of the body of the uterus in relation to the bladder (see Figure 1.4). When fully distended, the bladder is palpable in most people. The bladder in an adult, when filled to capacity, holds approximately 350–500 ml of urine under normal conditions.

The ureteral orifices in their normal position are located on the floor of the bladder in a triangular area known as the trigone (Figures 1.7A and 1.7B), so named for its configuration with the ureteral orifices comprising the base of the triangle and the bladder neck serving as

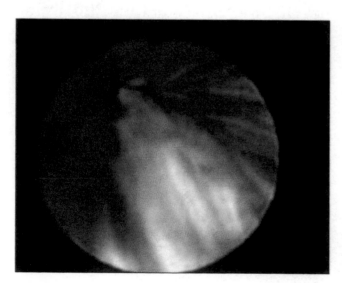

**Figure 1.5**
Endoscopic view of the female urethra. Noted the coapted folded appearance of the highly vascular mucosa.

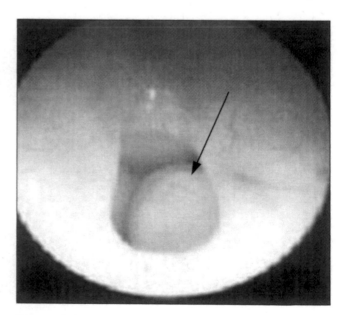

**Figure 1.6**
Urethral diverticulum with wide-open orifice and calculi (arrow) within the diverticulum. Urethral diverticula can cause symptoms of dysuria, dyspareunia and discharge or post-void dribbling, among others.

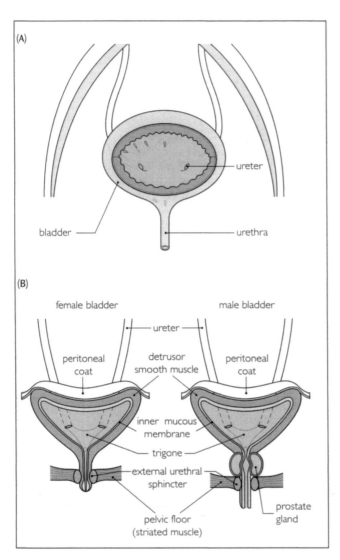

**Figure 1.7A**
Schematic of the pelvic organs with the ureteral orifices, labeled ureter, located within the bladder on the trigone.
**Figure 1.7B**
Comparison of the male and female urinary bladder.

the apex of the triangle. As the endoscope is passed into the bladder through the bladder neck, the scope must be directed laterally and posteriorly to identify the orifices. As mentioned previously, a large prostate can displace the ureteral orifices, especially when a large median lobe is encountered. Similarly, previous transurethral resection of the prostate or open pelvic surgery may have altered the anatomy. In a partially distended bladder, one can recognize the intertrigonal ridge connecting the two ureteral orifices.

The bladder is in close approximation to several important organs within the pelvis. The peritoneum and a portion of the intraperitoneal contents, namely the bowel, sit on the dome of the bladder. The uterus may slightly compress the cephalad portion of the bladder, which can be seen on plain film imaging. An obturator 'kick' can develop as a rapid and unexpected contraction of the adductor leg muscles when the obturator nerve is stimulated during resection of a lateral wall bladder tumor. The rectum is adjacent to the posterior bladder surface in a male, and the anterior vaginal wall is interposed between the bladder and rectum in the female pelvis.

# Ureter

The intrarenal collecting system is joined to the urinary bladder by the ureter, a completely retroperitoneal tubular structure (Figure 1.8). This is composed of both circular and longitudinal muscle fibers that enable the ureter to transport urine by peristalsis. The inner lining of transitional epithelium prevents absorption of fluid and electrolytes in the usual healthy state. Three natural points of narrowing exist: the ureteropelvic junction (UPJ), the ureterovesical junction (UVJ), and where the ureter crosses the common iliac vessels in the mid ureter. Urinary calculi will typically obstruct at one of these three locations if unable to pass spontaneously (Figure 1.9). Transitional cell carcinoma of the ureter can occur anywhere along the length of the ureter (Figure 1.10).

The ureter exits the renal pelvis at approximately the level of vertebral body L2. It proceeds vertically in the retroperitoneum along the lateral aspect of the transverse processes of the lower lumbar vertebrae to the sacrum. The ureter follows a path along the dorsal aspect of the retroperitoneum, crossing over the sacrum at the sacroiliac joint and into the true pelvis. Once in the pelvis, the ureter will course medially to enter the bladder just cephalad to the ischial spines. Figure 1.11 demonstrates these relationships as seen on intravenous urogram (A) and retrograde pyelogram (B).

Ureteropelvic junction obstruction (Figure 1.12), resulting in dilation of the renal pelvis and calyces with increased intrarenal pressures, can lead to renal insufficiency, calculus formation, recurrent infection, hematuria, and chronic pain. Causative factors include an aperistaltic segment of ureter, high insertion of the ureter on the renal pelvis, and crossing lower pole vessels, arteries, veins, or both (Figure 1.13). The location of the crossing vessels should be identified before an endopyelotomy is performed in order to avoid injury to these structures. Imaging modalities commonly utilized include computed tomography (CT) angiogram with three-dimensional reconstruction, endoluminal ultrasound (Figure 1.14), or, less commonly, plain angiography.

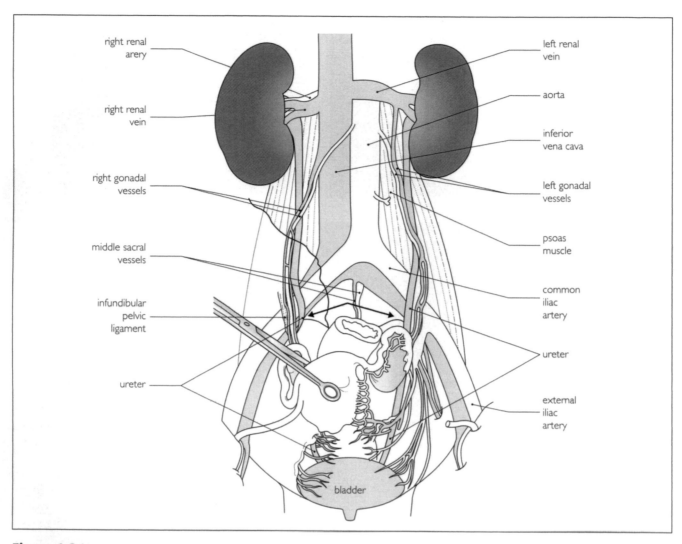

**Figure 1.8**
Diagram of the retroperitoneal organs. Note the ureters as they cross over the common iliac arteries (arrows) and then dive deep into the pelvis to enter the bladder posteriorly at the trigone (not shown).

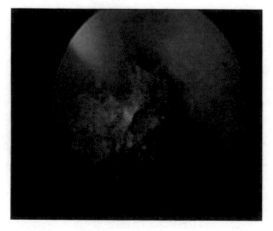

**Figure 1.9**
Endoscopic view of a calculus within the ureter being broken with the laser.

# Intrarenal collecting system

The kidneys are situated within the retroperitoneum encompassed by Gerota's fascia. They are oriented so that the lateral aspect of the kidney is rotated posteriorly. The intrarenal collecting system consists of the renal pelvis and calyces, lined with transitional epithelium. The normal urine volume for a calyx ranges from 2.5 to 5 ml (Figure 1.15). The renal pelvis is the structure most posterior to the renal hilum, with the renal artery situated between the vein (anterior) and pelvis. The 10–15 calyces divided between upper pole, lower pole, and mid-polar regions are oriented in an anterior and posterior direction. This is important for obtaining percutaneous access, which typically is reached through a posterior route to avoid intra-abdominal

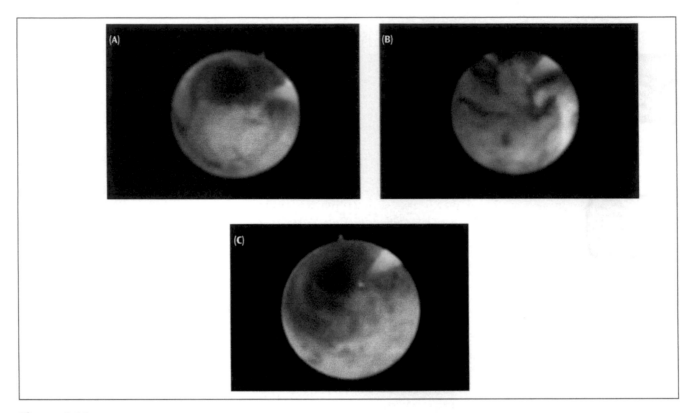

**Figure 1.10**
Intraluminal transitional cell carcinoma of the ureter amenable to holmium laser ablation: tumor prior to (A), during (B), and after (C) laser ablation.

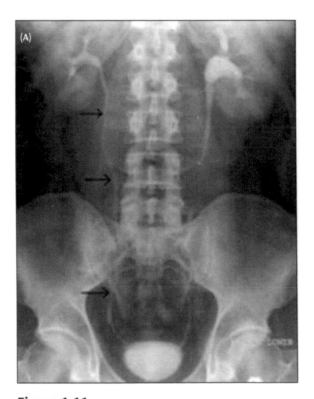
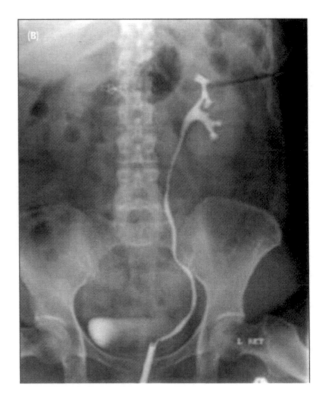

**Figure 1.11**
Intravenous urogram (A) and retrograde pyelogram (B) delineating the normal radiographic appearance and pathway of the ureter from the renal pelvis to the bladder.

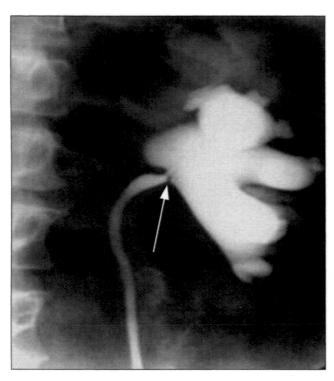

**Figure 1.12**
Left ureteropelvic junction obstruction. The ureter is of normal caliber and the intrarenal collecting system is markedly dilated proximal to the stricture.

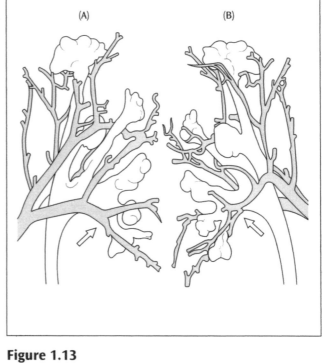

**Figure 1.13**
Casts of the intrarenal collecting system and vasculature demonstrating lower pole crossing vessels both ventrally (A) and dorsally (B).

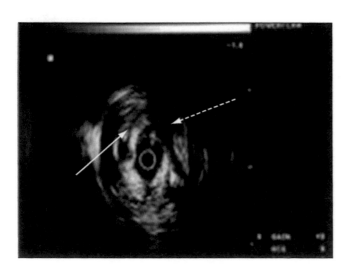

**Figure 1.14**
Endoluminal ultrasound revealing crossing vessels at the ureteropelvic junction. Large arrow indicates ureteral lumen and dashed arrow localizes the crossing vessel.

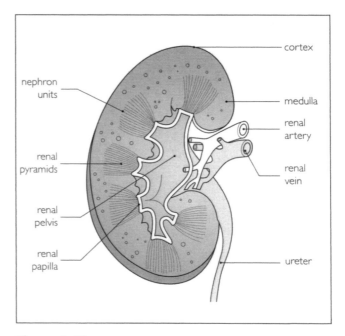

**Figure 1.15**
Schematic of intrarenal collecting system and vasculature of the renal hilum. The renal vein is the most anterior structure, followed by the renal artery and renal pelvis.

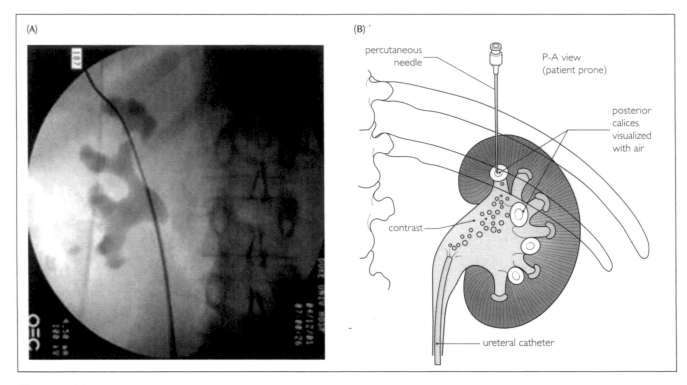

**Figure 1.16**
Percutaneous access is obtained through a posterior calyx with the patient in the prone position.

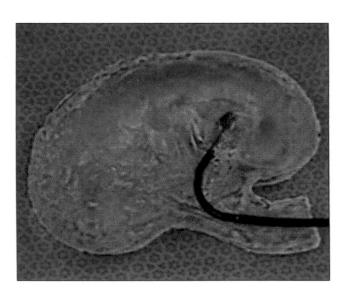

**Figure 1.17**
Plastic model of the renal collecting system demonstrating the ability of the flexible ureteroscope to access calculi within the lower pole.

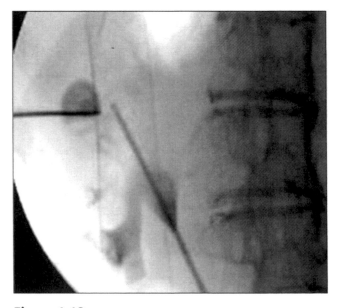

**Figure 1.18**
Access into a calyceal diverticulum can prove to be difficult in manipulating a wire through the stenotic infundibulum to achieve transureteral access.

contents (Figure 1.16). In both the upper and lower pole of the kidney are complex calyces, whereas the mid portion of the kidney has only simple calyces.

With the advent of the actively deflectable flexible ureteroscopes, complete inspection of the intrarenal collecting system can be performed routinely without much difficulty. Pathology not previously accessible not only can be visualized but also can be managed with lasers, baskets, or graspers (Figure 1.17). Stenosis of the infundibulum draining a calyx can lead to diverticulum formation and subsequent calculus formation, intermittent pain, hematuria, or infection (Figure 1.18). Difficulty can be experienced in attempting to access this stenotic infundibulum either from an antegrade or retrograde approach.

## Summary

A complete and clear understanding of the anatomic relationships of the parts of the urinary tract is necessary for performance of efficient and effective endourologic procedures. Knowledge of the various permutations, from both a radiologic and endoscopic point of view, is invaluable in allowing the urologist to perform these procedures safely.

# 2

# Urologic laparoscopic anatomy

Jaime Landman and John G Pattaras

## Introduction

The breadth of urologic pathology that can be managed via the laparoscopic approach continues to expand as technologies and surgical experience mature. Mounting evidence has demonstrated that for many urologic procedures pathology can be managed efficiently and effectively while significantly decreasing the pain and convalescence traditionally associated with ablative and reconstructive open urologic procedures.

The blossoming of laparoscopic surgery within urology has resulted in some challenges as the most common procedure, laparoscopic nephrectomy, remains technically demanding. Unlike our general surgery colleagues who commonly perform simple ablative procedures such as cholecystectomy, the urologic surgeon must traverse the learning curve of laparoscopic surgery on a steep and slippery slope.

One of the challenges of learning laparoscopic surgery remains the novel perspective on well-known anatomy. For thousands of years clinical anatomists (surgeons) have admired and described anatomy from the 'outside in.' Using direct vision, palpation, and an external perspective, the human body has been precisely characterized. Similarly, traditional medical education has focused on the teaching and learning of anatomy in this manner. Laparoscopic surgery, however, presents a novel perspective on a traditional science.

The laparoscopic surgeon must work in a two-dimensional world with limited haptic feedback. While initially counter-intuitive, limiting, and perhaps frustrating, the technology associated with laparoscopic surgery permits the experienced laparoscopic surgeon a view that may be considered superior to that of the traditional surgical approach. While generally still providing two dimensions, currently available laparoscopes provide excellent optics and lighting. The standard laparoscope provides the surgeon a well-lit surgical field and a magnification 12 times better than use of the naked eye. Having once mastered this technology, the surgeon experiences a wealth of exquisite anatomic detail that cannot be appreciated without technological enhancement. Superior visualization of structures allows some compensation for limited tactile feedback. The laparoscopic surgeon relies on detail such as alteration in the weave of suture material to determine tension during laparoscopic suturing.

While not intended to be an inclusive and complete anatomic description of urologic anatomy, this chapter will focus on assisting the experienced urologic surgeon to transition to the 'inside out' view of laparoscopy.

## Body surface anatomy

Successful laparoscopic surgery is based on trocar access. Like open surgery, the thoughtful choice of location and type of incision is crucial to surgical outcome. However, unlike traditional open incisions, trocar sites cannot be extended to provide superior exposure, and additional retraction cannot be placed to improve access.

Thoughtful trocar placement incorporates parameters that include the surgical objectives, anatomic considerations, and body habitus. While trocar placement templates are available for each procedure, trocar positioning must be individualized for each patient, the location of the pathology, and surgeon preference. Laparoscopic surgical experience will refine the ability of each surgeon to establish optimal access.

### Skin incision

At the present time, all trocar access requires a skin incision. Trocar incisions should be made along natural skin cleavage lines (Langer's). These lines define the prevailing arrangement of connective tissue fibers and are evident as crease lines in the skin (Figure 2.1). Incisions created along lines of Langer yield superior cosmetic results. The vast majority of urologic pathology is accessed via the torso

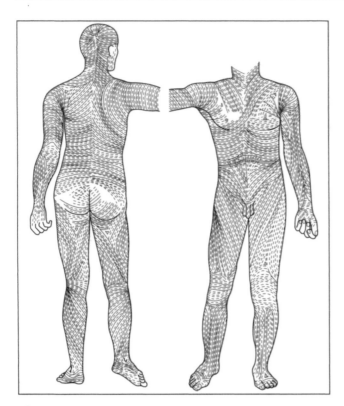

**Figure 2.1**
Langer's lines are natural skin cleavage lines.

where the lines of Langer run circumferentially around the torso. Thus, incisions should be made in a transverse direction to optimize healing.

The umbilicus is a common site for laparoscopic access. Trocar placement may be above or below the umbilicus, depending on the surgical target, and access should be made via a curvilinear incision. The incision itself should be as close to the umbilicus as possible, as healing will usually result in contraction that will yield an almost undetectable scar.

## Surface anatomy

Key surface landmarks for urologic laparoscopic access are the umbilicus, the anterior superior iliac spine, the costal margin, and the 12th rib. These important surface landmarks help the urologic surgeon to choose appropriate trocar access sites and orient the surgeon to the underlying visceral anatomy. Another important structure, the rectus abdominus muscle, may be difficult to appreciate by inspection or palpation. Consequently, the laparoscopic surgeon is obliged to estimate the location of the rectus margin. Moreover, abdominal access through the rectus abdominus muscle is a relative contraindication because the epigastric vessels run through the muscle, and potentially may be injured.

## Umbilicus

The umbilicus is an optimal site for laparoscopic access. Because the umbilicus is centrally located, it will usually provide an intuitive perspective for laparoscopic visual orientation. Cosmetically, it is a superior site, as a curvilinear incision made close to the umbilicus will frequently retract into the umbilicus. When the patient is in the supine position, the umbilicus is an excellent site for primary access to the peritoneal cavity because the peritoneum is closest to the skin at this point on the abdominal wall. The properitoneal layer of fatty tissue, which lies between the linea alba and the peritoneum, is thinnest at the level of the umbilicus. Moreover, the umbilicus is an excellent extraction site for intact removal of renal tumors.

In establishing umbilical access, special consideration should be given to the patient with an extremely obese or very thin body habitus. When Hurd and colleagues evaluated the relationship of the umbilicus to the aortic bifurcation using magnetic resonance imaging (MRI) and computed tomography (CT),[1,2] they assessed the effect obesity has on this relationship. In non-obese patients weighing less than 160 lb (73 kg), the umbilicus is a mean distance of 0.4 cm caudal to the aortic bifurcation, with a skin-to-peritoneum distance of 2 cm. In obese patients weighing between 160 and 200 lb (73 and 91 kg), the umbilicus is 2.4 cm caudal to the aortic bifurcation, with a skin-to-peritoneum distance of 2 cm. In obese patients weighing more than 200 lb (91 kg), the umbilicus is located 2.9 cm caudal to the bifurcation of the aorta, with a skin-to-peritoneum median distance of 12 cm. The authors concluded that Veress needle insertion in the non-obese patient should be at a 45° angle from the horizontal in order to reduce the risk of major abdominal vascular injury and properitoneal placement. Because of the increased distance to the peritoneum in the obese patient, and the caudal displacement of the umbilicus in relation to the aortic bifurcation, the Veress needle should be inserted at a 90° angle from horizontal to achieve intraperitoneal placement. In the overweight patient, an angle between 45° and 90° from horizontal will allow satisfactory intraperitoneal placement of the Veress needle.

## Anterior superior iliac spine

The anterior superior iliac spine is an excellent surface landmark as it is easily discernible even in the most obese patient. Many urologic procedures are performed with the patient in the lateral decubitus position. Trocar placement at a site just cephalad and medial to the anterior superior iliac spine is useful because this is a common left-handed working site for laparoscopic procedures. The anterior superior iliac spine is a site of attachment for the internal oblique, external oblique, and transversalis fascial layers. Penetration of the abdominal wall is facilitated at this site by the 'tenting-up' of the abdomen by this boney prominence.

## Costal margin

When the patient is in the lateral decubitus position, a similar 'tenting' effect is noted at the costal margin. Thus, another common primary trocar placement site is in the anterior axillary line below the costal margin. In the lateral decubitus position, this site is useful as a right-handed working trocar site. Primary access to the peritoneal cavity at this site is similarly facilitated by the 'tenting' effect of the attachment of the abdominal wall fascial layers to the costal margin. As the inferior edge of the liver may extend below the costal margin, care should be taken at this site to prevent liver laceration.

## Twelfth rib

Retroperitoneal access in the flank position is usually gained through an incision just caudal to the tip of the 12th rib. The 12th rib is usually discernible by palpation. In the very obese patient, the surgeon may estimate the location of the 12th rib. Digital palpation and dissection of superficial fatty layers through a small incision will allow localization of the 12th rib in the majority of patients and will facilitate properly positioned primary renal access.

## Body habitus/obesity

There are multiple physiologic and anatomic alterations that occur with obesity. Fat distribution will frequently alter the choice of access sites. Abdominal fat may be distributed primarily in the form of a pannus, or the patient may have a more even 'barrel-like' distribution of fat. The operating surgeon should assess fat distribution after the patient is properly positioned.

When the patient is in the lateral decubitus position, a large pannus may frequently fall medially, allowing the surgeon to enter laterally through a relatively thin abdominal wall. In these cases the umbilicus may fall far to the contralateral side and should not be utilized as an access site. Medial access may be obtained at any site lateral to the margin of the rectus abdominus muscle; the location of this margin must frequently be estimated. In contrast, the more evenly distributed 'barrel-like' body habitus may have little change in the position of the umbilicus relative to the midline.

Another anatomic consideration in the obese patient is the ability to tolerate pneumoperitoneum. For many pelvic procedures laparoscopic access to deep pelvic structures (i.e. bladder, pelvic lymph nodes, or prostate) may be

achieved only with a steep Trendelenburg position. In the obese patient the steep Trendelenburg position may result in an excessive weight of abdominal contents on the diaphragm, which may result in increased inspiratory pressures and hypercapnea. Decreasing insufflation pressures and reducing the steep Trendelenburg position may allow laparoscopic procedures to progress in some cases.

## Previous surgery/scars and adhesions

Abdominal scars from earlier surgery or trauma should be noted by the laparoscopic surgeon. Access sites for earlier laparoscopic procedures occasionally may be difficult to discern because small (<5 mm) trocar sites frequently result in subtle scar formation. Although laparoscopic access should be achieved with great care in all patients who have undergone abdominal surgery, previous laparoscopic procedures will have resulted in significantly less scar formation,[3] and surgical access in patients who have undergone prior laparoscopic surgery is usually uncomplicated.

In patients who have undergone open surgery, laparoscopic access is usually easy to obtain at a site distant from the surgical scar. Special attention should be given, however, to patients having undergone complicated procedures associated with infectious processes, significant inflammation, peritonitis, or urinoma formation. These patients will more frequently have significant diffuse and dense adhesions, which may make any access challenging and hazardous. The effect of previous abdominal surgery on perioperative outcomes in patients undergoing a renal/adrenal laparoscopic procedure via a transperitoneal approach was recently reviewed. The authors found that a previous open abdominal operation increased the risk of laparoscopic operative and major complications, which mostly resulted in increased length of hospital stay.[4] The ipsilateral location of the open prior surgical scar impacted the laparoscopic access complication rate.

Often, adhesions resulting from earlier procedures may be avoided by altering the surgical approach. After abdominal surgery, access to the kidney, ureter, and pelvic structures can frequently be obtained using an extraperitoneal approach. Similarly, patients who have had extraperitoneal surgery (i.e. percutaneous nephrolithotomy) can be approached transabdominally to avoid areas of heavy scarring.[5,6] Prior open abdominal or renal surgery had once been considered a relative contraindication to laparoscopic surgery in the past. Because of the likelihood of adhesion formation and perinephric scarring, there is a greater difficulty of obtaining access to the peritoneal cavity and surgical dissection. Chen et al.[6] retrospectively looked at 24 patients who had prior significant open or renal surgery. They were able to complete all secondary laparoscopic cases successfully and concluded that, with experience, laparoscopic urologic surgery can be performed in a safe timely manner.

# The retroperitoneum

Most urologic pathology is of extraperitoneal origin. Because adrenals, kidneys, ureters, prostate, and urinary bladder are all extraperitoneal structures, the anatomy of the retroperitoneum is particularly important to the urologic surgeon.

Laparoscopic transperitoneal anatomy is intuitive and comfortable for the urologic surgeon as the space is filled with easily identifiable fixed organs and structures, which can continuously orient the surgeon. In contrast, the retroperitoneum is characterized by fatty tissue, which initially is disorienting to the surgeon because anatomic landmarks are not always immediately visable. However, with the experience of a few cases, the retroperitoneal approach becomes more comfortable.

The retroperitoneal approach to the kidneys and upper urinary tract has been popularized by several endourologists.[7–9] Initial access is gained via a 1.5–2.0 cm incision created at the tip of the 12th rib, inferior or superior lumbar triangle (Figure 2.2). After blunt penetration of the lumbodorsal fascia, the retroperitoneal space is initially created by digital palpation. Using digital palpation at this site, the surgeon can identify the psoas muscle posteriorly and the lower aspect of Gerota's fascia (Figure 2.3). The psoas muscle is the most important landmark in the retroperitoneum. This muscle may be used for orientation both by digital palpation and laparoscopic vision.

The psoas muscle originates from the lateral aspects and transverse processes of the vertebral bodies and discs (T12 to L4) and has a characteristic appearance. Distally, the psoas muscle fuses with the iliac muscle to form the ileopsoas muscle. The longitudinal striations and tendon of the psoas muscle are easily visible through the fascia that invests this muscle. After developing the retroperitoneal space via blunt and/or balloon dissection, the ureter and gonadal vessels are evident as they transverse the 'lower cone' of Gerota's fascia. These structures are useful for orientation landmarks of the retroperitoneum.

Retroperitoneal fat has a characteristic appearance and typically will be easy to dissect bluntly with minimal bleeding. However, patients with a history of surgery or inflammatory responses in the retroperitoneum may have fibrosis of the retroperitoneal fat that may make blunt dissection challenging. Using the access site at the tip of the 12th rib, the surgeon can usually identify the peritoneum and bluntly mobilize it medially to provide additional

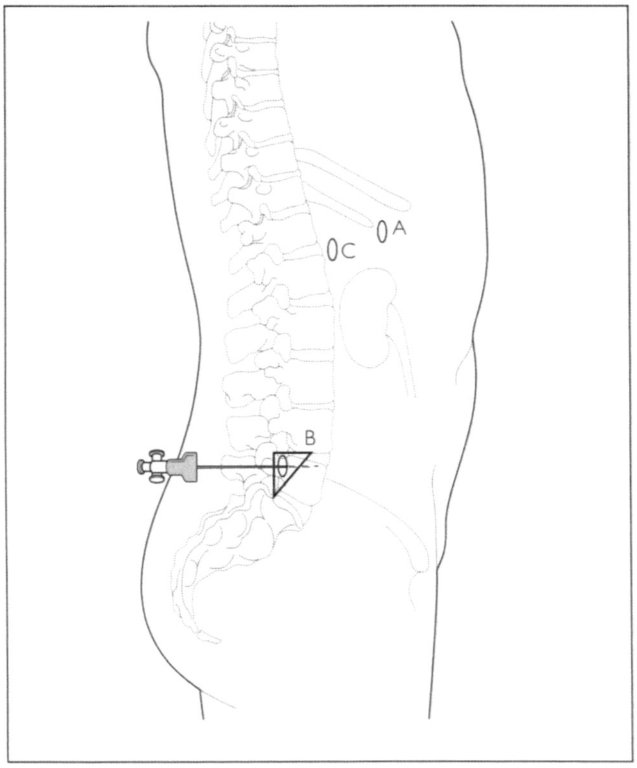

**Figure 2.2**
Initial access sites for retroperitoneoscopy: tip of 12th rib (A), inferior (B) or superior lumbar triangle.

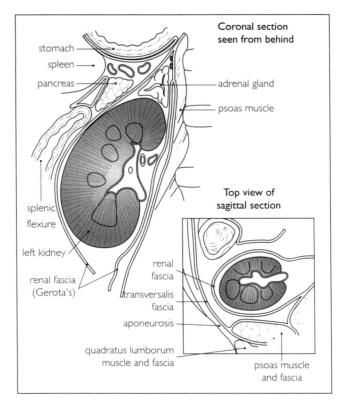

**Figure 2.3**
Both transverse and coronal sections of Gerota's fascia and the kidney delineates its relationship to adjacent organs and structures.

working space in the retroperitoneum for secondary trocar placement. Immediately after access, the renal hilar pulsations are frequently visible by slight cephalad orientation of the laparoscope. On the left side, the lumbar vein is the most posterior and the first vessel of the renal hilum to be visualized. Gentle dissection of the fat in this region will disclose the renal artery. From this viewpoint the renal vein usually can be found immediately behind the renal artery. Occasionally, the location of the renal vasculature is difficult to discern. In these cases the lower pole of the kidney within Gerota's fascia can be identified. The dissection can then proceed cephalad along the psoas muscle to identify the renal hilum, much like the transperitoneal approach to the renal hilum.

A major advantage to the retroperitoneal approach is the avoidance of complicated adhesions from prior transperitoneal surgery. One can approach the peritoneum from an initial retroperitoneal access (see Figure 2.2). This is a safe approach in which the peritoneum is carefully examined and entered at a point where it is thinnest. This allows lysis of adhesions and direct visual placement of intraperitoneal trocars. This form of access should be considered the approach of choice for the patient with a history of abdominal surgery undergoing laparoscopic renal surgery.[5]

Renal anatomy is familiar territory to all urologists. However, the magnification and excellent illumination afforded by the laparoscopic approach reveal a fine level of detail that is not appreciable with traditional open surgery. The anatomic relationships of the kidney with surrounding structures are easily appreciated via the transperitoneal approach (see Figure 2.3).

# Right kidney

In the flank position, gravity mobilization of the small intestine occurs and allows for visualization of the kidney within Gerota's fascia as a bulge under the ascending colon. Classically, the attachment of the colon to the abdominal wall has been inaccurately referred to as the 'Line of Toldt.' In fact, laparoscopic inspection reveals clearly that the ascending colon is attached to the abdominal sidewall via a thin mesentery. This mesentery is not a 'line,' but rather is a band that can range in width from several millimeters to several centimeters. Typically, the band is 1–2 cm in width and can be best appreciated by gently sliding a laparoscopic instrument lateral to the colon. The 'band of Toldt' is typically separate from the anterior surface of Gerota's fascia, and the two layers can be seen sliding over each other. Also, the band can be identified by characteristic linear capillaries that run from the abdominal sidewall to the lateral edge of the colon (see Figure 2.4). Initial careful dissection will allow the surgeon to enter the avascular plane between the colon and Gerota's fascia. Usually, this plane is most distinct, and thus technically easiest to establish, at the lower pole of the kidney.

Once the plane has been established, the colon and the colonic mesentery can be mobilized medially to expose the anterior surface of Gerota's fascia. The mesenteric fat has a distinct color and character. The mesenteric fat can be identified laparoscopically as much more distinctly yellow than Gerota's fascia. The mesentery is also more friable and has a tendency to bleed with manipulation. Even minor bleeding noted during the dissection of the plane between the colonic mesentery and Gerota's fascia should alert the surgeon that his plane of dissection is too medial. Superiorly, separation of the colon from Gerota's fascia can be challenging to dissect as the inferior edge of the liver commonly is draped over this area. Mobilization of the liver's edge and superior retraction of the liver are very helpful in identifying and dissecting upper pole structures. For adequate mobilization of the liver, incision of the triangular ligament connecting the lateral margin of the liver to the diaphragm is necessary. Incision of the triangular ligament should be performed with care to avoid diaphragmatic injury.

As the colonic mesentery is mobilized, the medial portion of the anterior Gerota's fascia becomes evident. As the dissection proceeds medially and posteriorly, the duodenum should become evident. Occasionally, it will appear that the vena cava has been identified. However, the duodenum will always be anterior to the vena cava. The surgeon should actively seek the duodenum after medial mobilization of the colon has been initiated. Usually the duodenum is quite obvious as a pink to purple bowel structure. Occasionally, the duodenum can be decompressed and confused with Gerota's fascia. Careful inspection to identify the duodenum will help avoid injury. The Kocher maneuver can be performed to gain access to the vena cava and renal vein. Using cold sharp dissection with scissors or the harmonic scalpel, which has minimal peripheral energy spread, is suggested to initiate duodenal mobilization, as there is little space between the duodenum and Gerota's fascia. After sharp incision of most lateral attachments of the duodenum to Gerota's fascia, there typically is only loose areolar tissue connecting these structures. Therefore, the surgeon can gently apply a blunt sweeping medial motion to complete the Kocher maneuver after the initial sharp mobilization. Attempting to bluntly push the duodenum off of Gerota's fascia without starting this dissection sharply may lead to duodenal injury.

Adequate mobilization of the duodenum and colon results in exposure of the lateral margin of the vena cava (Figure 2.5). Inferiorly, the gonadal vein is usually readily identified, inserting on the lateral aspect of the vena cava below the renal hilum. The gonadal vein may be sacrificed if necessary, but preservation of the gonadal vein should be attempted even with radical renal surgery. Transection of

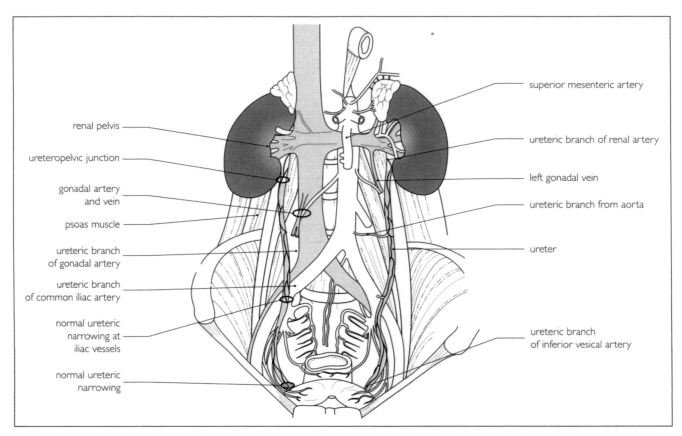

**Figure 2.4**
Anatomic relationship between kidney, ureter, psoas muscle and great vessels. Three areas of ureteral narrowing are demonstrated.

the gonadal vein in the male will occasionally result in testicular pain. While this pain is transient, sparing the gonadal vein is optimal. If significant bleeding is encountered during medial mobilization of the lower pole, it is likely that the surgeon has transected or avulsed the gonadal vein off of the vena cava. As the insertion of the gonadal vein into the vena cava is quite delicate, it has been referred to as 'the angle of sorrows.' Further lateral dissection of the lower pole of the kidney will reveal the inferior tail of Gerota's fascia, which rests on the psoas major muscle. Laparoscopically, the psoas major muscle is a useful anatomic landmark. Inspection of the psoas major muscle will reveal characteristic muscle bundles, the psoas tendon, and the genitofemoral nerve. Following the psoas major muscle will help delineate the lower pole of the kidney within Gerota's fascia. At the level of the lower pole of the kidney, the ureter can be identified lateral to the gonadal vein on the surface of the psoas muscle (Figure 2.4). The ureter is another structure that it is useful to identify before dissection of the renal hilum, as anterior and lateral traction on the ureter will help identify the location of the hilum. Although laparoscopic surgery results in oliguria, the ureter maintains its characteristic peristalsis, which is useful to distinguish the ureter from the gonadal vein.

After mobilization of the colon and duodenum, and dissection of the lower pole of the kidney, the lateral edge of the vena cava usually is easily identified. In thin patients with little retroperitoneal fat, the medial aspect of the vena cava, contralateral renal vein, and aorta are frequently discernible. Identification of the gonadal vein and ureter can be helpful in orienting the laparoscopic surgeon. Renal vein abnormalities such as duplication are uncommon, but are much more common on the right side. The right renal vein is usually located at the level of the inferior edge of the liver. Consequently, releasing the cephalad traction on the liver and inspecting its lower edge will provide a useful clue as to the location of the renal vein. Lumbar branches of the right renal vein are uncommon, and the right adrenal vein typically drains directly into the vena cava. Keeping these 'anatomic textbook' descriptions in mind, the laparoscopic surgeon should dissect the right renal vein with great care, as laparoscopic vascular control can be challenging.

The renal artery is located posterior to the renal vein (see Figure 2.5). The availability of high-quality imaging with CT and MRI scans is very helpful in preoperatively delineating the renal hilar anatomy. The renal artery is commonly posterior to the renal vein, but it may be directly behind, slightly cephalad, or slightly caudal to the renal vein. Imaging can also help identify early medial

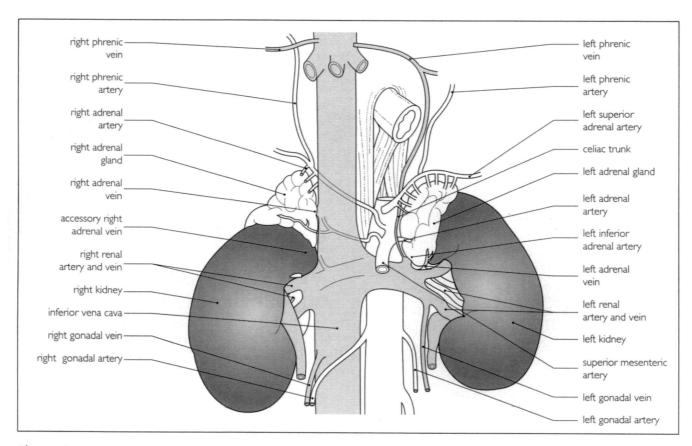

**Figure 2.5**
Blood supply of kidney and adrenal gland derived from the aorta and inferior vena cava.

branching of the main trunk of the renal artery. Complete dissection of the renal vein is occasionally helpful to identify the location of an elusive renal artery. Superior to the renal hilum the adrenal gland is positioned between the kidney and vena cava within a sheath of Gerota's fascia. Adrenal anatomy is described in the Adrenal glands section of this chapter. Posteriorly, the right Gerota's fascia is attached to the psoas and quadratus lumborum muscles by flimsy tissues.

Within Gerota's fascia the kidney is located under a variable layer of perinephric fat. Of interest, the amount of perinephric fat surrounding the kidney does not always correlate with the exterior appearance of the patient (see Figure 2.3). Careful inspection of CT or MRI scans can help the surgeon determine the amount of perinephric fat that will be present. In patients with a large amount of perinephric fat, a nephrectomy specimen for a small kidney may be quite large, and even very exophytic masses may be difficult to discern laparoscopically. Thus, the amount of perinephric fat has significant clinical impact on the level of difficulty associated with laparoscopic renal procedures. The perinephric fat is easily separable from the capsule of the kidney, and the renal capsule is usually separable from the renal parenchyma with minimal bleeding. In patients with a history of surgery, tumors with desmo-

plastic reactions, infections, or inflammatory processes, these planes may be quite adherent and difficult to separate.

# Left kidney

When the patient is in the lateral decubitus position, gravity mobilization of the small bowel results in exposure of the left kidney within Gerota's fascia as a mass under the descending colon. The 'line of Toldt' is identified as previously described. However, there is a physiologic adhesion in the left upper quadrant that anchors the left kidney to the abdominal wall. This adhesion is present in the majority of patients without a history of surgery or an abdominal inflammatory process. The adhesion is a condensation of the mesentery that anchors the spleen and upper pole of the kidney to the diaphragm and lateral abdominal wall. This adhesion is avascular, and its release initiates release of Gerota's fascia from the spleen, diaphragm, and anterior abdominal wall (see Figure 2.3). The colon appears to cover more of the surface area of the anterior portion of the kidney on the left side than on the right side.

Medial mobilization of the descending colon allows access to the plane between Gerota's fascia and the colonic mesentery. This natural plane between the mesentery of the descending colon and Gerota's fascia is most easily identified and entered along the lower pole of the kidney or just inferior to the kidney. The anterior and superior aspect of Gerota's fascia is attached to the spleen by the splenocolic ligament, which can be incised in order to fully mobilize the descending colon medially. Typically, release of the splenocolic ligament and medial mobilization of colon off of Gerota's fascia will result in medial mobilization of the tail of the pancreas (see Figure 2.3). Occasionally, however, the tail of the pancreas will remain adherent to the medial surface of Gerota's fascia. As it is not commonly identified during renal surgery, the tail of the pancreas may be mistaken for other structures such as reactive lymph nodes. The pancreas has a characteristic pale lobulated appearance that should be recognized by the urologic surgeon.

Medial mobilization of the descending colon and its mesentery inferiorly results in exposure of the psoas major muscle. Usually, the gonadal vein is identified along the medial aspect of the psoas major muscle (see Figures 2.4 and 2.5). On the left side, the gonadal vein is a very useful landmark because it enters directly into the left renal vein. The gonadal vein can most easily be exposed inferiorly; it is then traced up to its entry into the renal vein. If necessary, for very challenging dissections, the surgeon can carry the dissection down to the level of the inguinal ring in order to reliably identify the gonadal vein and trace it cephalad; this maneuver is particularly helpful in the morbidly obese patient with a large amount of retroperitoneal fat. Anteriorly, along the gonadal vein, there are invariably no tributaries so the surgeon has a safe plane of dissection all the way up to the insertion of the gonadal vein into the main renal vein. Once the gonadal vein has been identified, the ureter can usually be located, as it lies just posterior and lateral to the gonadal vein.

Tracing the gonadal vein cephalad reliably leads to its junction with the left renal vein (see Figures 2.4 and 2.5). It is much more challenging to control the renal vein on the left than the one on the right. Typically, the left renal vein has tributaries, including the gonadal vein inferiorly, one or more posterior lumbar veins that may enter the renal vein posteriorly, and the adrenal vein, which enters the superior edge of the renal vein medial to the insertion of the gonadal vein. Lumbar veins are short and easily disrupted. The lumbar veins may enter the renal vein directly posteriorly or may even join the gonadal vein near its insertion into the renal vein.

Inferior retraction of the superior border of the renal vein will usually expose the renal artery posteriorly. The left renal artery, similar to the one on the right, may lie immediately posterior, slightly cephalad, or slightly caudal to the renal vein (see Figure 2.5). Although dissection of the renal vein usually allows for rapid identification of the renal artery, preoperative imaging frequently is helpful in challenging cases for discerning the location of the renal artery relative to the renal vein. 'Fortunate' identification of the renal artery anterior to the renal vein should engender much suspicion on the part of the surgeon. Most likely, the arterial structure anterior to the left renal vein is the superior mesenteric artery (see Figure 2.5). This artery must be preserved during renal procedures as its sacrifice results in bowel ischemia. The adrenal gland is located just cephalad to the renal vein. The anatomy of the left adrenal gland is further described later in this chapter. As with the right kidney, there are only flimsy attachments between the posterior aspect of Gerota's fascia and the psoas and quadratus lumborum muscles.

# Adrenal glands

## Overview

The adrenal glands, like the kidneys, are paired retroperitoneal organs enveloped in Gerota's fascia and surrounded by perirenal adipose tissue. Adult adrenal glands weigh 4–8 g and on average are larger in women than in men. The adrenals lie superior to the kidneys and thus are sometimes referred as suprarenal glands. A layer of loose connective tissue stroma surrounds each gland and separates the adrenal capsule from its respective kidney. Embryologically, the adrenal and kidney develop separately, and if the kidney is ectopic or absent, the adrenal will be in the normal anatomic location. Occasionally, the adrenal gland will be fused with the kidney such that differentiation is difficult and can even be mistaken for a renal tumor.[10] Adrenalectomy for a fused gland may even require a partial nephrectomy.

The three classic layers of the cortex and their respective volumes are the outer zona glomerulosa (15%), the middle zona fasciculata (78%), and the inner zona reticularis (7%). Several steroids are produced from the adrenal cortex, but only a few are biologically active and clinically significant. Aldosterone is produced in the zona glomerulosa, while cortisol and corticosterone are produced in the zona fasciculata. The innermost zona reticularis produces the weak androgen dehydroepiandrosterone (DHEA) and some small amounts of glucocorticoids and estrogens.

The inner medulla is of neuroendocrine derivation. The medulla is derived from the ectodermal neural crest cells in the thoracic region. There is a migration ventrally around the developing aorta and adrenal vein. A group of these chromaffin cells invade the adrenal cortex and eventually are completely surrounded. Preganglionic sympathetic fibers synapse directly to these chromaffin cells, which form the adrenal medulla. Additional developing neuroblasts form the aortic glands or the glands of Zuckerkandl.

The glands of Zuckerkandl have no known function, are located laterally to the aorta at the level of the inferior mesenteric artery, and may be a site for extra-adrenal pheochromocytoma (paraganglioma) or neuroblastoma. The chromaffin cells of the adrenal medulla synthesize epinephrine, norepinephrine and dopamine in conjunction with the sympathetic nervous system.

Per gram of tissue, the adrenal receives one of the greatest percentages of cardiac output. The vasculature of the adrenals is split into the multi-vessel arterial system and a single large vein. The adrenal arteries are divided into three general sources: superior, medial, and inferior branches. The superior supply usually arises from the inferior diaphragmatic artery bilaterally; it is a small plexus of arteries that is difficult to visualize directly. The middle adrenal artery can arise from the aorta, renal artery, or the celiac trunk on the right. The inferior artery usually arises from the renal artery, an accessory renal artery, superior polar renal artery, or small branches from the upper ureteric arteries. There is an abundant branching of the adrenal arteries, leading to up to 50 small perforating vessels over the surface of the capsule. Adrenal venous drainage does not accompany the arterial supply.

The adrenals are true retroperitoneal organs that may be accessed both transperitoneally and retroperitoneally. The retroperitoneal approach is ideal for small tumor burdens such as adenomas. The transperitoneal approach, which may be more familiar to surgeons, is favored for larger pathologic glands such as large adenomas, pheochromocytomas and adrenocortical carcinomas, which may invade adjacent structures. Minimally invasive laparoscopic adrenalectomy has become the true gold standard approach since first performed by Gagner[11] and will be discussed in greater detail in Chapter 49.

## Right adrenal gland

Transperitoneal access to the right adrenal begins with a similar previously described dissection of the right kidney. Once the colon is reflected and the duodenum is kocherized, the inferior vena cava is identified. Following the vena cava superiorly leads to the gonadal vein insertion, which is just above the right renal vein. When the lateral border of the vena cava is followed, the main right adrenal vein can be bluntly dissected and visualized. It is a short wide vein found just superior to the renal vein, with an occasional accessory vein entering the inferior phrenic vein. This single, large vein, usually emerging from the adrenal hilum, is a very important surgical landmark. This right vein usually passes obliquely to open posteriorly and drain directly into the vena cava. Damage to this vessel is perhaps the greatest source of vascular injury in right-sided renal and adrenal surgery. The adrenal arterial supply is multi-faceted, as previously described. The arterial plexus is usually not clearly visualized but should be considered and handled with either clips or harmonic scalpel.

Once the vasculature is handled, the plane between the adrenal and kidney can be established. The right adrenal is a triangular suprarenal gland with its anterior surface interfacing with the liver, its posterior surface lying on the diaphragm and inferiorly lying on the upper pole of the kidney. The right adrenal is usually engulfed in Gerota's fascia and sandwiched medial to the upper pole of the kidney and lateral to vena cava (see Figure 2.4). The distinctive yellowish-gold tissue of the adrenal stands out even amidst the perirenal adipose tissue.

## Left adrenal gland

Transperitoneal access to the left adrenal once again follows access to the kidney. Medial mobilization of the colon is followed by blunt dissection of the renal vasculature. The spleen will completely fall away from the kidney when excised from its previously described lateral peritoneal attachments in addition to the separation of the splenorenal ligaments. The tail of the pancreas is near in proximity and will be identified at this point. The plane between the pancreatic tail and medial border of the adrenal is separated by mobilizing the left colon mesentery off of Gerota's fascia. Careful exposure of the long left renal vein is the key to the adrenal identification. The left adrenal vein, similar to the gonadal vein, drains directly into the left renal vein and is significantly longer than the right. The left adrenal vein exits the adrenal hilum inferiorly and passes over the anterior surface of the gland, merging with the inferior phrenic vein before entering the renal vein. The adrenal vein enters the renal vein on the superior aspect of the renal vein and medial to the gonadal vein (see Figures 2.4 and 2.5). The left adrenal vein is a crucial landmark for left adrenal surgery and once ligated may be used to identify the gland. Once this long vein is controlled and ligated, medial retraction will create a plane between the adrenal gland and kidney. The left adrenal gland is usually smaller than the right and interfaces with the stomach and pancreas anteriorly, the spleen superiorly, the diaphragm posteriorly, and the upper pole of the kidney inferiorly. The left adrenal gland is identified within Gerota's fascia and more superior to the kidney than its right counterpart. Once again the arterial anatomy is usually not clearly visualized, even with laparoscopic magnification.

## Ureters
### Overview

The ureters are paired muscular urinary conduits that travel from the kidney to the bladder and lie entirely in the retroperitoneal space. The ureter is described radiologically as three segments: *upper* (renal pelvis to upper border of sacrum); *middle* (down to lower border of sacrum); and *lower* or *pelvic* (extends to the bladder). From a surgical standpoint, the ureters are distinguished as the ureteropelvic junction, intermediate tract, and the ureterovesical junction. The ureters are tubular organs and are approximately 22–32 cm in length, varying directly with patient height and renal location. The average diameter of the ureter is 10 mm in the abdominal location and tapers to 5 mm in the pelvis. Microscopically, they are composed of three distinct layers (from outside to inside): the adventitial surface, the muscularis, and the internal uroepithelium. The adventia consists of a dense network of collagen and elastic fibers in which course the vasculature and neural supply. This layer is continuous proximally with the renal pelvic capsule and distally with the fibrinous tissue known as Waldeyer's sheath. The muscular layer is contiguous with the renal collecting system and bladder.

As a tubular extension of the renal pelvis, the ureter forms a gentle 'S' pattern from the kidney to the bladder. The ureters course along the anterior-medial surface of the psoas muscle embedded in a subserous fascia before encountering the genitofemoral nerve around the 4th lumbar vertebral body (see Figure 2.4). The gonadal vessels cross over the ureter from medial to lateral as the ureter enters the bony pelvis. The ureter continues toward the pelvic brim, turning medial to traverse over the external iliac vessels on the right and the common iliac vessel on the left. In the pelvis it courses medially and posteriorly to the medial umbilical ligament and enters the detrusor muscle just behind the superior vesicle artery.

## Vasculature

The ureter receives its multiple and variable blood supply in a segmental distribution, depending on its level (see Figure 2.5). From proximal to distal, the ureter receives vascular branches from the renal artery, gonadal artery, abdominal aorta, and common iliac artery and, finally, branches of the internal iliac artery. The iliac region of the ureter has the fewest direct arterial branches. The feeding arterial branches approach the ureter medially in the upper ureter and laterally after crossing the iliac vessels in the pelvis. Surgically, it is important to be aware of the apparent vascular course to the affected ureteral segment. Laparoscopic or endoscopic intervention should be limited to the contralateral area (i.e. lateral in the upper ureter and medial in the lower ureter). On reaching the ureter, the perpendicular arterial vessels turn and course longitudinally within the periureteral adventitia as an extensive plexus. Venous drainage follows the arterial supply.

## Access

Access to the ureter depends on the affected area (proximal or distal location). Access is generally similar to the lower pole kidney dissection, as previously described. From the transperitoneal perspective, the ureter is identified just posterior to the colon after it is reflected medially and courses along the psoas muscle. The ureter is usually intimately associated with the peritoneum and may at times be reflected with the colon. From the retroperitoneal approach, after balloon dilation, the ureter is located attached to the posterior aspect of the peritoneum and freed off the psoas muscle.

## Right ureter

Transperitoneal access to the right ureter follows the steps of renal access, as previously described. Reflection of the right colon and blunt dissection off the lower pole of the kidney is an ideal way to identify the abdominal ureter. Through the retroperitoneal adipose tissue, a gentle sweeping motion of a blunt instrument may initiate ureteral peristalsis. The right ureter leaves the renal pelvis and passes posterior to the second part of the duodenum, running along the lateral aspect of the inferior vena cava. A Kocher maneuver is necessary to access the upper ureter in a non-hydronephrotic system. At this point, the ureter encounters the gonadal vessel as it enters the inferior vena cava. The gonadal vein travels medial and parallel to the ureter, then crosses over and lateral to the gonadal vein. The right ureter descends towards the pelvis and is crossed by the right colic and ileocolic vessels. The right ureter is anteriorly associated with the terminal ileum, cecum, appendix, and the ascending colon. Transperitoneal right ureteral access can be complicated by adhesions from an earlier appendectomy or chronic appendicitis that makes the usually distinct planes difficult to find. A prior appendectomy or history of appendicitis may have caused variations in appendiceal/cecal vascular supplies, potentially leading to ischemia and secondary bowel perforation from vigorous colonic mobilization. Thus, caution must be exercised when performing the above maneuver.

## Left ureter

The left ureter leaves the renal pelvis, running lateral to the aorta and passing behind the left colic vessels. As with the right ureter, the left ureter runs parallel with and lateral to its respective gonadal vein and both pass under the pelvic mesocolon. The left ureter is anteriorly associated with the descending and sigmoid colons.

Important structures near the distal ureter in the male include the vas deferens, which crosses over the distal ureter medial to the middle and upper seminal vesicle before entering the urinary bladder. This is well-visualized transperitoneally in laparoscopic seminal vesicle surgery. In the female, the ureter traverses the posterior aspect of the ovarian fossa, then goes under the inferior part of the broad ligament lateral to the cervix. The uterine artery crosses over the juxtavesical portion of the ureter before it enters the urinary bladder. This becomes a common area of ureteral injury during emergent or radical hysterectomies. Access to the pelvic ureter may require that these structures be identified and divided.

## Pathology

The ureters are small tubular organs that can be misidentified in pathologic or even non-pathologic conditions. Midline retroperitoneal masses, such as massive lymphadenopathy, aortic aneurysms, or sarcomas, may laterally deviate the ureters. The disease process of retroperitoneal fibrosis or post-chemotherapy tumors may contract and pull the ureters medially. Several other pathologic entities, such as ureteropelvic junction obstruction or a circumcaval ureter that may lead to hydronephrosis, are associated deviations from normal anatomy.

## Ureteropelvic junction obstruction

Accessory crossing arterial and venous vessels contribute to secondary ureteropelvic junction (UPJ) obstructions. Crossing vessels are a significant cause of UPJ obstruction and are more frequently the source in adolescents and adults than in the pediatric age group. An anterior crossing vessel may cause UPJ obstruction in between 25 and 67% of cases and may lead to a failed endopyelotomy or, worse, hemorrhage.[12,13] Because arterial crossing vessels supply the lower pole of the kidney as end vessels, they must be preserved at all costs. Venous vessels may be solitary or run parallel to an artery and may be sacrificed, but ureteroplasty should also be performed in addition to focal upper ureterolysis.

## Circumcaval ureter

Circumcaval (or retrocaval) ureter is a rare embryologic condition found on the right side. An anomalous embryologic development of the inferior vena cava (IVC) results in circumcaval ureter. The lack of regression of the fetal posterior cardinal vein causes the IVC to develop anterior to the ureter and displace it medially. If this obstruction is below the 3rd lumbar vertebrae, the result is ureter obstructed by kinking. The overall incidence is *unknown*

and is not symptomatic in every case. Contemporary diagnosis is usually based on three-dimensional volume rendering computed tomography (3D-CT) with intravenous contrast and diuretic radionucleotide renography.[14]

Indications for reconstruction of the circumcaval ureter include recurrent infection, obstruction, and flank pain. The course of the right ureter is deviated immediately medial to the UPJ, passing posterior to the vena cava before swinging laterally over the vena cava and coursing down toward the urinary bladder. A procedure similar to a dismembered pyeloplasty is used to correct this congenital anomaly.

## Retroperitoneal fibrosis

Retroperitoneal fibrosis or Ormand's disease is a non-malignant inflammatory condition that encases the ureters and great vessels. Retroperitoneal fibrosis has been linked to the migraine medication methysergide or may develop iatrogenically. The fibrous encasement of the ureter may lead to a physiologic obstruction of the ureters by inhibiting peristalsis. The resulting inhibition of peristalsis leads to obstruction, which in turn leads to hydronephrosis, pain, and deterioration of renal function. Computed tomography showing a retroperitoneal mass engulfing the retroperitoneal organs routinely makes diagnosis. The radiographic hallmark of this process on intravenous urography (IVU) or retrograde ureteropyelography (RUPG) is hydronephrosis without ureteral dilation, and severe deviation of the mid-ureters towards the midline. No intrinsic obstructive process is noted on RUPG, and stent placement is easily performed without the need for ureteral dilation. There are reports of unilateral fibrosis, but this should be considered a bilateral process. Secondary retroperitoneal fibrosis may be caused by inflammatory bowel disease, endometriosis, radiation therapy, or post-chemotherapy changes. Bilateral ureteral lysis is curative, but must be coupled with a biopsy of the fibrosis tissue to rule out malignancy.

## Retroperitoneal lymph nodes
### Overview

Clinically, retroperitoneal lymph node anatomy is important for oncologic surgery. Testicular carcinoma is the one true urologic oncologic disease in which a retroperitoneal lymph node dissection (RPLND) is curative as well as important in diagnostic staging for additional medical therapy. There continues to be a debate whether extended node dissection with radical nephrectomy is necessary because of the poor prognosis when local lymph nodes are involved with cancer. The testes embryologically develop as retroperitoneal organs before their descent. Thus, they obtain their blood supply and lymphatic drainage from the retroperitoneal vascular structure. A clear knowledge of lymph node anatomy is mandatory before contemplating laparoscopic or open RPLND surgery. The spermatic cord carries all of the vascular and lymphatic structures of the testis through the inguinal canal deep to the peritoneum from its origin at the retroperitoneal vessels. The retroperitoneal lymph nodes can be divided into three major groupings. The main retroperitoneal lymph node chains are named by their relationship to the great vessels (Figure 2.6). The left para-aortic nodes extend from the left ureter to the midline of the aorta. The right paracaval nodes extend from the right ureter to the midline of the inferior vena cava. The remaining nodes, extending from the midline of the aorta to the midline of the inferior vena cava, are called the interaortocaval nodes.

From the observations of Donahue et al, the retroperitoneal drainage of each testis has been mapped.[15] The right testis drains predominantly to the interaortocaval nodes, with significant drainage to the paracaval nodes below the renal hilum. There is a small but significant number of early metastases to the left para-aortic nodes. The left testis drains predominantly to the para-aortic nodes (including nodal tissue above the renal hilum) and there is some significant drainage to the interaortocaval nodes. In the left side, unlike the right side, there is relatively no drainage or associated early metastases in the paracaval region.

With this knowledge, modified RPLND templates have been determined to spare the morbidity of bilateral sympathetic nerve damage (Figure 2.7). Sparing one of the sympathetic chains allows unilateral innervation for the preservation of competent ejaculatory function. Damage to both the right and left sympathetic chains may lead

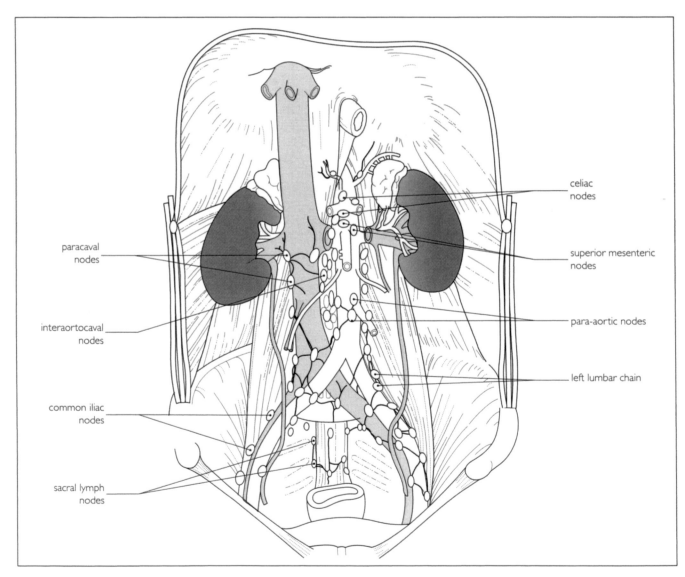

**Figure 2.6**
Retroperitoneal lymph node chains: paracaval (PC), interaortocaval (IAC), and para-aortic (PA).

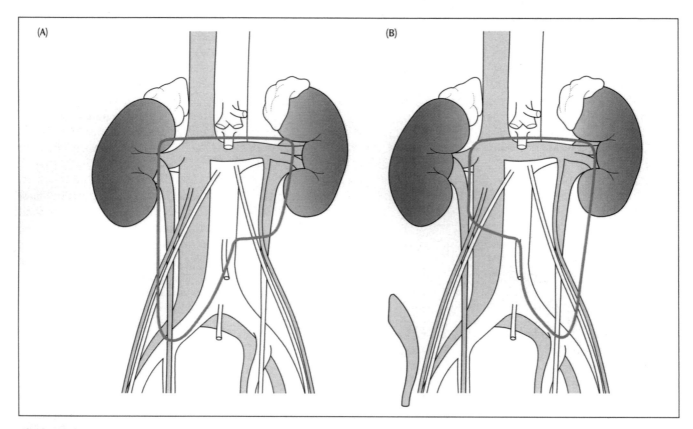

**Figure 2.7**
Left (A) and right (B) modified RPLND templates.

to retrograde ejaculation and secondary infertility. In template dissections, the lateral border consists of the ipsilateral ureter, superior border, the ipsilateral renal vein, and the inferior margin, the end of the ipsilateral spermatic cord, and the bifurcation of the common iliac artery on the contralateral side.

## Right access

Retroperitoneal node dissection is best approached through a transperitoneal route. The patient should be in left lateral decubitus 45° to facilitate the gravitational retraction and allow access to the entire abdomen for possible open conversion. Extended mobilization of the right and transverse colons should be paramount as the initial approach to the nodal tissue. Freeing the hepatic flexure must not be limited and should include dissection medially and superiorly along the mesenteric root to the ligament of Treitz. The cecum should be mobilized, more extensively than in renal/ureteral surgery. The template borders, as described above, should all be dissected and identified. The right renal hilum should be first evaluated with dissection of the renal vein and ureter after the duodenum is medially relocated (Kocher). The left renal vein is located superiorly to the right vein and should be

dissected as laterally as possible. The traditional 'split & roll' technique should start on the vena cava. The origin of the right gonadal vein is carefully identified and ligated. In inflammatory conditions such as enlarged adenopathy or post-chemotherapy situations, the gonadal vein can be identified medial to the ureter at the level of the lower pole of the kidney and followed cephalad. Mobilizing the nodal tissue laterally frees up the vena cava for the interaortocaval dissection. There are small perforating veins draining the lymphatics encountered at this point. The true right template may be limited medially if the right and transverse colonic attachments have not been mobilized sufficiently. The interaortocaval dissection is extended caudal and to the right of the inferior mesenteric artery, ending inferiorly at the iliac bifurcation on the right.

## Left access

Starting with the patient in a 45° right lateral decubitus position, the transperitoneal approach once again mimics extended access to the kidney. The left colon and splenic flexure should be adequately mobilized, allowing complete access to the medial aspect of the aorta. The tail of the pancreas is seen near the medial portion of the upper pole of the left kidney, and blunt dissection medially will facilitate cephalad template dissection. The long left renal vein can be followed to the vena cava and defines the upper template limits. The lateral ureter margin can be identified sitting on the psoas muscle. Once again the lateral nodal packet should be dissected first (para-aortic chain). The ligation of the left gonadal insertion on the inferior location of the renal vein is a good starting place. Once again, the caudal limit is the iliac bifurcation, and the inferior mesentery artery is the marker for bilateral node dissection. Staying on the ipsilateral side of the inferior mesenteric limits the potential of harming both of the sympathetic chains.

# Pelvic lymph nodes

## Introduction

The initial use of prostate-specific antigen (PSA) as an adjunct for screening resulted in an increased detection of prostate cancer. Since the late 1980s the majority of patients with clinically diagnosed prostate cancer have had stage T1c disease. Prior to PSA and use of clinical staging nomograms, the lack of epidemiologic, radiologic, or physical evidence made the diagnosis of metastatic disease a difficult task. Despite significant refinements in the anatomic approach to the radical retropubic or perineal prostatectomy, they both remain operative procedures with significant morbidity. Radiation modalities have also improved over time with conformal external beam and interstitial brachytherapy delivering lethal doses to the cancer with decreased morbidity to the surrounding structures. Postoperative complications of radical prostatectomy and radiation include urinary incontinence, erectile dysfunction, and fecal incontinence. This significant morbidity mandates that a conservative approach be entertained when a patient is suspected of having metastatic disease. Therefore, one of the goals of laparoscopic pelvic lymphadenectomy (laparoscopic pelvic lymph node dissection) is to exclude select high-risk patients with positive pelvic lymph nodal involvement from non-curative local regional therapy.

Since the establishment of LPLND as a viable procedure in patients with documented prostate cancer, the indications have broadened to include bladder malignancies, penile cancer and urethral cancer. The refinement of equipment and the increasing number of laparoscopically trained surgeons make this minimally invasive approach to staging pelvic lymphadenectomy ideal for suspect patients prior to definitive regional therapy. The combination of a decade of widespread PSA screening and better definitions of the risks of metastatic disease have led to a dramatic decline of stage migration and a decline for LPLND prior

to definitive treatment. The increased laparoscopic skills of the urologist and the acceptance of laparoscopic radical prostatectomy will drive a resurgence of LPLND being performed at the same time.

There are several groups of pelvic lymph nodes located around the iliac artery and vein. There are usually 4–6 common iliac nodes located up to the bifurcation. The external iliac nodes are a group of 8–10 nodes located laterally, medially and, occasionally, anteriorly. The internal iliac nodes surround the artery and are a group of 2–4 nodes (Figure 2.8). The obturator lymph nodes are the ones most commonly dissected for prostate cancer. These are considered to be the initial source for lymphatic drainage of the prostate. These are one or two nodes located in the obturator foramen under the external iliac vein and in close proximity to the obturator neurovascular bundle. Lymphatic dissection should be concentrated on the group of nodes associated with the offending cancerous organ. Extended pelvic node dissection can be performed for bladder, penile, and proximal urethral carcinoma.

## Access

The approach for pelvic node dissection can be via a transperitoneal or extraperitoneal route. The extraperitoneal approach has several advantages. Through a midline anterior approach, both pelvic sites can be dissected without entering the peritoneal compartment. The peritoneum acts as a bowel retractor, allowing for a more direct approach to the nodal tissue. Another advantage is the familiarity of the extraperitoneal approach to urologists. In

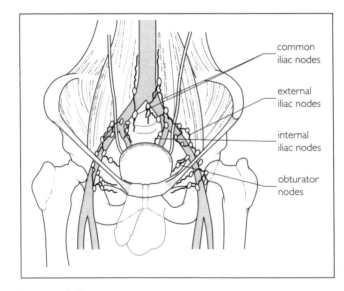

**Figure 2.8**
Pelvic lymph node groups.

the transperitoneal approach, the lateral sidewall with iliac vessels is carefully identified and the peritoneum is opened longitudinally and parallel to the iliac artery, allowing entrance to the extraperitoneal space. Access to either side can be performed by employing midline trocar sites, and the dissection is similar. Open retropubic prostatectomy traditionally involves the extraperitoneal approach and allows access to the nodal tissue up to the iliac bifurcation. Preperitoneal dissection can be performed bluntly, and pulsations of the iliac artery allow a quick localization of the desired target location. The limits of obturator node dissection include the external iliac vein anteriorly, Cooper's ligament inferiorly, the hypogastric artery and pelvic muscular sidewall laterally, and the bifurcation of the common iliac artery cranially. The large external iliac vein is followed caudal to the pubic bone. Circumflex accessory veins can be encountered and are a potential hemorrhage source. Incising the perivenous tissue allows access to the nodal tissue inferior to the vein and superior to the obturator neurovascular bundle. The perforating vascular and small lymphatic supply to the pelvic nodes is anterior and posterior, with few or no attachments medially and laterally. Care must be taken not to injure the large obturator nerve, which serves as the innervation for ipsilateral lower extremity adduction.

## Urinary bladder

The urinary bladder is perhaps one of the most identifiable extraperitoneal organs. In recent years, laparoscopic cystectomy has established itself as a feasible, minimally invasive approach for oncologic surgery. A purely laparoscopic approach, which includes the urinary diversion, at present, is a lengthy procedure. The combination of laparoscopic cystectomy and extracorporeal reconstructive surgery is an acceptable compromise that allows smaller incisions and a quicker recovery time.

The urinary bladder is a hollow muscular organ whose sole purpose is to act as a reservoir. In simplest terms, the bladder fills over time, stores urine, and empties in a co-ordinated fashion. When full, the bladder is situated above the pubic ramus, along the anterior abdominal wall, and in severe cases of urinary retention can extend to the umbilicus. As the urinary bladder empties, there is a descent of the bladder dome under the pubic symphysis towards the fixed portion, the trigone. In the female, the superior surface of the bladder is intimately associated with the peritoneum, whereas in the male the entire posterior wall from dome to trigone lies on the peritoneum.

Microscopically, there are distinct layers of the urinary bladder similar to those of the ureter. The watertight uroepithelium is first surrounded by an underlying layer of connective tissue, then bands of linear and circular bands

of muscularis, which is covered by a serosal layer. The superior-most area of the bladder, the dome, is attached to the urachal remnant via a short fibrous cord called the urachus. The urachus should be removed en bloc during radical cystectomy because uroepithelial bladder cancer, squamous cell carcinoma, or adenocarcinoma may be present. Urachal adenocarcinoma is a rare malignancy that is often difficult to detect; it should be managed similar to bladder carcinoma.

## *Vascular supply*

The internal iliac artery supplies the urinary bladder. Branches of the anterior division of the internal iliac artery include the superior, middle, and inferior vesical arteries. The first branch of the anterior division is one of the main gluteal arteries, which could lead to claudication if inadvertently ligated (Figure 2.9). Small, less-important branches of the obturator, inferior gluteal, and, in the female, uterine and vaginal vessels also contribute to the abundant vascular supply of the urinary bladder. The bladder pedicles approach the bladder from a posterior and lateral approach. A posterior intraperitoneal approach to the bladder results in a delineation of both the lateral and posterior vascular supply, which is easily amenable to ligation using a laparoscopic endo-vascular stapling device.

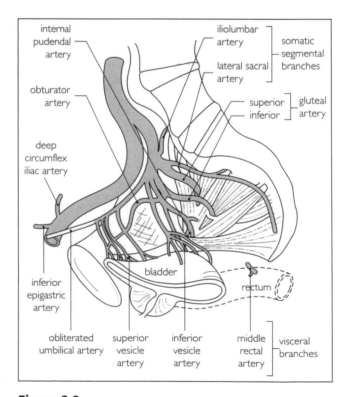

**Figure 2.9**
Blood supply of male bladder.

In the male, the bladder extends from the urachus to the dome, then widens to form the bladder proper before funneling and approaching the trigone and bladder neck. The urothelium extends in continuity as the urethra surrounded by the prostate under the pubic bone, then surrounded by corpus spongiosum it traverses the penis. On the superior surface of the male bladder, there is the peritoneal interface and the site for intraperitoneal rupture. Posteriorly, the bladder sits on the peritoneum, which in turn lies on the sigmoid colon and proximal rectum. The ureters enter in a posteriolateral location, being crossed by the ipsilateral vas deferens, prior to becoming transmural. Dissection and clipping of the distal ureter during cystectomy affords direct access to the posterior and lateral bladder vascular pedicles. The vasa deferentia traverse the posterior aspect of the bladder, crossing over the ureter, and then become the ductus deferentes before merging with the base of the seminal vesicles. The ejaculatory ducts exit this junction, running through the prostate, before becoming the ejaculatory ducts at the verumontanum.

The female bladder has completely different anatomic relationships. The peritoneum interfaces from the bladder dome, down to the posterior wall (Figure 2.10). The reflection of peritoneum interposes between the bladder and uterus and is known as the 'pouch of Douglas'. An anteverted uterus and proximal anterior vagina lie on the posterior bladder wall and therefore are considered part of the radical female cystectomy specimen.

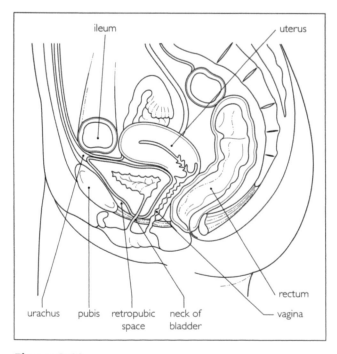

**Figure 2.10**
Sagittal section of female pelvis, demonstrating anatomic relation of pelvic structure with the bladder.

# Prostate

The anatomy of the prostate is surgically challenging because of the position of the gland deep in the pelvis in close proximity to critically important surrounding structures. The rectum, external urethral sphincter, neurovascular bundles, bladder neck, and dorsal venous complex make laparoscopic extirpation of the prostate gland challenging. Although with current technology laparoscopic prostate surgery remains technically demanding, the ability to work in a small space, deep in the pelvis, and with excellent illumination, makes the laparoscopic approach very appealing. The rapid expansion and dissemination of laparoscopic radical prostatectomy is inevitable, but the procedure will require advances in surgical skills and adjunctive technologies, including digital imaging, surgical robotics and, perhaps, anastomotic suturing devices.

Prostatic anatomy has been redefined by the transperitoneal approach to the laparoscopic radical prostatectomy popularized by Guillonneau and Vallancien.[16] The transperitoneal approach affords the urologist the comfort of familiar anatomic structures and landmarks. When the patient is placed in the Trendelenburg position, the peritoneal contents move cephalad by gravity retraction. Inspection of the operative field will reveal familiar structures anteriorly, including the lateral and medial umbilical ligaments. The urinary bladder is easily identified by locating the Foley catheter in the midline. The internal spermatic rings can be clearly identified with the vas deferens exiting posteromedially and the spermatic vessels entering anterolaterally. Lateral to the medial umbilical ligaments, pulsations of the external iliac arteries can be appreciated through the peritoneum. In thin patients, the outline of the iliac arteries can also be seen. The external iliac veins are usually compressed by standard insufflation pressures, but they are reliably located medial to the external iliac artery.

Using steep Trendelenburg positioning and instrument retraction, the surgeon can identify two pelvic 'arches'. The superficial 'arch' is the transverse vesical fold, and the deep 'arch' is the vesicosacral (sacrogenital) fold. The sigmoid colon can be seen posterior to the lower arch. Incision of the peritoneum just posterior to the deep pelvic arch in the midline will reveal the vas deferens in the midline. Immediately lateral to the vas deferens, the seminal vesicles can be identified with a characteristic white lobular appearance (Figure 2.11). The ureters are located lateral to the seminal vesicles and typically are a more robust tubular structure. If there is any question as to which structure has been identified, the vas deferens can be identified exiting the internal spermatic ring and dissected out to the midline incision.

Cephalad traction on the seminal vesicles and the vas deferens will expose Denonvilliers' fascia. This fascia has a glistening white appearance and can be incised to expose

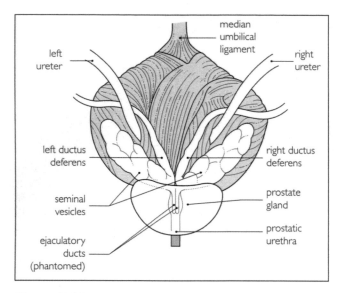

**Figure 2.11**
The posterior view of the bladder and prostate delineating the relationship of seminal vesicles, ureters, and ductus deferentes.

the perirectal fat. Depending on the individual patient's anatomy, the plane between the prostate gland and the rectum sometimes can be developed via this approach. Occasionally, the rectum appears oriented in a more anterior-posterior direction, precluding antegrade dissection to the apex of the prostate. With the transperitoneal approach, the anterior surface of the prostate can only be exposed by mobilizing the bladder. The margins of the bladder are easily identified by instillation of fluid via the Foley catheter. In the midline, the urachus and dome of the bladder are typically more cephalad than is anticipated. Once the bladder has been anteriorly mobilized, the anterior surface of the prostate is easily identifiable. The symphysis pubis is an excellent laparoscopic landmark, as it is quite hard and can easily be appreciated even with the limited tactile sensation afforded by laparoscopic instrumentation.

The endopelvic fascia investing the prostate is covered with a layer of fibroadipose tissue that can be bluntly dissected free and separated from the fascia. Once the fatty tissue is removed, the endopelvic fascia appears white and glistening. Frequently, a small defect in the endopelvic fascia can be appreciated between the lateral aspects of the puboprostatic ligaments and the fascia investing the prostate. Incision of the endopelvic fascia exposes the pubococcygeus component of the levator ani muscle complex laterally and the lateral edge of the prostate medially. In the midline, the superficial dorsal venous veins are relatively subtle because of standard insufflation pressure. The superficial dorsal veins can be controlled easily and safely with bipolar or ultrasonic energy. The branches of the dorsal vein complex are diffuse in their distribution; small

branches may pass medially or laterally to the puboprostatic ligaments. The excellent illumination and magnification of laparoscopy allow the laparoscopic surgeon to identify and avoid these structures. In fact, standard insufflation pressures create a tamponade effect and greatly reduce the venous bleeding associated with ligation and transaction of the dorsal vein complex. The urethra lies immediately posterior to the dorsal venous complex. A distinct 'notch' is identifiable as the urethra exits the apex of the prostate. Again, the magnification and decreased bleeding associated with the laparoscopic approach allows for accurate transection of the urethra with preservation of the external urethral sphincter. The rectourethralis muscle connects the posterior aspect of the urethra and the rectum. The fibers of this muscle are distinct and can be transected to separate the posterior aspect of the apex of the prostate and the urethra from the rectum.

Typically, during open prostate procedures, the bladder anterior neck is identified by palpation. Laparoscopically, the location of the bladder neck can be reliably determined by gently sweeping the fibroadipose tissue off the anterior surface of the prostate in a cephalad direction. At the level of the bladder neck the fatty tissue becomes adherent to the bladder and gives a distinct visual clue as to the location of the bladder neck. Sharp and blunt dissection in the plane between the prostate and bladder neck reveals a relatively avascular plane. Frequently, the urethra can be distinctly identified, and bladder neck preservation is facilitated by the laparoscopic approach. Early retrovesical dissection facilitates transection of the posterior bladder neck as the retrovesical space is easily identified. Anterior traction on the previously dissected vasa deferentia and seminal vesicles allows for posterior dissection of the prostate off the perirectal fat.

The neurovascular bundles may have a variable course but usually are located at the 5 and 7 o'clock positions on the prostate. As the neurovascular bundles run towards the apex of the prostate, their course moves anteriorly. At the apex of the prostate the neurovascular bundles are located at the 3 and 9 o'clock positions immediately lateral to the urethra (Figure 2.12). Incision of the lateral prostatic fascia and gentle posterior dissection will expose the lateral prostatic pedicle, which can be secured with clips or harmonic scalpel, thus avoiding and preserving the neurovascular bundle.

## Conclusion

Intimate knowledge and thorough understanding of genitourinary anatomy are the foundations of all urologic laparoscopy. This is an enhanced visual approach to anatomic dissection with limited haptic feedback as opposed to open surgery (with its limited visual with full

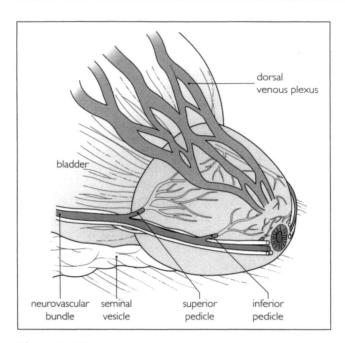

**Figure 2.12**
Superior lateral view of prostate and its neurovascular
bundle.

haptic feedback). Thus, laparoscopic visual details of
anatomy enables the laparoscopist to approach all urologic
disease processes.

# References

1.  Hurd WH, Bude RO, Delancey JO, et al. Abdominal wall char-
    acterization by magnetic resonance imaging and computed
    tomography. The effect of obesity on laparoscopic approach.
    J Reprod Med 1991; 36:473.

2.  Hurd WW, Bude RO, DeLancey JO, et al. The relationship
    of the umbilicus to the aortic bifurcation: implications for
    laparoscopic techniques. Obstet Gynecol 1992;
    80:48.

3.  Pattaras JG, Moore RG, Landman J, et al. Incidence of post-
    operative adhesion formation after transperitoneal genito-
    urinary laparoscopic surgery. Urology 2002; 59(1):37–41.

4.  Seifman BD, Dunn RL, Wolf JS. Transperitoneal laparoscopy
    into the previously operated abdomen: effect on operative
    time, length of stay and complications. J Urol 2003; 169:
    36–40.

5.  Chen RN, Moore RG, Cadeddu JA, et al. Laparoscopic renal
    surgery in patients at high risk for intra-abdominal or
    retroperitoneal scarring. J Endourol 1998; 12(2): 143–7.

6.  Cadeddu JA, Chan DY, Hedican SP, et al. Retroperitoneal
    access for transperitoneal laparoscopy in patients at high
    risk for intra-abdominal scarring. J Endourol 1999;
    13(8):567–70.

7.  Gaur DD. Laparoscopic operative retroperitoneoscopy: use of
    a new device. J Urol 1992; 148:1137.

8.  McDougall EM, Clayman RV, Fadden PT. Retro-
    peritoneoscopy: the Washington University Medical School
    Experience. Urology 1994; 43:446.

9.  Capelauto CC, Moore RG, Silverman SG, Kavoussi LR.
    Retroperitoneoscopy: anatomic rationale for direct retro-
    peritoneal access. J Urol 1994; 152:2008.

10. Fromer DL, Birkhoff JD, Hardy MA, et al. Bilateral intrarenal
    adrenal glands in cadaveric donor kidneys resembling renal
    cell carcinoma on intraoperative frozen section. J Urol 2001;
    166:1820.

11. Gagner M, Lacroix A, Bolte E, et al. Early experience with
    laparoscopic approach for adrenalectomy. Surgery 1993;
    114:1120.

12. Sampaio FJB, Favorito LA. Ureteropelvic junction stenosis:
    vascular anatomical background for endopyelotomy. J Urol
    1993; 150:1787.

13. Gupta M, Smith AD. Crossing vessels at the ureteropelvic
    junction: do they influence endopyelotomy outcomes? J
    Endourol 1996; 10:183.

14. Pienkny AJ, Herts B, Streem SB. Contemporary diagnosis of
    retrocaval ureter. J Endourol 1999; 13:721.

15. Donahue JP, Maynard B, Zachary JM. The distribution of
    nodal metastasis in the retroperitoneum from nonsemino-
    matous testis cancer. J Urol 1982; 128:315.

16. Guillonneau B, Vallancien G. Laparoscopic radical prostatec-
    tomy: initial experience and preliminary assessment after 65
    operations. Prostate 1999; 39(1):71–5.

# 3

# Endourologic instrumentation and equipment

## Michael J Conlin

Endourology is a relatively new urologic field, and it has undergone significant change over the last two decades. Continued improvements in the design and manufacture of endoscopes and working instruments and refinement of our endoscopic techniques have increased the variety of upper urinary tract conditions that can be treated endoscopically. The rapid progress in endoscope and working instrument design can be attributed to significant cooperation between urologists and manufacturers.

Familiarity with available nephroscopes, ureteroscopes, and working instruments can equip the practicing urologist to treat a variety of upper urinary tract problems using minimally invasive techniques.

## Rigid ureteroscope development

Hugh Hampton Young first performed rigid ureteroscopy in 1912.[1] During cystoscopy of a 2-month-old child with posterior urethral valves and massively dilated ureters, he was able to pass a 9.5F (French units) pediatric cystoscope through the ureter to the renal pelvis and visualize the calices. Although this was the first ureteroscopy, it wasn't until the late 1970s that Goodman and Lyon separately reported routine rigid ureteroscopy.[2,3] Goodman reported using an 11F pediatric cystoscope to perform ureteroscopy in three adults. One of these patients had a distal ureteral tumor which was fulgurated. Lyon et al reported ureteral dilation with Jewett sounds prior to ureteroscopy with an 11F pediatric cystoscope in five adults.

Useful rigid ureteroscopes could not have been developed without the work of Harold Hopkins and his development of the rod lens system in the 1960s.[4] Until then, endoscopic telescopes were manufactured with small lenses separated by relatively large air spaces. The lenses were fragile and could easily become misaligned. The light transmission and optical quality were also poor by modern standards. Hopkins reversed the lenses and air spaces, so the majority of the telescopes were occupied by glass. Glass has a higher refractive index, resulting in better image and light transmission. The smaller air spaces functioned as the lenses. The result was more durable telescopes with improved optical quality and light transmission.

Wolf Medical Instruments developed the first endoscope specifically designed for ureteroscopy in 1979. This 13F endoscope was similar to pediatric cystoscopes, but its longer length (23 cm) permitted further excursion into the ureter of adult men and women.[5] This scope was designed for inspection only, and larger sheaths of 14.5 and 16F were required to perform stone extraction or other therapeutic procedures. These sheaths allowed passage of the relatively limited tools available for stone removal, including catheters, loops, and baskets. A longer ureteroscope of 39 cm, which could reach the renal pelvis, was developed with Perez-Castro and introduced by Karl Storz in 1980.[6] The longer length permitted inspection of the renal pelvis. Although these early ureteroscopes were useful, they required significant ureteral dilation. Further miniaturization was needed.

Significant advances in fiberoptics led to the development of flexible ureteroscopes, actually prior to routine rigid ureteroscopy. The development of flexible fiberoptics is discussed later in the chapter. Incorporation of fiberoptic image bundles and light bundles into rigid ureteroscopes resulted in smaller ureteroscopes while still maintaining excellent image quality. The first fiberoptic rigid ureteroscope was developed by Candela and reported by Dretler and Cho in 1989.[7] With a tip of 7.2F and two working channels of 2.1F, ureteral dilation was often unnecessary. All modern rigid ureteroscopes incorporate these fiberoptic improvements. Simultaneous improvements in working instruments and lithotripsy devices have made rigid ureteroscopy the standard of care for distal ureteral stones.

# Characteristics of rigid ureteroscopes

Although larger rod lens rigid ureteroscopes are available, most endourologists agree that the smaller fiberoptic ureteroscopes are less traumatic, less often require ureteral dilation, and are equally effective. These scopes have tips with diameters of 7F or less, and working channels greater than 3F. Working channels can be larger single or two smaller separate channels. There are significant advantages to having separate working channels. These include the ability to irrigate through one unrestricted channel while a working instrument occupies the other. Separate working channels also permit passage of a lithotripsy device through one channel to fracture a stone that cannot be disengaged from a basket in the other channel. With a single channel this can be difficult because of friction between the two working instruments. Eyepieces are commonly 'in line' with the ureteroscope, which allows easy introduction of the scope (Figure 3.1). Offset eyepiece design (Figure 3.2) permits a straight working channel for the use of more rigid working instruments (such as ultrasonic and pneumatic lithotripsy probes). With the more widespread use of the holmium laser for ureteroscopic lithotripsy, the need for ureteroscopes with offset eyepieces has decreased. Table 3.1 shows the specifications of the currently available fiberoptic rigid ureteroscopes.

Larger ureteroresectoscopes (11.5F) can be useful for large distal ureteral tumor resection (Figure 3.3). Some urologists prefer this instrument for ureteroscopic endopyelotomies.[8] Preoperative ureteral stenting is necessary in this setting to allow passage of the ureteroresectoscope to the ureteropelvic junction.

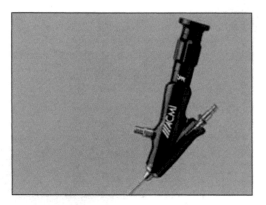

**Figure 3.2**
USA Series™ MRO™-6 MICRO operating ureteroscope. (Courtesy of Circon ACMI, Stamford, Connecticut.) The offset eyepiece is designed for physician comfort and the straight working channel gives added control for use of rigid operating instruments such as ultrasonic and pneumatic lithotripsy probes.

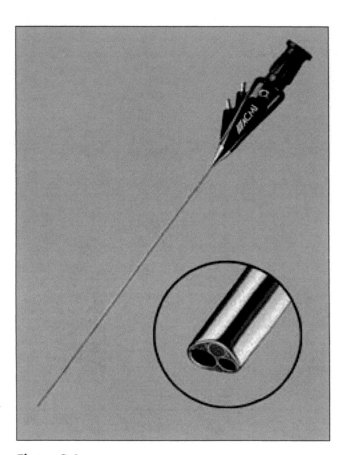

**Figure 3.1**
ACMI™ USA Series™ MICRO-6® semi-rigid ureteroscope. (Courtesy of Circon ACMI, Stamford, Connecticut.) Small ureteroscope with two large working channels for diagnostic and therapeutic procedures. It reduces patient trauma and operative time for procedures with minimal or no dilation and general anesthesia. It is also ideal for either laser or electrohydraulic intracorporeal lithotripsy.

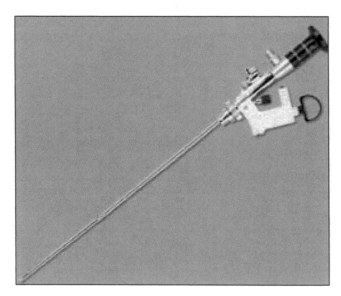

**Figure 3.3**
Rigid ureteroresectoscope. (Courtesy of Circon ACMI, Stamford, Connecticut.)

**Table 3.1** Fiberoptic rigid ureteroscopes (data supplied by manufacturers)

| Model | Eyepiece | Diameter (F) | Working length (CM) | Channels | Channel size (F) | Field of view (degrees) | Angle of view (degrees) | Focusing ocular |
|---|---|---|---|---|---|---|---|---|
| **Circon ACMI (Stamford, Connecticut)** | | | | | | | | |
| MR6 | Standard | 6.9/8.3/10.2 | 33 (MR6); 41 (MR6L) | 2 | 2.3; 3.4 | 65 | 5 | Yes |
| MR9 | Standard | 9.4/10.2/12.6 | 33 (MR9); 42 (MR9L) | 2 | 2.1; 5.4 | 65 | 5 | Yes |
| MRO6 | Angled offset | 6.9/8.3/10.2 | 33 (#633); 42 (#642) | 2 | 2.3; 3.4 | 65 | 5 | Yes |
| MRO7 | Angled offset | 7.7/9.2/10.8 | 33 (#733); 42 (#742) | 1 | 5.4 | 65 | 5 | Yes |
| MRO742-A | Angled offset | 7.7/9.2/11.2 | 42 | 1 | 5.4 | 65 | 5 | |
| **Olympus America (Lake Success, New York)** | | | | | | | | |
| A2940A; A2941A | Angled | 6.4/7.8 | 43 (A2940A); 33 (A2941A) | 1 | 4.2 | 88 | 7 | No |
| A2942A | Angled | 8.6/9.8 | 43 | 1 | 6.6 | 88 | 7 | No |
| A2948A; A2949A | Straight | 6.4/7.8 | 43 (A2948A); 33 (A2949A) | 1 | 4.2 | 88 | 7 | No |
| **Karl Storz Endoscopy (Culver City, California)** | | | | | | | | |
| 27400CK/CL | Movable/angled | 7.5/9/10.5 | 34 (CK); 43 (CL) | 2 | 2.4; 3.5 | 80 | 0 | Yes |
| 27410SK/SL | Straight | 7.5/9/10.5 | 34 (K); 43 (L) | 2 | 2.4; 3.5 | 80 | 0 | No |
| 27410CK/CL | Angled | 7.5/9/10.5 | 34 (K); 43(L) | 2 | 2.4; 3.5 | 80 | 0 | No |
| 27430K/L | Angled | 8/9/10.5/11 | 34 (K); 43 (L) | 2 | 2;4 | 80 | 0 | No |
| 27401K/L | Movable/angled | 10/10.5/12/13 | 34 (K); 43 (L) | 2 | 3; 5.5 | 80 | 0 | Yes |
| 27411K/L | Angled | 10/10.5/12/13 | 34 (K); 43(L) | 2 | 3; 5.5 | 80 | 0 | No |
| 27023SA/SB | Straight | 10/10.5/12/13 | 34 (SA); 43(SB) | 2 | 3; 5.5 | 80 | 0 | No |
| **Richard Wolf Medical Instruments (Vernon Hills, Illinois)** | | | | | | | | |
| 8721 | Standard | 4.5/6 | 31 | 1 | 2.5 × 3.6 (oval) | 73 | 0 | No |
| 8702; 8712 | Standard | 6/7.5/8.5 | 31 (8702); 42.5 (8712) | 1 | 4.2 × 4.6 (oval) | 73 | 0 | No |
| 8702.523; 8702.524 | Parallel offset | 6/7.5/8.5 | 31.5 (8702.523); 43 (8702.524) | 1 | 4.2 × 4.6 (oval) | 73 | 0 | No |
| 8702.533; 8702.534 | Angled | 6/7.5/8.5 | 31.5 (8702.533); 43 (8702.534) | 1 | 4.2 × 4.7 (oval) | 73 | 0 | Yes |
| 8707, 8703 | Standard | 8/9.8 | 31 (8707); 42.5 (8703) | 1 | 5.2 × 6.2 (oval) | 74 | 10 | No |
| 8705; 8719 | Offset | 8/9.8 | 31 (8719); 42.5 (8705) | 1 | 5.2 × 6.2 (oval) | 74 | 10 | No |
| 8704 | Offset | 8.5/11.5 | 31 | 1 | 6.2 × 8.2 (oval) | 74 | 10 | No |

# Flexible ureteroscope development

The history of flexible endoscopy is closely tied to the development of flexible fiberoptics. When light travels through a medium such as glass, internal reflection of the light occurs at the interface between that medium and its surroundings. This physical property of internal reflection which allows bending of light within flexible glass was first reported by Tyndall in 1854.[9] This technique of image transmission using internal reflection was patented in 1927. Current medical fiberoptic technology is based upon this physical property first demonstrated nearly 150 years ago.

Molten glass can be drawn or pulled into small-diameter fibers. These fibers will uniformly transmit light from one end to the other proportional to the light input. When the fibers are bundled randomly (such as the 'light bundle' within flexible endoscopes) and connected to a light source, they provide excellent light transmission for illumination. When the fibers are bundled with identical fiber orientation at each end (i.e. coherent), the single dots of light will coalesce to transmit images. 'Cladding' each individual fiber of glass with a second layer of glass of a different refractive index will improve the internal reflection and light transmission. This cladding process was developed and reported by Curtiss and Hirschowitz in 1957.[9] These men later reported the first use of a flexible gastroscope, which was used to visualize a duodenal ulcer. Cladding the fibers also improves the durability of the image bundles. The mesh-like appearance of the image from flexible endoscopes is due to the lack of light transmission through this cladding. The quality of the image obtained depends upon the number of fibers and how closely they are packed within the image bundle. Improvements in image bundle manufacture have allowed closer packing of more fibers, resulting in improved images, smaller outer diameters, and larger working channels in both rigid and flexible endoscopes.

Early flexible ureteroscopy, reported by Marshall in 1964 and later by Takagi et al and Bush et al, actually predated the first reports of routine rigid ureteroscopy.[10–12] Marshall reported passage of a 9F flexible endoscope through a 26F cystoscope into the ureter. A ureteral stone was visualized, but because there was no deflecting mechanism or working channel, little else could be done. These early prototype flexible ureteroscopes could only be used for visualization of the upper urinary tract. Because of these limitations, flexible ureteroscopy did not achieve widespread acceptance.

Takagi and coworkers reported their use of a flexible ureteroscope with deflecting tip allowing visualization of the calyces in 1971.[12] They and other urologists continued to improve flexible ureteroscopic techniques, such as the use of ureteral guide tubes and the use of diuresis for improved visualization. However, the interest of urologists and endoscope manufacturers remained focused on rigid ureteroscopy, and rapid improvements in rigid ureteroscopes dominated the 1980s. Access to much of the upper urinary tract for fragmentation of calculi was possible with these rigid endoscopes. When the limitations of the rigid ureteroscopes became apparent, there was renewed interest in flexible ureteroscope development. The later addition of active deflection, larger working channels, and effective working instruments 3F and less made possible the diagnosis and treatment of many more upper urinary tract problems than was possible with rigid ureteroscopes alone.

# Characteristics of flexible ureteroscopes

The basic components of flexible ureteroscopes include the optical system, deflection mechanism, and working channel (Figure 3.4). The optical system consists of the flexible fiberoptic image and light bundles. Improvements in the image bundles have been discussed in the preceding

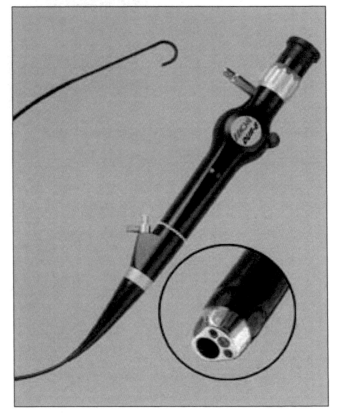

**Figure 3.4**
USA Series™ DUR™-8 durable flexible ureteroscope system. (Courtesy of Circon ACMI, Stamford, Connecticut.) A flexible ureteroscope has a dual deflection that facilitates access to the proximal ureter and the renal pelvis; it allows complete intrarenal access, including the lower pole calyces.

section. Small lenses attached to the proximal and distal ends of the image bundle create a telescope with image magnification, increased field of view, and focusing ability. By changing the axis of the optical system at the tip of the scope, the angle of view of the ureteroscope can be changed to improve early visibility of any working instruments passed out the working channel.[13] Another recent design modification is the splitting of the light bundle distally to provide more than one point of light transmission. This permits a more centrally placed working channel as well as better distribution of the light within the field of view.

The deflection mechanism is an integral part of flexible ureteroscopes (Figure 3.5). It permits complete maneuverability within the intrarenal collecting system.[14] Most deflecting mechanisms consist of control wires running down the length of the ureteroscope attached on the proximal end to a manually operated lever mechanism. Distally, the wires run through movable metal rings to the distal tip where they are fixed. Moving the lever up or down will pull the control wire and move the tip. When the tip moves in the same direction as the lever, the deflection is said to be 'intuitive' (i.e. down is down and up is up). Most modern flexible ureteroscopes allow both up and down deflection in a single plane.[15] This plane of deflection is marked by the reticle seen as a notch within the field of view of the ureteroscope (Figure 3.6). The active deflection mechanism frequently wears out with repeated use, requiring repair. Improvements in the design of the deflecting mechanism with each new generation of flexible ureteroscopes should improve durability.

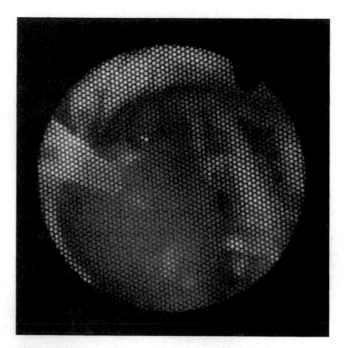

**Figure 3.6**
Endoscopic image of renal stone, guide wire, and laser fiber seen through a flexible ureteroscope. A reticle is seen at 1 o'clock.

Modern flexible ureteroscopes permit down deflection of approximately 180°. Bagley and Rittenberg measured the angle between the major axis of the ureter and the lower pole infundibulum (ureteroinfundibular angle) in 30 patients.[16] They reported the average angle to be 140°, with a maximum of 175°. Active deflection of the ureteroscope of 180° should allow visualization of the lower pole in most patients. However, reaching into the lower pole calyx with the tip of the ureteroscope can still be difficult. Active deflection occurs only at the distal tip of the ureteroscope, and the deflected segment may not be long enough to reach the lower pole calyx. The secondary, passive deflection mechanism addresses this problem. All flexible ureteroscopes have a more flexible segment of the ureteroscope due to a weakness in the durometer of the sheath, located just proximal to the point of active deflection. By passively bending the tip of the ureteroscope off of the superior margin of the renal pelvis, the point of deflection is moved more proximally on the ureteroscope, effectively extending the tip of the ureteroscope. When passive deflection is used, the lower pole calyx can be reached in over 90% of patients. Significant hydronephrosis can limit the ability to engage passive secondary deflection and reach the lower pole.

The first ureteroscope incorporating active secondary deflection was developed by Circon ACMI (Stamford, Connecticut). In addition to active primary deflection of 185° down and 175° up, there is a second control lever for active secondary deflection of 165° (Figure 3.7). This ureteroscope should enable the urologist to reach the lower

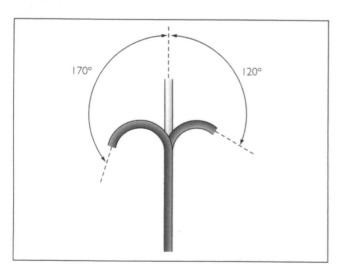

**Figure 3.5**
Flexible uretero-fiberscope. (Courtesy of Olympus America, Lake Success, New York.) The deflection mechanism is an integral part of a flexible ureteroscope. Active deflection of the ureteroscope allows visualization of the lower pole in most patients.

pole even under conditions when access with passive secondary deflection is not possible (Figure 3.8).

All currently available flexible ureteroscopes have working channels of at least 3.6F size. This allows use of

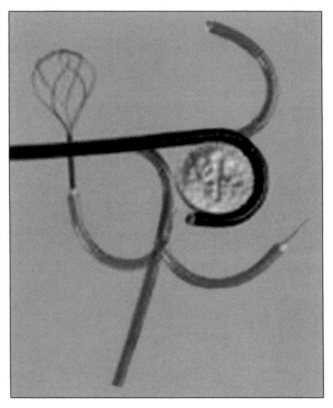

**Figure 3.7**
USA Series™ DUR™-8 Elite durable flexible ureteroscope system with primary and secondary deflection. (Courtesy of Circon ACMI, Stamford, Connecticut.) This ureteroscope provides an active secondary deflection. In addition to active primary deflection of 185° down and 175° up, there is a second control level for active secondary deflection of 165°.

instruments up to 3F, while still permitting adequate irrigation. When working instruments are used, higher pressure irrigation will be necessary to compensate for the effectively smaller irrigation channel. This higher pressure irrigation can be delivered using a pressurized irrigation bag, roller pump, or hand-held syringes. The specifications of currently available flexible ureteroscopes are detailed in Table 3.2.

Rigid and especially flexible ureteroscopes are very delicate instruments and need to be handled accordingly. Any damage to the working channel, deflecting mechanism, or fibers within the image bundle can render the ureteroscope useless. Ureteroscopes, including the working channel, should be cleansed with warm water and a nonabrasive detergent after each use. Sterilization of ureteroscopes can be performed by gas (ethylene oxide), soaking in a glutaraldehyde solution, or by using the Steris system (Mentor, Ohio).[17] The Steris system provides automated washing and rinsing of the endoscopes in a peracetic acid solution.

## Nephroscopes

Percutaneous nephrostolithotomy developed from early experience with antegrade pyelography in the early 1950s. Percutaneous nephrostomy was described by Goodwin et al in 1955 for the relief of hydronephrosis.[18] Surgical nephrostomy tube placement was largely replaced by percutaneous nephrostomy placement in the mid 1970s. In 1976, Fernstrom and Johannson placed a nephrostomy tube to remove a renal calculus.[19] It was the refinement of the percutaneous nephrostomy procedure that led to the development of percutaneous nephroscopy and nephrostolithotomy in the 1980s.

Percutaneous nephrostolithotomy is most commonly performed to remove large volumes of stone. Currently,

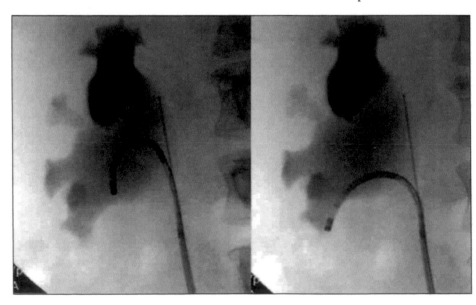

**Figure 3.8**
Inability to access the lower pole with primary deflection (left), but the lower pole is easily accessed using active secondary deflection (right).

**Table 3.2** *Flexible ureteroscopes*

| | Manufacturer/Model | | | | | | |
|---|---|---|---|---|---|---|---|
| | Circon-ACMI | | | Olympus | Karl Storz | Richard Wolf | |
| Parameter | AUR-7 | DUR-8 | DUR-8 elite | URF-P3 | 11274AA | 7330.072 | 7325.172 |
| Tip diameter (F) | 7.5 | 6.75 | 6.75 | 6.9 | 7.5 | 7.4 | 6.8 |
| Shaft diameter (F) | 7.5 | 8.6 | 8.6 | 8.4 | 8.0 | 9.0 | 7.5 |
| Working length (cm) | 65 | 65 | 65 | 70 | 70 | 70 | 70 |
| Channel size (F) | 3.7 | 3.6 | 3.6 | 3.6 | 3.6 | 4.5 | 3.6 |
| Active deflection up (degrees) | 100 | 175 | 175 | 180 | 120 | 130 | 130 |
| Active deflection down (degrees) | 160 | 185 | 185 | 100 | 170 | 160 | 160 |
| Location of passive deflection (cm from tip) | 7.5 | 7.5 | Active secondary deflection | 4.0–7.0 | 5.0 | 6.0 | 6.0 |
| Angle of view (degrees) | 0 | 12 | 12 | 0 | 6 | 0 | 0 |
| Field of view (degrees) | 80 ± 5 | 80 ± 5 | 80 ± 5 | 90 | 90 | 65 | 65 |
| Depth of field (mm) | 2–40 | 2–40 | 2–40 | 1–50 | 2–50 | 2–40 | 2–40 |
| Magnification | 30× | 30× | 30× | 52× | 40× | 50× | 50× |

the most effective intracorporeal lithotripsy energy for quickly removing large volume of stone is ultrasonic. Rigid nephroscopes are built with this in mind. The ultrasonic lithotripsy probes used for percutaneous applications are 3.5–4 mm in diameter and rigid. The working channels of rigid nephroscopes must be straight and large enough to accommodate these probes. Most rigid nephroscopes use rod lens technology, which provides superior optics. The eyepiece is offset to allow a straight working channel (Figure 3.9). Irrigation delivered through the large working channel is generally excellent, with some nephroscopes incorporating continuous flow designs. Flexible cystoscopes are frequently used as nephroscopes (Figure 3.10). Flexible nephroscopy combined with holmium laser lithotripsy and tipless baskets for fragment removal have decreased the need for multiple percutaneous accesses in most cases.

## Guide wires

Guide wires are essential to endourologic procedures (Figure 3.11). They are used for many portions of these procedures, including establishment of percutaneous access, ureteroscopic access, straightening of the ureter, a guide for dilation of the ureter or percutaneous tract, and for stent placement. There are many different guide wires available, differing in diameter, rigidity, tip design, materials, and coating. The choice of the most appropriate wire will depend upon the task involved, and the patient's anatomy and upper urinary tract problem being confronted.

The most common guide wire design is a solid core stainless steel wire around which an outer wire is wrapped. Nitinol (nickel–titanium alloy) inner wires give guide wires a kink-resistant construction. Because of nitinol's 'memory' quality, reliable angling of the tip is possible. Many newer wires have a nitinol core wire and a polyurethane outer cover. When coated with a hydrophilic polymer, these exceptionally slippery wires are useful for negotiating around impacted ureteral calculi, tortuous ureters, and ureteral strictures (Figure 3.12). The hydrophilic-coated wires are too slippery to be reliable safety wires, because of their tendency to slide out of the patient. When these wires are used for initial access, they are exchanged for a standard safety wire. New hybrid designs incorporating a hydrophilic tip with a standard Teflon (polytetrafluoroethylene; PTFE)-coated shaft may serve as both the access and safety wires for these difficult access cases.

Guide wires for urology range in diameter from 0.018 to 0.038 inches, the most commonly used being 0.038 inches in diameter. Lengths vary from 80 to 260 cm (centimeters). The most useful length for endourology is 145 cm. The tips

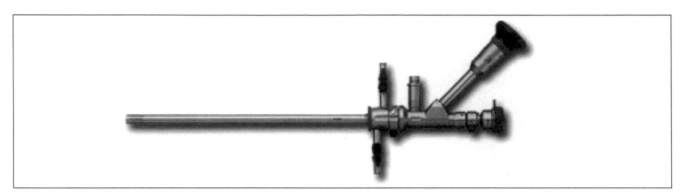

**Figure 3.9**
Percutaneous nephroscope. (Courtesy of Olympus America, Lake Success, New York.) The offset eyepiece allows a straight working channel.

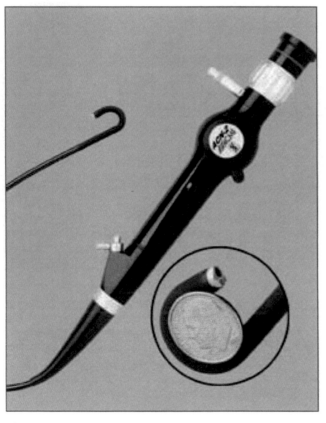

**Figure 3.10**
USA Series™ ACN™-2 Flexible CystoNephroscope. (Courtesy of Circon ACMI, Stamford, Connecticut.) The flexible nephroscope allows access to the different calyces via one percutaneous site and thus decreases the need for multiple percutaneous accesses in most cases.

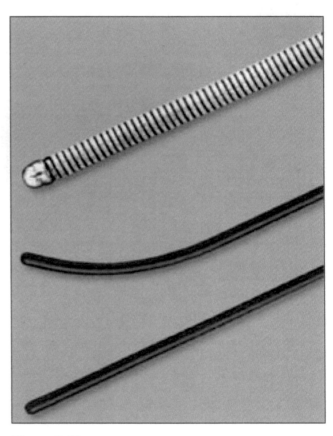

**Figure 3.11**
Guide wires. (Courtesy of Circon ACMI, Stamford, Connecticut.) Many guide wires are available, differing in diameter, rigidity, tip design, materials, and coating.

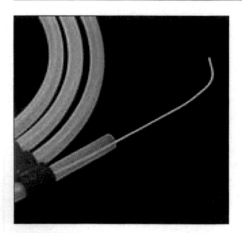

**Figure 3.12**
Roadrunner PC® wire guides with Slipcoat™ hydrophilic coating. (Courtesy of Cook Urological, Spencer, Indiana.) This guide wire has a nitinol core wire and a polyurethane outer cover coated with a hydrophilic polymer. This slippery guide wire is very useful for negotiating around impacted ureteral calculi, tortuous ureters, and ureteral strictures.

of these wires are generally 'floppy' for 1–3 cm. Bentson and Newton wire designs have flexible tips of up to 15 cm, and are seldom used today. Some wires have a movable core wire which can be partially withdrawn to increase the length of the flexible tip. Other variable characteristics in guide-wire construction include the distal tip design and the wire stiffness. The distal tip can be straight, angled, or 'J' tipped. The rigidity of the wires can be varied by changing the diameter and design of the inner core wire. Stiffer wires are useful for straightening out tortuous ureters, and dilating long percutaneous tracts in obese patients.

The choice of the most appropriate guide wire for the endourologic task at hand can mean the difference between success and failure. Despite all of these advances in wire design and construction, an 0.038-inch diameter straight, flexible tip, Teflon-coated, stainless steel wire is still the best choice for most cases.

## Dilation devices

Ureteral dilation is less necessary for ureteroscopy with the advent of the newer, smaller-diameter ureteroscopes.[20] Ureteral dilation can be accomplished passively with indwelling stent placement. More commonly, ureters are dilated with dilating catheters (Figure 3.13) or balloons (Figure 3.14). Ureteral dilating catheters are hydrophilic-coated polyurethane catheters, tapered from a 6F tip to 12F shaft, and are passed over a wire to dilate the ureter.[21] Ureteral balloon dilators are also passed over a wire, have a low profile of 3–8F, and dilation diameters of 12–30F. Dilation of the ureter beyond 15–18F is rarely necessary for routine ureteroscopy. Balloons can have maximum

inflation pressures of 8–20 atmospheres, depending upon the design and the material used for balloon manufacture. Zero-tip design ureteral balloon dilators are useful for dilating immediately adjacent to an impacted ureteral calculus. Ureteroscopic balloon dilators are 3F in size, can be inflated to 12F, and are passed directly through the ureteroscope. They are used to dilate under direct vision such as dilation of stenotic infundibula and calyceal diverticular necks. Once inflated, these ureteroscopic balloons often cannot be removed through the ureteroscope. The ureteroscope must be removed with the balloon.

The most common dilation devices for percutaneous tracts are the disposable Amplatz dilators (Figure 3.15), and balloon dilators (Figure 3.16). The Amplatz dilators are tapered tip catheters sequentially passed over a wire in increasing sizes. The balloon dilation systems are faster and simpler to use and don't require multiple passes over the wire. The Amplatz dilators are better than the balloon dilators for dilating scar tissue from previous renal surgery.

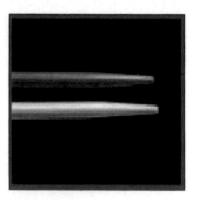

**Figure 3.13**
Ureteral dilators. (Courtesy of Cook Urological, Spencer, Indiana.) Dilators are used for dilation of the ureter prior to ureteroscopy and/or stone manipulation.

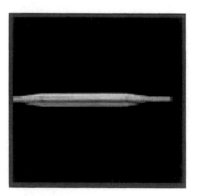

**Figure 3.14**
Balloon ureteral dilator. (Courtesy of Cook Urological, Spencer, Indiana.) A ureteral dilation balloon catheter is used for transluminal dilation of ureteral strictures or ureteral dilation prior to ureteroscopy or stone manipulation. It has radiopaque markers that indicate the proximal and distal ends of the balloon.

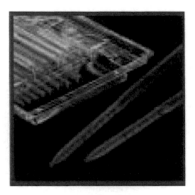

**Figure 3.15**
Amplatz renal dilator set. (Courtesy of Cook Urological, Spencer, Indiana.) This set allows sequential dilation of a tract to the kidney for percutaneous access. The tips of the catheters are tapered to pass over a wire in increasing sizes.

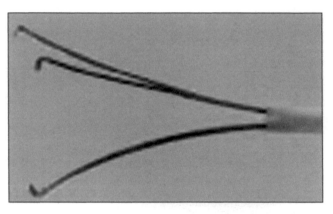

**Figure 3.17**
Grasping forceps. (Courtesy of Circon ACMI, Stamford, Connecticut.) A grasping forcep for stone removal with a ureteroscope.

## Stone retrieval devices

Essentially, any working instrument 3F or less in size can be used through the ureteroscope. These include a variety of stone graspers and baskets, electrodes, cup biopsy forceps, and intraluminal lithotripsy devices. Three-pronged stone-grasping forceps are the safest instruments for removing calculi with the flexible ureteroscope (Figure 3.17). They permit disengagement of calculi that have been found to be too large to be safely removed from the ureter. In fact, their grasp is weak enough to release the stone if too much force is applied. This is critical when performing flexible ureteroscopy because there is no second channel to permit fragmentation of an unyielding stone trapped within a basket. Rigid ureteroscopes with two working channels have this added degree of safety, permitting more routine use of baskets. The components of stone baskets include the control handle, the control wire, the sheath, and the basket itself. Stone baskets are available in the usual helical and flat-wire designs, and can also vary in the

number and type of wires used. Two sheathing materials are available, Teflon and polyimide. Polyimide is a very durable but stiff material and will limit deflection of the flexible ureteroscope. Teflon does not limit deflection as much as polyimide. Newer hybrid designs incorporate Teflon at the tip and polyimide in the shaft, to emphasize the advantages of each material. Helical baskets can be made with three-, four- or double-wire designs with six or more wires (Figure 3.18A,B). The double-wire designs have improved opening strength, which may facilitate removal of impacted calculi. Helical baskets have round wires, and unlike flat-wire baskets, are safe to rotate within the ureter. They are opened above the stone and pulled down while rotating the basket to engage the stone.

Flat-wire baskets are nonhelical and are designed to have larger spaces between the wires to allow engagement of larger stones (Figure 3.19A,B). Most are constructed with four wires. They were originally designed for percutaneous use, where, by filling the calyx when opened, they can more

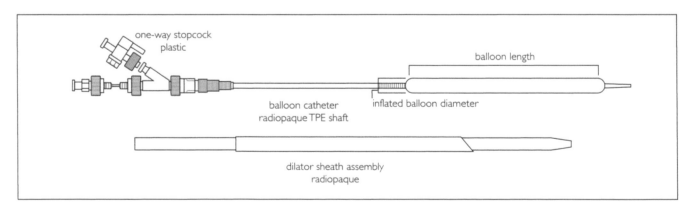

**Figure 3.16**
Nephrostomy tract dilator set. (Courtesy of Cook Urological, Spencer, Indiana.) The balloon dilator is used to dilate the musculofascial tract, renal capsule and parenchyma during percutaneous procedures. Radiopaque markers are placed at the proximal and distal ends of the balloon. A radiopaque dilator/sheath is fitted to the balloon catheter to allow coaxial placement.

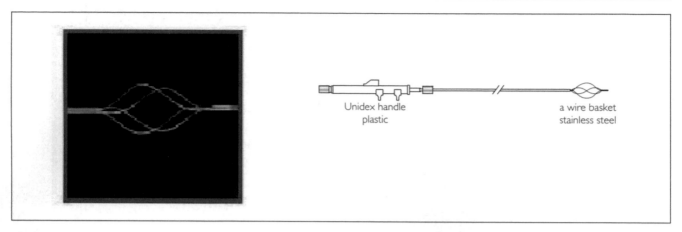

**Figure 3.18A,B**

Helical stone extractor. (Courtesy of Cook Urological, Spencer, Indiana.) Helical baskets are made with three-, four-, or double-wire designs with six or more wires. The double-wire designs have improved opening strength, which may facilitate removal of impacted calculi.

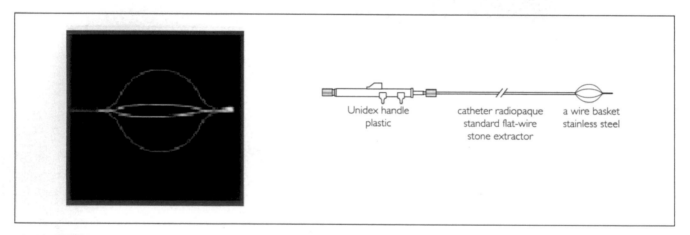

**Figure 3.19A,B**

Flat-wire stone extractor. (Courtesy of Cook Urological, Spencer, Indiana.) Flat-wire baskets are nonhelical and are designed to have larger spaces between the wires to allow engagement of larger stones.

easily engage calyceal stones. When used for ureteral calculi a flat-wire basket should be opened alongside rather than above the stone. They are also useful for the biopsy of papillary ureteral tumors.[22]

Stone basket diameters vary in size from 1.9 to 7.0F, with baskets for ureteroscopy 3.0F or less, and larger sizes for percutaneous nephrostolithotomy. A new addition is the tipless, nickel–titanium (nitinol) stone basket (Figure 3.20). The soft nitinol wires have memory, maintain their shape, resist kinking, and therefore open safely and reliably. This basket is particularly useful for percutaneous applications, but because it may permit safer disengagement of larger calculi, may also be used within the intrarenal collecting system through the flexible ureteroscope. Other basket designs such as the Parachute (Figure 3.21) (Boston Scientific, Natick, Massachusetts) and the SurCatch™ (Figure 3.22) (Circon ACMI, Stamford, Connecticut) have more wires exposed on the distal end of

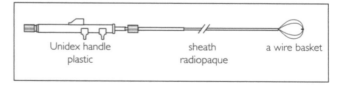

**Figure 3.20**

N-Circle nitinol tipless stone extractor. (Courtesy of Cook Urological, Spencer, Indiana.) A nitinol stone basket is useful in the intrarenal collecting system with a flexible ureteroscope because of its softness and its ability to disengage from a stone.

the basket, making them effective for removing multiple small fragments.

The latest development in stone retrieval devices is the Stone Cone (Figure 3.23) (Boston Scientific, Natick, Massachusetts).[23] This is a 3F device with a distal coil that can be deployed above the stone prior to fragmentation to help prevent stone migration. Following fragmentation of

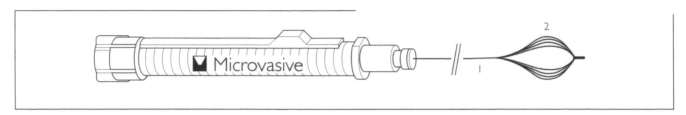

**Figure 3.21**
Microvasive Leslie Parachute™ stone retrieval device. (Courtesy of Boston Scientific, Natick, Massachusetts.) The unique basket geometry allows efficient capture and retention of multiple stone fragments.

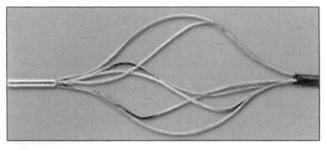

**Figure 3.22**
Sur-Catch™ paired-wire basket. (Courtesy of Circon ACMI, Stamford, Connecticut.) This basket has large proximal openings to facilitate stone entry while crossed distal wires capture fragments to prevent escape.

the stone, it is withdrawn to remove fragments. Any fragments too large to remove safely will be left behind because the coil simply unravels around the stone. Further experience with this device should demonstrate its clinical usefulness.

Other devices are available for ureteroscope use. Small 3F cup biopsy forceps can be used to biopsy sessile tumors (Figure 3.24). Electrodes are available in various shapes including pencil point, ball point, angled, and straight tips (Figure 3.25). These are used for fulguration and incision procedures such as endoureterotomy and endopyelotomy.

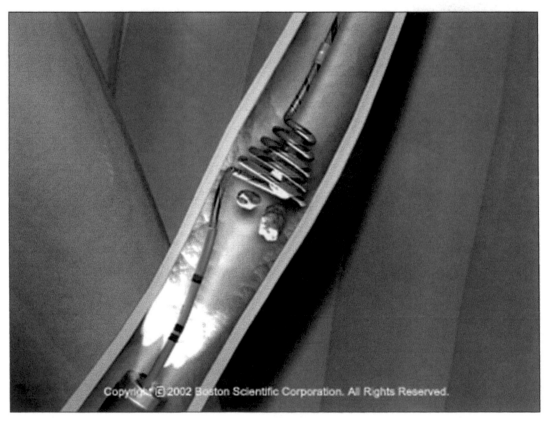

**Figure 3.23**
Microvasive Stone Cone™ nitinol retrieval device. (Courtesy of Boston Scientific, Natick, Massachusetts.) The Stone Cone nitinol retrieval coil is designed to sweep multiple stone fragments.

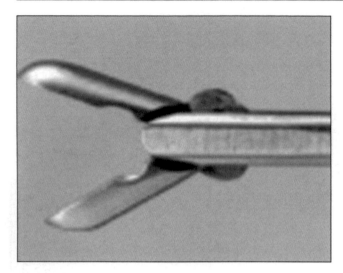

**Figure 3.24**
Flexible biopsy cup. (Courtesy of Circon ACMI, Stamford, Connecticut.) Ureteroscopic biopsy forceps are used to biopsy upper tract lesions.

## Additional equipment

Fluoroscopy is a critical tool during endourologic procedures, and is needed for initial ureteral and percutaneous access, monitoring during the endoscopy, and stent and/or nephrostomy tube placement. Although tables designed for urologic endoscopy with fixed fluoroscopy units are available, mobile C-arm fluoroscopy units are preferable. C-arm fluoroscopy units allow greater mobility, improved image quality, and less radiation exposure for the surgeon because the X-ray source is below the patient rather than above. Modern C-arm fluoroscopy units incorporate digital enhancement of the image and last image-hold technology to minimize radiation exposure to the patient and surgeon. Older units without these features should not be used. Urologic endoscopy tables allow fluoroscopy of the entire abdomen, positioning of the patient in lithotomy, and should support at least 500 lb (227 kg) of patient weight. Additional features such as the ability to position the patient in the prone split-leg position for percutaneous procedures are also desirable.

## Conclusions

This chapter has only scratched the surface of available devices used for endourologic procedures. Detailed knowledge about instruments and their relative advantages and problems can be the difference between success and failure. Endourologists are only as good as their instruments, and appropriate choice and use of these devices can contribute greatly to improved patient outcomes.

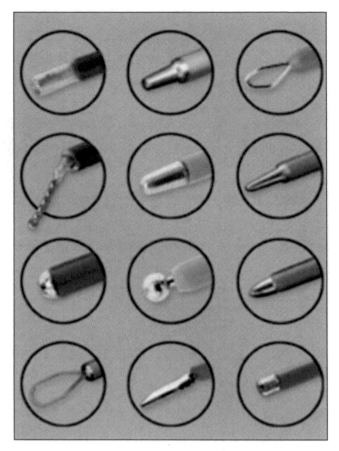

**Figure 3.25**
Flexible electrodes. (Courtesy of Circon ACMI, Stamford, Connecticut.) Different shapes of electrodes are available for fulgurations and incisions with the ureteroscope.

## References

1. Young HH, McKay RW. Congenital valvular obstruction of the prostatic urethra. Surg Gynecol Obstet 1929; 48:509.

2. Goodman TM. Ureteroscopy with pediatric cystoscope in adults. Urology 1977; 9:394.

3. Lyon ES, Kyker JS, Schoenberg HW. Transurethral ureteroscopy in women: a ready addition to the urological armamentarium. J Urol 1978; 119:35–6.

4. Hopkins HH. British patent 954,629 and US patent 3,257,902, 1960.

5. Lyon ES, Banno JJ, Schoenberg HW. Transurethral ureteroscopy in men using juvenile cystoscopy equipment. J Urol 1979; 122:152–3.

6. Perez-Castro EE, Martinez-Piniero JA. Transurethral ureteroscopy – a current urological procedure. Arch Esp Urol 1980; 33:445.

7. Dretler SP, Cho G. Semirigid ureteroscopy: a new genre. J Urol 1989; 141:1314–6.

8. Thomas R, Monga M, Klein EW. Ureteroscopic retrograde endopyelotomy for management of ureteropelvic junction obstruction. J Endourol 1996; 10:141–5.

9. Barlow DE. Fiberoptic instrument technology. In: Tams TR, ed. Small animal endoscopy. St Louis: CV Mosby, 1990.

10. Marshall VF. Fiberoptics in urology. J Urol 1964; 91:110.

11. Bush IM, Goldberg E, Javadpour N, et al. Ureteroscopy and renoscopy: a preliminary report. Chic Med Sch Q 1970; 30:46–9.

12. Takagi T, Go T, Takayasu H, Aso Y. Fiberoptic pyeloureteroscope. Surgery 1971; 70:661–3.

13. Higashihara E, Minowada S, Kameyama S, Aso Y. Angled optical axis for central viewing of endoscopic accessories. J Endourol 1990; 4:361.

14. Bagley DH. Flexible ureteroscopy. Semin Urol 1989; 7:7–15.

15. Grasso M, Bagley D. A 7.5/8.2 F actively deflectable, flexible ureteroscope: a new device for both diagnostic and therapeutic upper urinary tract endoscopy. Urology 1994; 43:435–41.

16. Bagley DH, Rittenberg MH. Intrarenal dimensions. Guidelines for flexible uteropyeloscopes. Surg Endosc 1987; 1:119–21.

17. Gregory E, Simmons D, Weinberg JJ. Care and sterilization of endourologic instruments. Urol Clin North Am 1988; 15:541–6.

18. Goodwin WE, Casey WC, Woolf W. Percutaneous trocar (needle) nephrostomy in hydronephrosis. JAMA 1955; 157:891.

19. Fernstrom I, Johansson B. Percutaneous pyelolithotomy. A new extraction technique. Scand J Urol Nephrol 1976; 10:257–9.

20. Bagley DH. Expanding role of ureteroscopy and laser lithotripsy for treatment of proximal ureteral and intrarenal calculi. Curr Opin Urol 2002; 12:277–80.

21. Gaylis F, Bastuba M, Bidair M, Friedel W. Ureteral dilation using a tapered dilator: a cost-effective approach. J Endourol 2000; 14:447–9.

22. Bagley DH. Ureteroscopic laser treatment of upper urinary tract tumors. J Clin Laser Med Surg 1998; 16:55–9.

23. Dretler SP. The stone cone: a new generation of basketry. J Urol 2001; 165:1593–6.

# 4

# Laparoscopic instrumentation and equipment

Stephen V Jackman and Jay T Bishoff

The advancement of laparoscopic surgical technique goes hand in hand with the development of laparoscopic instrumentation. Only the surgeon's imagination and the willingness of industry to produce innovative equipment limit the development and application of new devices. In this chapter we describe the current state of the art in laparoscopic instrumentation with the goal of increasing surgeons' knowledge of the devices available to assist them in their laparoscopic surgical procedures. Many instruments, although not essential, are advantageous in condensing the learning curve, shortening procedure times, and improving outcomes.

## Access

A significant number of complications during laparoscopic surgery occur at the time of initial access to the peritoneal cavity.[1] The traditional method of Veress needle insufflation followed by blind insertion of a cutting trocar is being replaced by numerous more controlled and theoretically safer techniques. These include use of dilating-tip trocars, visual obturators, and variations on the open Hasson technique. Balloon inflation may be used to rapidly develop the retroperitoneal or retropubic spaces.

Blind-cutting trocars offer rapid access to the peritoneal cavity. Their sharp blades require less force than blunter options. However, their safety has been questioned for initial port placement, especially in the non-virgin abdomen. Even utilizing these trocars during secondary trocars placed under direct internal vision, the risk of laceration of body wall blood vessels and muscle exists. Transillumination of the abdominal wall is seldom useful for locating blood vessels, except in thin patients. Finally, cutting trocars $\geq 10$ mm make incisions in the fascia that require closure. For these reasons, dilating-tip or non-bladed trocars were developed. Many manufacturers offer versions of this style of trocar (Figure 4.1). The tips are typically cone-shaped, often with laterally placed fins to assist in the dilation. The fins can vary from sharp to dull. Advantages include smaller fascial openings after port removal that do not require closure and a higher likelihood of pushing aside rather than lacerating blood vessels and

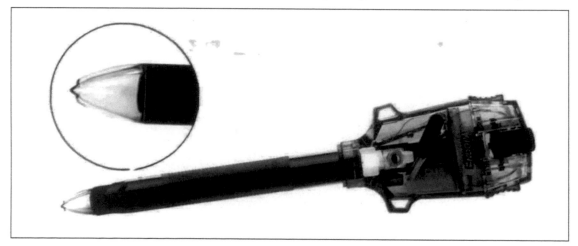

**Figure 4.1**
The 10/12 mm bladeless trocar with tip close-up (Ethicon Endo-Surgery, Cincinnati, Ohio). (Composite of photos courtesy of Ethicon Endo-Surgery.)

muscle.[2] This technology may be combined with direct visualization as described below. Disadvantages include a higher insertion force and increased difficulty penetrating compliant structures such as the peritoneum and bladder.[3]

Visual obturators or direct-view trocars are systems combining sheath, cutting, or dilating elements and laparoscope. These systems allow direct visualization of the layers and blood vessels of the body wall during entry. These devices are typically used after insufflation. However, with experience, they may be used for both initial access and insufflation. Two disposable instruments in this category are the Visiport RPF Optical Trocar (USSC, Norwalk, Connecticut), shown in Figure 4.2, and the Optiview Non-bladed Obturator (Ethicon Endo-Surgery, Cincinnati, Ohio), (shown in Figure 4.3). The Visiport uses a trigger-activated cutting blade to enter the abdomen, whereas the Optiview has two dilating fins. The Optiview requires more pressure and rotation to enter the abdomen but

retains the advantages of non-bladed instruments, including smaller fascial defects that may not require closure. The EndoTIP system (Karl Storz GmbH & Co. KG, Tuttlingen, Germany) is a reusable threaded screw-in trocar that allows visualization and also incorporates a dilating tip.

Arguably the safest method for entrance to the peritoneal cavity is by the open Hasson technique. Open access is particularly important in children, in whom standard-sized laparoscopic trocars may be more likely to damage vital structures. Disadvantages of the Hasson technique include the need for a larger incision, more cumbersome trocar systems that may leak gas if not well-secured, and increased difficulty in obese patients. The Step System (formerly InnerDyne, Inc.; now USSC, Norwalk, Connecticut) is a modification of this method that solves some of these problems (Figure 4.4). Through a small skin incision, the fascia and peritoneum are opened 2–3 mm

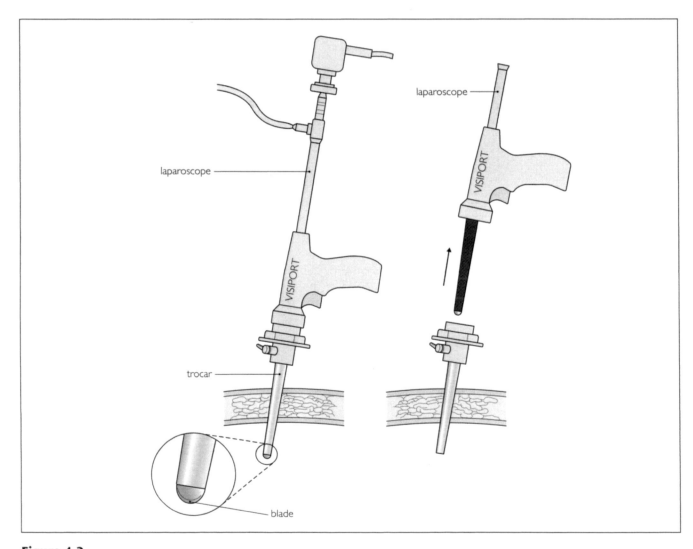

**Figure 4.2**
The Visiport (USSC, Norwalk, Connecticut) uses a recessed blade that extends out of the end of the obturator as the surgeon fires a trigger.

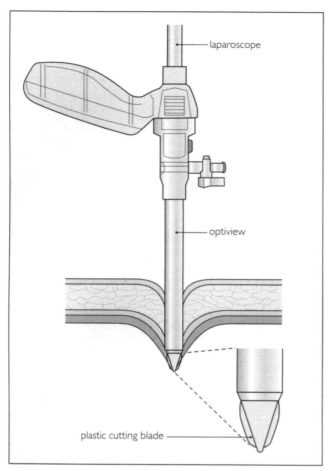

**Figure 4.3**
The Optiview (Ethicon Endo-Surgery, Cincinnati, Ohio) uses two sharpened plastic fins on the tip of the trocar.

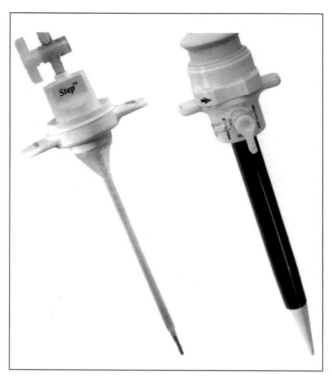

**Figure 4.4**
The Step System (USSC, Norwalk, Connecticut). The mesh sleeve can be placed in an open fashion or used with a Veress needle as shown. The cannula and dilator is then passed through the sleeve. (Photos courtesy of United States Surgical, a division of Tyco Healthcare.)

under direct visualization. The mesh sleeve is then inserted and dilated with a rigid cannula and dilator to the desired size (5–12 mm). This radial dilation both fixes the sheath in place and seals the peritoneal cavity, preventing gas leakage. The access may also be conveniently upsized if needed by inserting a larger rigid sheath and dilator. The entire system can also be used over a Veress needle. However, the advantages of open insertion are lost. The fascial defect left after removing a Step trocar has been shown to be 50% smaller than that associated with a conventional cutting trocar.[4] Overlying tissue and muscle planes return to their preoperative location after removal and provide further closure of the wound. A prospective randomized trial in 250 patients showed that the Step system results in significantly less intraoperative cannula site bleeding and fewer postoperative wound complications than conventional cutting trocars.[5] Furthermore, no port-site hernias were seen despite not closing any of the Step port sites.

Another modification of the Hasson technique for access to non-peritoneal locations is use of a balloon to rapidly develop the space. This was initially done using a red-rubber catheter with a glove finger secured to the end. More convenient commercial products that perform the same task are now available. A useful combination of balloon and visual obturator, the Preperitoneal Distention Balloon System (PDB; formerly Origin Medsystems; now USSC, Norwalk, Connecticut) or Spacemaker II Balloon Dissector (formerly GSI, Inc.; now USSC, Norwalk, Connecticut) is available to allow direct observation during space creation (Figure 4.5). A balloon-tipped or Hasson trocar is required to seal the initial incision. The Blunt-tipped Trocar (USSC, Norwalk, Connecticut) is a significant advance over the standard Hasson trocar. It has a balloon at the distal end to hold it in place and a sliding foam ring proximally to seal it to the abdomen. This allows full 360° motion without leakage in a small footprint device.

## Retraction

Prolonged retraction of organs such as the liver and bowel is often necessary for access to the operative site. When adequate gravity retraction is not possible, numerous

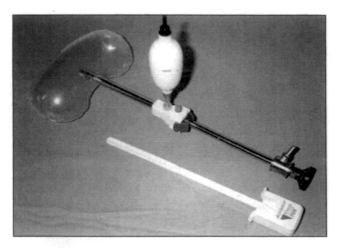

**Figure 4.5**
The PDB System (USSC, Norwalk, Connecticut). The retroperitoneal space can be balloon developed under direct vision.

instruments are available. The ideal retractor would fit through a small trocar, hold the target organ securely and atraumatically, remain exactly where it was placed, and be either reusable or inexpensive. Most current instruments accomplish the first two conditions with reasonable success. They are typically variations on the design of a straight 5 or 10 mm instrument that transforms into a wider configuration once inserted.

An innovative reusable device is the Diamond Flex 80 mm Angled Triangular Liver Retractor (Genzyme Surgical Products Corp., Tucker, Georgia) (Figure 4.6). This long multi-jointed instrument passes through a 5 mm port and then transforms into a rigid triangular shape after its knob is tightened. Other sizes and configurations exist.

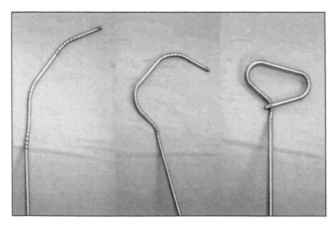

**Figure 4.6**
The Diamond Flex 80 mm Angled Triangular Liver Retractor (Genzyme Surgical Products Corp., Tucker, Georgia) fits through a 5 mm cannula and converts to a rigid angled triangular shape.

Disadvantages include the initial expense and the metal construction that does not hold organs as securely as some disposable fabric devices. The PEER retractor (Jarit Surgical Instruments, Hawthorne, New York) is another reusable device that opens to provide retraction in a variety of situations. It is available in 5 and 10 mm sizes.

Fan retractors are available from several manufacturers in either a reusable or disposable form. They typically fit through a 10 mm port and 'fan' open into a triangular shape. Other common variations include balloons and fabric that expand after insertion. One significant disadvantage of the previously described instruments is that they require an assistant to reliably hold them in position. This introduces the human factors of fatigue and inattention, which can cause lack of retraction, often at the worst possible moment. In addition, the assistant takes up space at the side of the table and can hinder the optimal movement and positioning of the surgeon. Several mechanical instrument holders have been developed to take the place of the assistant. The instrument is then positioned and locked in place by one of several methods. The basic Martin Arm (Mick Radio-Nuclear Instruments, Inc., Mount Vernon, New York) is a multi-jointed stainless steel arm that requires each joint to be positioned and hand-tightened. The Unitrac Retraction System (Aesculap, Center Valley, California) is an advanced version of the Martin Arm that uses compressed air to allow pneumatic locking and unlocking with a single button (Figure 4.7). The Endoholder (Codman Inc., Cincinnati, Ohio) is an innovative device with a flexible gooseneck that can be quickly bent into position.[6] The TISKA Endoarm is a system developed to assist with trocar and instrument positioning (TISKA Endoarm, Karl Storz, Endoskope, Tuttlingen, Germany). This device maintains the position of the trocar sheath at a fixed point at the trocar puncture site, while instruments or laparoscopes are changed or removed. Routine laparoscopic needs such as tissue retraction can easily be performed with this system. When combined with a robotic camera holder, these instrument holders permit many procedures to be done completely without assistance.

## Hand-assist devices

The merits of hand-assisted laparoscopy (HAL) vs pure laparoscopy in urology are a matter of significant current debate. Proponents point to the proven ability to decrease operative times, allow performance of complex procedures, and aid in resident teaching.[7] This is achieved with a slight increase in postoperative pain but no significant increase in recovery times.[8] The issue of cost can be balanced by shorter operating room times and decreased need for other disposables such as trocars and entrapment

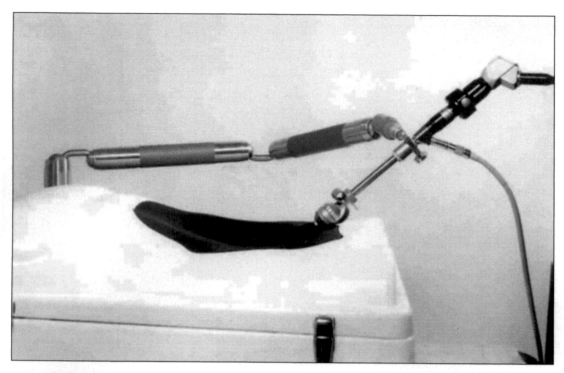

**Figure 4.7**
The Unitrac Retraction System (Aesculap, Inc., Center Valley, California) is locked in place with compressed air. It can hold various instruments for retraction. (Photo courtesy of Aesculap, Inc.)

bags. Furthermore, injuries related to Veress needle and initial trocar access should be eliminated, as all of the HAL devices except the Pneumo Sleeve can be used for primary insufflation. The GelPort and Lap Disc also allow airtight passage of the laparoscope to visually direct subsequent port placement.

Opponents object to hand-assisted techniques because they are not actually minimally invasive since HAL requires an incision large enough to allow placement of the surgeon's hand into the abdomen. The same complex cases are being done 'purely laparoscopically' by experts, often in shorter times than those reported in hand-assisted series. These experts argue that use of the hand is a 'crutch' rather than a 'bridge' to improved surgical ability.[9] Other disadvantages of HAL include device failure, air leakage, hand pain and fatigue with extended dissection or tight incisions, decreased view and working room due to the intra-abdominal placement of the surgeon's hand, and cosmetic concerns created by the larger incision.

Currently, there are six FDA-approved devices available for HAL surgery (Table 4.1). They all incorporate two basic features: an airtight seal between the device and the incision and a second seal between the device and the surgeon's arm (Figure 4.8). In general, devices using adhesive to seal the incision require a larger footprint and may offer more interference with choice of port-site locations. They also will not provide a reliable seal when placed so that the adhesive is near the umbilicus. An Ioban drape (3M Health Care, St. Paul, Minnesota) may be helpful in improving the durability of the adhesive seal. Regardless of the device chosen, some gas leakage can be expected, especially in longer operations. A high-flow or dual insufflation system is desirable.

Little data exist comparing the different HAL devices. A recent prospective evaluation of three HAL devices (HandPort, Intromit, and Pneumo Sleeve) showed highest overall satisfaction with the Intromit.[10] It was easier to exchange hands or lap pads with the Intromit or HandPort than with the Pneumo Sleeve. The HandPort was the easiest to set up but also had the highest failure rate. Surgeons are encouraged to try several devices before selecting one for routine use.

## Hemostasis

Some of the most significant advances in laparoscopic instrumentation have been achieved in hemostasis. Excessive bleeding from even small venous vessels can

**Table 4.1** *Hand-assisted laparoscopic devices*

|  | Pneumo Sleeve | Omniport | HandPort | GelPort | Intromit | Lap Disc |
|---|---|---|---|---|---|---|
| Company | Weck Closure Systems, Research Triangle Park, North Carolina | Weck Closure Systems, Research Triangle Park, North Carolina | Smith & Nephew, Inc., Andover, Massachusetts | Applied Medical, Rancho Santa Margarita, California | Applied Medical, Rancho Santa Margarita, California | Ethicon Endo-Surgery, Cincinnati, Ohio |
| Seal to incision | Adhesive | Inflation/wound retractor | Inflation/wound retractor | Wound retractor | Adhesive | Wound retractor |
| Seal to arm | Sleeve | Inflation | Sleeve | Gel | Inflation | Iris |
| Cost | $495 | $440 | $375 | $725 | $495 | $440 |

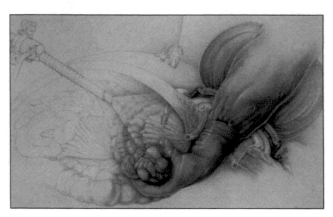

**Figure 4.8**
The Pneumo Sleeve (Weck Closure Systems, Research Triangle Park, North Carolina) in cross section showing the airtight seals between the device and abdominal wall and the device and the surgeon's arm. (Photo courtesy of Weck Closure Systems.)

quickly obscure the surgical field, making it difficult to find the correct planes of dissection. The availability of new delivery systems for electrocautery, ultrasound, clips, staples, clamps, and fibrin products has allowed laparoscopy to approach open surgery in even the most challenging cases.

## *Electrocautery*

Monopolar electrocautery has been the mainstay for hemostasis of small vessels during dissection. In the monopolar circuit the active electrode is in the surgical site and the return electrode is the grounding pad. Consequently, the current passes through the body of the patient to complete the circuit. The waveform can be continuous or intermittent (cut or coagulation) and is low current with high voltage.

When monopolar electrocautery is used, the current is not localized to the visible portion of the instrument. Since only 15% of the entire length of the electrocautery instrument is seen with the laparoscope at any given time, injuries from stray energy can occur out of the surgeon's field of view.[11] More than half of laparoscopic bowel injuries reported in the literature result from monopolar electrocautery.[12] Application of monopolar electricity to duct-like strands of tissue attached to the bowel, even during a short burst of energy, can result in tissue death at the bowel segment.[13] Unrecognized bowel injuries can also occur from the use of monopolar electrocautery when stray energy is released from unrecognized breaks in the integrity of the insulated coating or from capacitive coupling along the shaft of the monopolar instruments or trocar.

The occurrence of cautery injury can be minimized through the use of active electrode monitoring (AEM) devices or insulation scanners for monopolar instruments and bipolar electrocautery. The Electroscope AEM system (Electroscope, Inc., Boulder, Colorado) includes a unique set of laparoscopic instruments that are simultaneously connected to a standard electrocautery machine and to a separate device that continuously searches for stray energy escaping along the shaft of the instrument. When stray energy is detected, the AEM system deactivates the electrosurgical generator before injury can occur. The integrity of the insulated coating on the shaft of laparoscopic instruments can also be determined on the back table, prior to placing the instrument into the patient, using the InsulScan (Medline Industries, Inc., Mundelein, Illinois). Both disposable and reusable instruments can be tested for visually undetectable holes in the insulation sheath.

In bipolar electrocautery, the active electrode and the return electrode functions are performed at the site of surgery between the tips of the instrument. The waveform is continuous, low current, and low voltage. Since the flow of current is restricted between the contact points of the instrument tip, only the tissue grasped is included in the electrical circuit, minimizing the risk of injury from stray surgical energy. Thermal injury can be prevented by vigilant surveillance of monopolar contact points during dissection.

The Ligasure is a specialized electrosurgical generator/instrument system that has been developed (Valleylab, Boulder, Colorado) to reliably seal tissue and blood vessels up to 7 mm in diameter during laparoscopic or open surgery. The electrical generator delivers a continuous waveform of low-voltage, high-current flow and pulsed electrosurgical energy to tissue between the jaws of the instrument. The tissue is under a predetermined amount of pressure set by the unique locking jaws of the instrument. The vessel lumen is obliterated as collagen and elastin in the vessel wall fuse to form a permanent seal. The seal zone is then divided with standard laparoscopic scissor. The newest version (Ligasure Atlas, Valleylab, Boulder, Colorado) is a 10 mm instrument that incorporates a blade in the jaws of the instrument to divide the obliterated tissue safely.

## Argon gas coagulation

Argon gas enhanced coagulation is useful in partial nephrectomy and in the treatment of injury to the liver and spleen. This system uses the properties of electrosurgery and a stream of argon gas to improve the delivery of the electrosurgical current. Argon gas is noncombustible and inert, making it a safe gas to use in the presence of electrosurgical current. The argon gas is ionized by the electrical current, making it more conductive than air. The highly conductive stream of argon gas provides an efficient pathway for delivering the current to tissue, resulting in hemostasis. The flow of argon gas also disperses blood, improving visualization during coagulation. During argon beam coagulation, the pressure inside the abdomen can quickly rise above the preset level. Consequently, an insufflation port should be opened during coagulation and the intra-abdominal pressure carefully monitored.

## Ultrasound

A relatively new tool for laparoscopic dissection uses ultrasonic energy to achieve precise cutting and coagulation. Three devices are currently available (The UltraCision System, Ethicon Endo-Surgery, Cincinnati, Ohio; The AutoSonix System, USSC, Norwalk, Connecticut; and SonoSurg, Olympus America, Inc., Melville, New York). Energy is delivered using a laparoscopic 5 mm or 10 mm handpiece with a shaft tuned to conduct the ultrasonic vibration at the rate of approximately 55,000 cycles/s. The vibration causes heat, which is more precisely located at the vibrating tip, and, at 50–100°C, is much lower than conventional electrocautery. Different tip configurations are available, including hooks, shears, and blunt probes. As the tissue is compressed between the jaws of the shears, blood vessels are occluded and the vibration causes intracellular water vaporization. Proteins are denatured in the tissue and protein coagulum forms, sealing blood vessels while tissue is divided. Hemostasis and division of tissue occur at temperatures less than conventional cautery, without the wide dispersion of heat, creating a small band of tissue necrosis. Water vapor is emitted in the abdomen instead of smoke. While the cords are reusable for all three systems, only the Olympus SonoSurg offers an autoclaveable, reusable handpiece.

## Temporary vessel occlusion

Laparoscopic partial nephrectomy is now possible due to instruments that allow temporary occlusion of the renal hilar vessels. Two manufacturers offer bulldog clamps that are endoscopically applied through a 10 mm trocar. The jaws range in size from 17 to 45 mm, and come in curved and straight configurations (Klein Surgical Systems, San Antonio, Texas; Aesculap, Inc., Center Valley, Pennsylvania) (Figure 4.9). A 5 mm laparoscopic Statinsky clamp is also available but requires the placement of an additional trocar (Klein Surgical Systems, San Antonio, Texas).

## Surgical clips

Occlusive clips are useful for small veins and arteries, and have become standard equipment in most laparoscopic cases. As in open surgery, clips provide a rapid alternative for hemostasis. Most endoscopic clips today are made of titanium, and vary in size from 5 to 12 mm. Nonabsorbable polymer locking clips are also available and offer the advantage of being radiolucent (Weck Closure

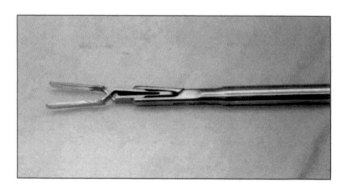

**Figure 4.9**
Laparoscopic bulldog clamp and applier (Klein Surgical Systems, San Antonio, Texas).

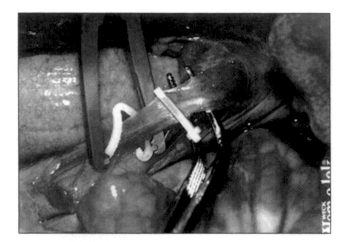

**Figure 4.10**
Hem-o-lok polymer clips (Weck Closure Systems, Research Triangle Park, North Carolina). (Photo courtesy of Weck Closure Systems.)

Systems, Research Triangle Park, North Carolina) (Figure 5.10). However, each clip is loaded separately on a reusable 10 mm applier. There are absorbable clips, and some research shows no difference in adhesion formation between metallic and absorbable clips.[14]

Most laparoscopic clip appliers are single use and multi-load, carrying between 15 to 30 clips per unit (Table 4.2). The ability to fire multiple clips without exiting the abdomen to reload can save significant time and decrease blood loss. In general, the diameter of the shaft depends on the size of clips. The Endoclip (USSC, Norwalk, Connecticut) 5 mm shaft single-use clip applier can deliver a slightly larger clip than other 5 mm clippers: its hinged jaws are normally retracted within the shaft, but upon squeezing the handles they advance and expand and a clip is automatically loaded. Most disposable clip appliers have 360° rotating shafts, allowing the handle of the instrument

to rest comfortably in the hand while placing the tips around the target tissue at an ideal angle. Right angle clip appliers (USSC, Norwalk, Connecticut) are also available and can offer a visual advantage in situations where the tips of straight appliers are not well seen.

## Tacking staples

The laparoscopic biting stapler was originally developed for laparoscopic hernia repair with mesh, but these devices are also useful in refashioning the peritoneum in laparoscopic ureterolysis and fixing mesenteric defects in bowel resections. Much like the staplers used for skin wound closure, laparoscopic staplers fire titanium staples with sharp ends that enter the tissue and then undergo deformation into a rectangular shape. Most contemporary devices are single use and multi-load, with 15–30 staples/unit. A 360° rotating shaft allows accurate placement of the staple. Some devices also come with a 60–65° distal articulating head, which permits tacking hard-to-reach areas like the anterior abdominal wall and deep pelvis.

## Linear staplers

Laparoscopic linear staplers are essential for rapid, safe intracorporeal tissue division and reapproximation of visceral structures. With a squeeze of a handle, these devices deploy multiple, closely spaced parallel rows of titanium staples. Staples come in three different 'loads' – thin/vascular, medium, and large/thick – and are color-coded for easy recognition. Thin staples penetrate tissue to a depth of 2–2.5 mm, deform to an exaggerated b-shape, and form a reliably hemostatic staple line. These staples are

| **Table 4.2** *Clip appliers (multi-load, single use)* | | | | | |
|---|---|---|---|---|---|
| | Ligaclip Allport | Ligaclip ERCA | Right Angle AccuClip | Endoclip 5 mm | Endoclip II |
| Company | Ethicon | Ethicon | USSC | USSC | USSC |
| Port size | 5 mm | 10 and 12 mm | 8 mm | 5 mm | 10 mm |
| Clips | 20 | 20 | 20 | 12 | 20 |
| Clip sizes | Medium, medium/large | Medium, medium/large, large | Medium/large | Medium/large | Medium/large, large |
| Clip load | Automatic | Automatic | Automatic | Separate lever | Automatic |
| Cost | $288 | $218 | $210 | $327 | $236 |

Ethicon = Ethicon Endo-Surgery, Cincinnati, Ohio; USSC = USSC, Norwalk, Connecticut

ideal for rapid division of vascular pedicles. Medium-to-large staples are 3.0–4.8 mm thick in their closed form, and are useful in securing thicker tissues like bowel, bladder, and ureter. The larger staples do not fold to the same tight shape as small staples and should not be used for primarily hemostatic ligation. Staplers today allow the same instrument to fire between 8 and 25 separate loads before stapler disposal.

Linear staplers can be broadly classified into cutting and non-cutting. Cutting versions deploy loads with six intercalated parallel rows of staples. As the staples are fired, a knife follows closely behind and incises the tissue between the staples, leaving three rows of staples on each side. The staple line extends past the range of the cutting knife by one or two staples to avoid incising non-secured tissue. Once the staples are fired, a safety feature on all devices prevents accidental re-deployment of the cutting knife until a new load with staples is in place. Non-cutting staplers simply fire three to four parallel rows of staples, and are useful for closing enterotomies and repairing bladder injuries.

Laparoscopic linear cutting staplers are further distinguished by the length of their staple line (30/35, 45, and 60 mm), and whether their firing heads are articulated or not (Table 4.3). An articulating head gives a greater range of motion from a fixed trocar but also adds to the price. All devices offer a rotating shaft, which allows proper visualization of the tips during firing. On most models, a replacement load consists of a fresh six rows of staples but uses the same knife and anvil inherent to the actual stapling device. The Endo GIA Universal linear cutting stapler is a universal firing device that accommodates both articulating and non-articulating loads of varying lengths (30, 45, and 60 mm) (USSC, Norwalk, Connecticut). The stapler is unique in that the jaws, anvil, and knife are inherent to the load and not part of the actual base unit; i.e. each re-load comes with a new knife. Also, this system allows the surgeon to use loads (articulating or fixed) of varying lengths without having to open a new stapler. The minimum-size limitation posed by the width of the staple load requires use of a 10 mm or larger port for all currently available staplers.[15]

## Loop ligation

Loop ligatures are valuable in securing an already transected pedicle. A length of suture with a pre-formed sliding, locking knot is passed intracorporeally. The structure to be ligated is then retracted through the loop with a grasper, and the loop cinched down with a knot pusher. Two loop ligature systems are available with both 0 and 2-0 plain gut, chromic gut, polyester, and synthetic absorbable varieties (Surgitie, USSC, Norwalk, Connecticut; Endoloop, Ethicon, Cincinnati, Ohio). The plastic knot pusher is only available in one length, and may be too short to reach the target site if the wrong port is chosen. Two hands are needed to cinch the knot, requiring an assistant to grasp the tissue and hold it still.

## Fibrin products

Fibrin tissue adhesive (FTA) has gained widespread acceptance in a variety of surgical procedures as an adhesive,

| **Table 4.3** *Linear staplers* | | | | | | |
|---|---|---|---|---|---|---|
| | Endopath ETS | Endopath ETS/flex articulating | Endopath EZ45: cutter | Multifire Endo GIA 30 | Multifire Endo TA | Endo GIA Universal |
| Company | Ethicon | Ethicon | Ethicon | USSC | USSC | USSC |
| Port size | 12 mm | 12 mm | 18 mm | 12 mm | 12 mm | 12 and 15 mm |
| Staple size | 2.5, 3.5, and 4.1 mm | 2.5, 3.5, and 4.1 mm | 3.8 and 4.5 mm | 2.0, 2.5, and 3.5 mm | 2.5 and 3.5 mm | 2.0, 2.5, 3.5, and 4.8 mm |
| Staple length | 35 and 45 mm | 35 and 45 mm | 45 mm | 30 mm | 30 mm | 30, 45, and 60 mm |
| Rotating shaft | Yes | Yes | Yes | Yes | Yes | Yes |
| Articulating | No | Yes | No | No | No | Yes |
| Cost | $399 | $498 | $495 | $433–500 | $433–500 | $433–500 |

Ethicon = Ethicon Endo-Surgery, Cincinnati, Ohio; USSC = USSC, Norwalk, Connecticut.

sealant, hemostatic agent, or carrier for growth factors or antibiotics. Fibrin products have been used in many different urologic procedures to assist with hemostasis and tissue adhesion.[16,17] FTA can also be valuable in treating complications of laparoscopic surgery, including spleen and liver injury, urinary fistula formation, and wound dehiscence.[18] Presently, FTA is made from autologous preparations using a patient's own blood or from homologous sources using a single donor or pooled samples.

Concentrates of coagulation factors are known for their adhesive and coagulation properties. In addition, fibrin in surgical wounds promotes healing by supplying a network for the growth of fibroblasts and activating macrophages.[19] Surgeons have prepared their own fibrin sealants for many years. However, these locally prepared products are not standardized and the sources of fibrinogen are not virally inactivated. Commercially available blood-derived products are now available for topical application to control bleeding and seal tissue. The basic principle is the same for these kits. Human thrombin and fibrinogen are applied separately to a bleeding site, resulting in formation of a layer of fibrin that controls the bleeding and seals tissue. Eventually, the fibrin film is reabsorbed.

Commercial preparations reproduce the final stage of coagulation, resulting in their adhesive, hemostatic, and healing effects through the polymerization of fibrin chains with collagen of adjacent or damaged tissue. These fibrin sealants are made from different combinations of fibrinogen and thrombin derived from human plasma and fibrinolysis inhibitor, a substance of bovine origin. As part of normal coagulation, fibrinogen undergoes proteolysis by the enzyme thrombin to form a fibrin monomer that polymerizes into fibrin strands, making up a major component of the actual clot. Thrombin also activates clotting factor XIII, promoting cross-linking of the fibrin monomer to stabilize the fibrin network. Thrombin is found in the plasma as an inactive precursor – prothrombin. After proteolysis, the active enzyme thrombin is formed. Proteolysis occurs as a result of tissue damage to cell membranes (extrinsic pathway) or trauma to the blood vessel walls, exposing collagen (intrinsic pathway), which results in the activation of thrombin followed by fibrin clot formation. The clotting time of fibrin sealant is dependent on the concentration of thrombin in the sealant.

Commercial fibrin sealants are typically packaged as freeze-dried concentrates of human fibrinogen and thrombin in separate containers. The powders are reconstituted and bovine fibrinolysis inhibitor (aprotinin) is added to the liquid fibrinogen. When the fibrinogen and thrombin solutions are mixed, they become active, forming a clot of adhesive (Haemacure Corp., Sarasota, Florida; Tisseel, Baxter Healthcare Corporation, Glendale, California). Another product currently available uses the patient's own plasma mixed with bovine thrombin and

bovine collagen (CoStasis, US Surgical, Norwalk, Connecticut) but is FDA approved for hemostasis alone and not for tissue sealing or tissue adhesion.

The American Red Cross has developed a lyophilized fibrinogen and thrombin product that is combined on a prepackaged absorbable backing (similar to a $4 \times 4$ sponge) or a powder spray. The $4 \times 4$ bandage is designed to be applied directly to the wound in open cases, while the powder formulation is readily delivered laparoscopically.[20–23] When these products contact the surgical site or blood, they are activated and rapidly form a dense synthetic clot. The lyophilized formulation is currently under investigation and not FDA approved for human use.

Since fibrin sealants commonly consist of human and bovine products, there is a theoretical risk of viral transmission, anaphylaxis, and coagulopathy. Viral transmission is of great concern since pooled human plasma is used to make the sealant. Donor screening, heat treatment of tissue, and solvent/detergent treatment seem to be effective in maintaining the safety of these products by preventing the transmission of HIV, Epstein–Barr virus, cytomegalovirus, and hepatitis.[24] However, four patients are known to have been infected with parvovirus B19 following treatment with fibrin sealant.[25,26] Infection with parvovirus B19 is usually asymptomatic or may present with a minor febrile illness. Rarely, transient aplitic crisis with rapid red blood cell turnover can occur. There is an isolated report of a patient who developed rash, bronchospasm, and circulatory collapse following use of fibrin sealant to close an enterocutaneous fistula. A complete investigation showed her to have aprotinin-specific antibodies, which were the most likely cause of the severe anaphylactic reaction.[27] Fibrin sealants are designed for topical use and are not designed for systemic injection. Intravenous injection could result in systemic activation of the coagulation cascade and fatal thrombosis. No systemic effects have been reported using sealants on surgical bleeding sites.

## Suture assist

Given the complexity of suturing in the laparoscopic environment, the majority of early laparoscopic urologic cases were extirpative and required little to no reconstruction. Unique demands to be overcome include a fixed center of motion, limited needle and suture handling ability, lack of three-dimensional perspective, and intracorporeal knot tying. Today, with the increasing interest in laparoscopic radical prostatectomy, more urologists are becoming proficient in free-hand suturing. This technique is applicable to most situations and offers the greatest flexibility with respect to suture and needle choices as well as the angle at which a needle may be held. For special circumstances and for those less experienced in free-hand techniques, several instruments have been developed to facilitate laparoscopic suturing.

The EndoStitch (USSC, Norwalk, Connecticut) is an innovative device that passes a small needle back and forth between jaws, allowing both running and interrupted suturing techniques without the need to worry about reloading the needle. It also facilitates rapid intracorporeal knot tying (Figure 4.11). Limitations of the EndoStitch include its 10 mm width and short dull needle that cannot be passed through thick tissue and is more traumatic than a similar-sized swedged-on suture. The needle can only be passed perpendicularly from jaw to jaw and may require excess tissue manipulation for proper suture placement. Finally, the device is disposable and reloads are costly, adding to the expense of a case. Despite these disadvantages, the EndoStitch has been used very successfully, even in cases requiring delicate reconstruction such as laparoscopic pyeloplasty.[28]

The Suture Assist (Ethicon Endo-Surgery, Cincinnati, Ohio) is a 5 mm instrument designed to place a pretied knot quickly after using either the device or a needle driver to place a single or figure-of-eight throw. Running sutures

are not possible without using an alternative knot-tying method for the second knot. Like the EndoStitch, the Suture Assist is disposable and relies on reloads.

A newer 5 mm instrument, the Sew-Right SR5 (LSI Solutions, Rochester, New York), uses two built-in needles to place a simple suture precisely through even relatively thick tissue. Advantages include its 5 mm size and needle passage parallel to the device, which may be better for some applications. With tenacious tissue, if the needle deviates or does not fully penetrate the tissue, it may miss or not engage the suture at the distal jaw. Again, this is a disposable instrument and only a single simple suture may be placed per load.

A final device, the Quik-Stitch (Pare Surgical, Englewood, Colorado) is available in 3, 5, 10, and 12 mm versions. This system consists of a proprietary needle driver passed through a spool containing a pretied knot. A single or figure-of-eight suture is placed or passed, followed by release, setting, and advancement of the knot. The device and needle driver are reusable, making it economical. Straight, curved, and blunt needles are available on absorbable and nonabsorbable sutures.

Intracorporeal knot tying, especially the second knot of a running suture, can be complicated. This is due to the short suture length often available for tying, the need to tie a single strand to a loop, and difficulty in maintaining constant tension on a knot. Two instruments are available to assist with this task. The Lapra-Ty (Ethicon Endo-Surgery, Cincinnati, Ohio) places a resorbable polyglycolic acid clip on the tail or tails of a suture to secure a running or simple suture. This allows precise tensioning of the suture with another instrument during 'tying'. The instrument is reusable and clips come six to a pack, making it economical. A concern is that a large number of clips may incite an inflammatory reaction or fistula. It is therefore most valuable for the final 'knot' of running sutures.

A second 'knot-tying' instrument is the Ti-Knot TK5 (LSI Solutions, Rochester, New York). This device is designed to replace extracorporeal knot tying. Once the two suture ends have been brought out through the trocar, they are snared and fed through a titanium cylinder at the end of the device. While holding the sutures under the proper tension, the instrument is advanced to the closure site and fired. This crimps the titanium knot onto the suture and trims the extra. Advantages promoted by the manufacturer include precise tensioning, one-step suture tying and cutting, and titanium's nonreactivity. Disadvantages are the need for extracorporeal loading of the suture into the device and the costs of a disposable instrument.

With experience, surgeons will find most suturing and knot tying is best done with a simple needle driver and curved graspers. However, the above instruments may be useful early in one's experience and in special circumstances.

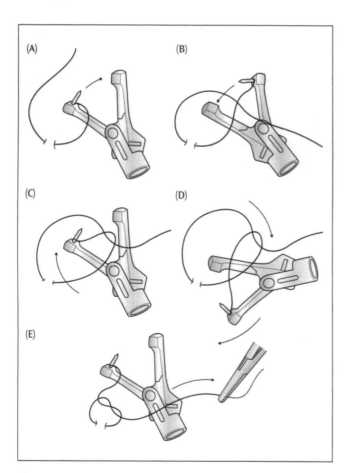

**Figure 4.11**
Knot tying with the EndoStitch (USSC, Norwalk, Connecticut).

# Tissue retrieval

Anyone who has struggled to place an organ or tissue in a bag can immediately appreciate new advances in retrieval technology. The Endocatch (USSC, Norwalk, Connecticut) is a self-opening bag, which comes in several sizes, including 10 mm and 15 mm. Once the instrument is placed through a trocar or directly through the skin, the inner core handle slides forward, advancing the bag. A metal band automatically opens the bag and can be used to scoop up the tissue to be removed. A separate string is pulled, closing the bag and tearing it away from the metal ring. The ring is pulled back into the handle and the device removed, leaving the closed bag and string in the working space. The current bags are not strong enough to withstand automated tissue morcellation, but are useful when intact removal of specimens is required.

If the specimen is to be morcellated, a LapSac (Cook Urological, Inc., Spencer, Indiana) fabricated from a double layer of plastic and nondistendable nylon must be used. This device has been shown to withstand morcellation and remain impermeable to bacteria and tumor cells.[29] In the past, placing large specimens in the LapSac was often a consuming and frustrating experience. Using several simple tricks the bag can now be modified to allow rapid entrapment of specimens. A stiff hydrophilic wire can be double passed through the holes in the LapSac, creating a rigid opening. The bag and wire can be rolled up and inserted through an 11 mm trocar site with the trocar removed. Replacing the trocar alongside the protruding ends of the wire allows the pneumoperitoneum to be reestablished. The modified LapSac opens easily and the rigid wire maintains the mouth of the sac open. Once the specimen is entrapped, the wire can be pulled from the holes in the sac and the mouth of the sac brought out through a trocar site.

# Morcellation

At the conclusion of any extirpative laparoscopic procedure, the organ must be removed from the patient. When malignancy is not involved and an incision is otherwise not required, morcellation and removal through the largest port site is ideal. This requires entrapment in a suitably sized pouch and mechanical reduction in size to allow passage through the port site. Morcellation of malignant lesions continues to be controversial.[30,31] There is clear cosmetic benefit and possibly a small decrease in postoperative morbidity with morcellation. Computed tomography (CT) has been proven to be an effective tool for planning surgery and predicting pathologic findings.[32] To date, there have been no reports of peritoneal seeding or local tumor recurrence in the renal fossa following laparoscopic nephrectomy with specimen morcellation. There have been two reports of trocar site seeding after radical nephrectomy. In one of the two patients it is likely that he had metastatic ascites at the time of nephrectomy.[33,34] No study to date has directly compared morbidity between use of morcellation vs use of an incision for specimen removal. One study compared pain and hospital stay in patients after morcellation vs those requiring conversion to an open procedure by subcostal incision.[35] Not surprisingly, there was less narcotic analgesic use and a shorter stay in the morcellation group. A more equal comparison would be that of HAL nephrectomy vs laparoscopic nephrectomy with morcellation. This has not shown a morbidity advantage for morcellation.[8] On the other hand, there has been only one reported port-site recurrence.[36] This was not clearly related to a morcellation accident but occurred at the appropriate port site. Finally, pathologic staging is rarely needed for treatment decisions after nephrectomy for renal cell carcinoma given excellent CT staging and the lack of effective adjuvant treatment options. This is not the case for transitional cell carcinoma, where morcellation is not recommended. In either case, prognostic information is lost with morcellation.

Once the decision has been made to morcellate an organ, it must first be placed in an impermeable bag (LapSac, Cook Urological, Inc., Spencer, Indiana). Once closed, the strings of the bag are removed through the chosen port site, removing the trocar at the same time. The area is then carefully draped with towels to prevent tumor contamination. The simplest, cheapest, and quickest option is to extend the fascial incision to 20 mm to allow manual fragmentation and extraction of the tissue using a combination of ring forceps, Kocher clamps, etc. The laparoscope should be used throughout this process to visually confirm bag integrity from inside the abdomen. The advantage of this technique is that it creates relatively large pieces of tissue and with the addition of India ink may allow preservation of much staging and margin information.[37]

Several instruments have been developed in an attempt to assist in the morcellation process, specifically to eliminate the need for port-site enlargement. Each is a combination of a rotating cylindrical blade with a mechanism for drawing the tissue into the device (Table 4.4). None is ideal and only one ex-vivo comparison trial exists, which attempts to quantitate morcellation time, bag integrity, and mean specimen weight.[38] Three morcellators were tested on human-sized kidneys without any perirenal tissue. This showed that the standard high-speed electrical laparoscopic (HSEL) morcellator (Cook Urological, Inc., Spencer, Indiana) performed the task acceptably in approximately 15 min. It was also the most economical. The Steiner morcellator (Karl Storz, Culver City, California) was twice as fast and provided specimen fragments 5 times larger (about 3 g), which may be more useful for pathologic evaluation. The Gynecare X-Tract (Ethicon

**Table 4.4** *Comparison of laparoscopic tissue morcellators*

|  | HSEL | Steiner electromechanical | Gynecare X-Tract | RIWO CUT |
|---|---|---|---|---|
| Company | Cook Urological, Inc., Spencer, Indiana | Karl Storz, Culver City, California | Ethicon Inc., Somerville, New Jersey | Richard Wolf Medical Instrument Corp., Vernon Hills, Illinois |
| Mechanism | Suction | Forceps | Forceps | Forceps |
| Blade | Recessed | Protrudes ~2 mm | Recessed with manual blade guard | Reusable bare blade, no sheath |

Inc., Somerville, New Jersey) and RIWO CUT (Richard Wolf Medical Instrument Corp., Vernon Hills, Illinois) devices are likely to perform similarly, given their modes of action. The modified electrical prostate morcellator (Coherent, Sturbridge, Massachusetts) was slow and expensive. A recommendation was additionally made that the use of a shortened trocar may provide increased safety by protecting the bag neck from heat and mechanical stress.

In conclusion, if the choice is made to morcellate a specimen, no current device offers a large advantage over the manual method. The Cook morcellator is currently unavailable. Use of one of the other morcellators may be time- and cost-efficient in high-volume programs and when already available in the operating room, usually as part of the gynecology instrumentation.

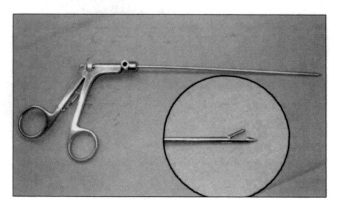

**Figure 4.12**
Berci fascial closure device (Karl Storz GmbH & Co. KG, Tuttlingen, Germany) with tip close-up.

## Closure

Exiting the abdomen consists of visually controlled port removal and purging the carbon dioxide gas. Port sites 10 mm in size or larger have traditionally been closed to prevent port-site hernias. These have been reported to happen in up to 3% of cases.[39] Despite newer-style trocars that may not require fascial closure up to 12 mm, most surgeons continue to close ports $\geq$ 10 mm in adults and 5 mm sites in children.

Conventional open suture closure of port sites can be difficult, especially in obese patients. Multiple instruments have been developed to simplify and expedite this task. Most follow the same basic principle of suture passage through the fascia and into the peritoneal cavity under direct vision followed by suture retrieval with a second pass through the opposite side of the fascia. The Carter–Thomason needle-point suture passer (Inlet Medical Inc., Eden Prairie, Minnesota) and Berci fascial closure device (Karl Storz GmbH & Co. KG, Tuttlingen, Germany) are two commonly used nondisposable instruments based on this model (Figure 4.12). Both have a sharp beak which punctures the fascia and then opens to

capture or release the suture. The EndoClose (USSC, Norwalk, Connecticut) is a similar disposable device. Its rigidity is less and suture capture opening smaller, making it somewhat more difficult to use.

## Robotic-assisted surgery

Once a mere fantasy, robotic-assisted surgery is now reality. Currently available robots vary in complexity and degree of involvement in the procedure. Simple robots are used for laparoscope holding and direction, while others are more directly involved in tissue manipulation at the surgeon's direction. The automated endoscopic system for optimal positioning or AESOP robotic device (Computer Motion, Inc., Santa Barbara, California) was the first FDA-cleared surgical robot. The AESOP system attaches to the side of the operating room table and incorporates a 7-degree of freedom robotic arm to hold and position the endoscope during laparoscopic surgery. The robot is voice-activated, allowing control by the operating surgeon, eliminating unintentional movement, and ensuring a stable surgical image (Figure 4.13).

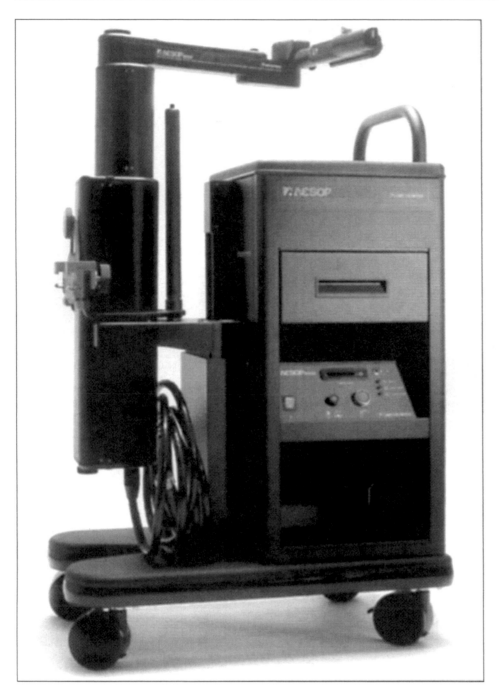

**Figure 4.13**
The AESOP robot (Computer Motion, Inc., Santa Barbara, California). (Photo courtesy of Computer Motion, Inc.)

Currently two robotic systems are FDA-cleared for tissue manipulation during laparoscopic surgery. Since the surgeon actually performs the procedure with the assistance of the mechanical device, these systems are not purely robotic. The ZEUS robotic surgical system (Computer Motion, Inc., Santa Barbara, California) consists of a surgeon's control console and three table-mounted robotic arms (Figure 4.14). Two arms are used for instrument manipulation and one for control of the endoscope. The da Vinci Surgical System (Intuitive Surgical, Inc., Mountain View, California) is a master–slave system that uses robotic technology with 3-dimensional visualization (Figure 4.15). The surgeon operates while seated at a console, viewing the surgical field. At the

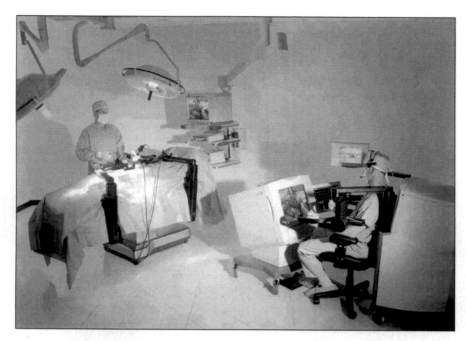

**Figure 4.14**
The ZEUS robotic surgical system (Computer Motion, Inc., Santa Barbara, California). (Photo courtesy of Computer Motion, Inc.)

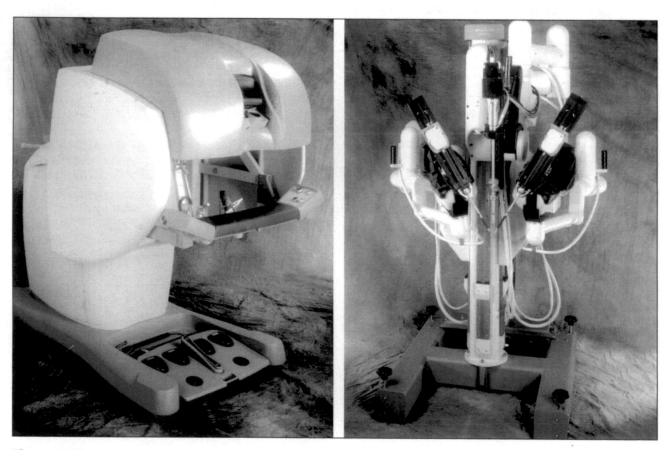

**Figure 4.15**
The da Vinci Surgical System (Intuitive Surgical, Inc., Mountain View, California) consists of the surgeon console and the patient side cart that provides the two robotic arms and one endoscope arm. (Photos courtesy of Intuitive Surgical, Inc.)

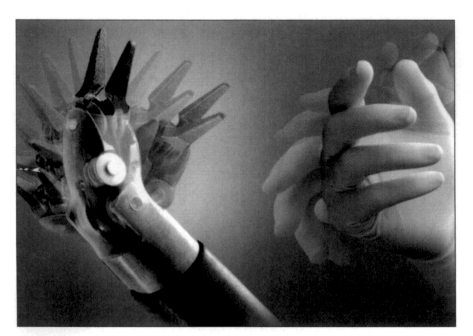

**Figure 4.16**
The 7 degrees of freedom Endowrist (Intuitive Surgical, Inc., Mountain View, California) end-effector of the da Vinci Surgical System. (Photo courtesy of Intuitive Surgical, Inc.)

patient's side, three robot arms position and maneuver the Endowrist endoscopic instruments and laparoscope with a wide range of movements and 360° maneuverability through laparoscopic trocars. The instruments are capable of delivering 7 degrees of freedom, like the human wrist (Figure 4.16). The surgeon's movements are translated into movements of the instruments, allowing precise dissection, manipulation, and suturing. The da Vinci Surgical System has received FDA market clearance for use in performing many different laparoscopic procedures. In the field of urology, it has received FDA clearance for use in radical prostatectomy, and several different studies have shown the feasibility of its use in this procedure.[40–42]

Robotic assistance has the potential to enhance the surgeon's capabilities. The machine translates the surgeon's movements into more steady and precise results at the end of laparoscopic instruments. With these new devices there is potential to decrease the learning curve associated with traditional laparoscopic surgery where instrument movements and degrees of freedom are limited. Motion scaling allows for more precise movements from the surgeon's hand. Intention and resting hand tremor are considerably diminished compared with open surgery, but are virtually eliminated with robotics.

# References

1. Bhoyrul S, Vierra MA, Nezhat CR, et al. Trocar injuries in laparoscopic surgery. J Am Coll Surg 2001; 192:677–83.

2. Liu CD, McFadden DW. Laparoscopic port sites do not require fascial closure when nonbladed trocars are used. Am Surg 2000; 66:853–4.

3. Bohm B, Knigge M, Kraft M, et al. Influence of different trocar tips on abdominal wall penetration during laparoscopy. Surg Endosc 1998; 12:1434–8.

4. Bhoyrul S, Mori T, Way LW. Radially expanding dilatation. A superior method of laparoscopic trocar access. Surg Endosc 1996; 10:775–8.

5. Bhoyrul S, Payne J, Steffes B, et al. A randomized prospective study of radially expanding trocars in laparoscopic surgery. J Gastrointest Surg 2000; 4:392–7.

6. Dunn MD, McDougall EM, Clayman RV. Laparoscopic radical nephrectomy. J Endourol 2000; 14:849–55.

7. Wolf JS. Hand-assisted laparoscopy. Pro. Urology 2001; 58:310–12.

8. Wolf JS, Moon TD, Nakada SY. Hand assisted laparoscopic nephrectomy: comparison to standard laparoscopic nephrectomy. J Urol 1998; 160:22–7.

9. Gill IS. Hand-assisted laparoscopy: Con. Urology 2001; 58:313–17.

10. Stifelman M, Nieder AM. Prospective comparison of hand-assisted laparoscopic devices. Urology 2002; 59:668–72.

11. Grosskinsky CM, Hulka JE. Unipolar electrosurgery in operative laparoscopy. Capacitance as a potential source of injury. J Reprod Med 1995; 40:549–52.

12. Bishoff JT, Allaf ME, Kirkels W, et al. Laparoscopic bowel injury: incidence and clinical presentation. J Urol 1999; 161:887–90.

13. Saye WB, Miller W, Hertzman P. Electrosurgery thermal injury: myth or misconception. Surg Laparosc Endosc 1991; 4:223–8.

14. Ling FW, Stovall TG, Meyer NL, et al. Adhesion formation associated with the use of absorbable staples in comparison to other types of peritoneal injury. Int J Gynecol Obstet 1989; 30:361–6.

15. Tierney AC, Nakada SY. Laparoscopic stapling and reconstruction. In: Bishoff JT, Kavoussi LR, eds. Laparoscopic retroperitoneal surgery. Philadelphia: WB Saunders, 2000: 33–56.

16. Shekarriz B, Stoller ML. The use of fibrin sealant in urology. J Urol 2002; 167:1218–25.

17. McDonough RC, Morey AF. Urologic applications of fibrin sealant bandage. In: Lewandrowski KU, Tantolo DJ, Gresser JD, Yaszemski MJ, Altobelli DE, eds. Tissue engineering and biodegradable equivalents: scientific and clinical applications. New York: Marcel Dekker, 2002.

18. Canby E, Morey AF, Jatoi I, et al. Fibrin sealant treatment of splenic injury during open and laparoscopic left radical nephrectomy. J Urol 2000; 164:2004–5.

19. Leibovich SJ, Ross R. The role of macrophages in wound repair. Am J Pathol 1975; 78:71–100.

20. Cornum RL, Morey AF, Harris R, et al. Does the absorbable fibrin adhesive bandage facilitate partial nephrectomy? J Urol 2000; 164:864–7.

21. Morey AF, Anema JG, Harris R, et al. Treatment of grade 4 renal stab wounds with absorbable fibrin adhesive bandage in a porcine model. J Urol 2001; 165:955–8.

22. Cornum R, Bell J, Gresham V, et al. Intraoperative use of the absorbable fibrin adhesive bandage: long term effects. J Urol 1999; 162:1817–20.

23. Perahia B, Bishoff JT, Cornum RL, et al. The laparoscopic hemi-nephrectomy: made easy by the new fibrin sealant powder. J Urol 2002; 167:suppl 2 (abst).

24. Greenhalgh DG, Gamelli RL, Lee M, et al. Multicenter trial to evaluate the safety and potential efficacy of pooled human fibrin sealant for the treatment of burn wounds. J Trauma 1999; 46:433–40.

25. Morita Y, Nishii O, Kido M, Tsutsumi O. Parvovirus infection after laparoscopic hysterectomy using fibrin glue hemostasis. Obstet Gynecol 2000; 95:1026.

26. Hino M, Ishiko O, Honda K, et al. Transmission of symptomatic parvovirus B19 infection by fibrin sealant used during surgery. Br J Haematol 2000; 108:194–5.

27. Scheule AM, Beierlein W, Lorenz H, Ziemer G. Repeated anaphylactic reactions to aprotinin in fibrin sealant. Gastrointest Endosc 1998; 48:83–5.

28. Bauer JJ, Bishoff JT, Moore RG, et al. Laparoscopic versus open pyeloplasty: assessment of objective and subjective outcome. J Urol 1999; 162:692–5.

29. Urban DA, Kerbl K, McDougall EM, et al. Organ entrapment and renal morcellation: permeability studies. J Urol 1993; 150:1792–4.

30. Bishoff JT. Laparoscopic radical nephrectomy: morcellate or leave intact? Definitely morcellate! Rev Urol 2002; 4:34–7.

31. Kaouk JH, Gill IS. Laparoscopic radical nephrectomy: morcellate or leave intact? Leave intact. Rev Urol 2002; 4:38–42.

32. Shalhave AL, Leibovitch I, Lev R, et al. Is laparoscopic radical nephrectomy with specimen morcellation acceptable cancer surgery? J Endourol 1998; 12:255–7.

33. Fentie DD, Barrett PH, Taranger LA. Metastatic renal cell cancer after laparoscopic radical nephrectomy: long-term follow up. J Endourol 2000; 14:407–11.

34. Castilho LN, Fugita OE, Mitre AI, Arap S. Port site tumor recurrences of renal cell carcinoma after videolaparoscopic radical nephrectomy. J Urol 2001; 165:519.

35. Walther MM, Lyne JC, Libutti SK, Linehan WM. Laparoscopic cytoreductive nephrectomy as preparation for administration of systemic interleukin-2 in the treatment of metastatic renal cell carcinoma: a pilot study. Urology 1999; 53:496–501.

36. Fentie DD, Barrett PH, Taranger LA. Metastatic renal cell cancer after laparoscopic radical nephrectomy: long-term follow-up. J Endourol 2000; 14:407–11.

37. Meng MV, Koppie TM, Duh QY, Stoller ML. Novel method of assessing surgical margin status in laparoscopic specimens. Urology 2001; 58:677–81.

38. Landman J, Collyer WC, Olweny E, et al. Laparoscopic renal ablation: an in vitro comparison of currently available electrical tissue morcellators. Urology 2000; 56:677–81.

39. Bowrey DJ, Blom D, Crookes PF, et al. Risk factors and the prevalence of trocar site herniation after laparoscopic fundoplication. Surg Endosc 2001; 15:663–6.

40. Abbou CC, Hoznek A, Salomon L, et al. Laparoscopic radical prostatectomy with a remote controlled robot. J Urol 2001; 165:1964–6.

41. Binder J, Kramer W. Robotically-assisted laparoscopic radical prostatectomy. BJU Int 2001; 87:408–10.

42. Sung GT, Gill IS. Robotic laparoscopic surgery: a comparison of the da Vinci and Zeus systems. Urology 2001; 58:893–8.

# 5

# The physiology of laparoscopic genitourinary surgery

J Stuart Wolf Jr

Laparoscopy may be minimally invasive, but in some ways it is more physiologically stressful on the patient than open surgery. During laparoscopy with gas insufflation, the patient is exposed to physiologic derangements that may be unfamiliar to the operating surgeon. Fortunately, there is now available considerable clinical and experimental research directed towards the physiology and pathophysiology of gas insufflation, and the knowledgeable practitioner can successfully manage most of the physiologic effects of laparoscopy. Prior to the development of operative laparoscopy, diagnostic laparoscopy carried a low 0.6 – 2.4% complication rate, and only a third of these could be attributed to physiologic problems.[1] In one large survey of operative laparoscopy (laparoscopic cholecystectomy), one-half of the mortality was due to non-technical ('physiologic') causes.[2] The main purpose of studying this topic is to avoid these physiologic complications.

Most of the work on this topic has concerned intraperitoneal insufflation of gas to produce pneumoperitoneum. Many of the phenomena that have been described likely pertain to gas insufflation into the preperitoneal and retroperitoneal spaces as well; where important differences exist, this will be pointed out, but otherwise the term 'pneumoperitoneum' is used to refer to any gas insufflation for pelvic, abdominal, or retroperitoneal laparoscopy

## Hemodynamic considerations

Laparoscopy affects hemodynamics in both stimulatory and inhibitory manners. The mechanical effect of the pneumoperitoneum and the absorption of the carbon dioxide ($CO_2$) are the primary determinants of hemodynamic changes associated with laparoscopy. Volume shifts due to positioning of the patient for laparoscopy play a role in some situations. These divisions are useful clinically because each component can be varied independently,

allowing the surgeon to alter the patient's hemodynamic response during laparoscopy.

## Physiology
### Effects of increased intra-abdominal pressure

Insufflation of gas elevates the intra-abdominal pressure, which subsequently increases the systemic vascular resistance. This is a direct compressive phenomenon, primarily affecting the sphlanchnic circulation (Figure 5.1),[3] in both capillaries and capacitance vessels, and in both the venous and arterial systems.[4–9] Blood flow to all abdominal and retroperitoneal viscera except the adrenal gland is diminished at 20 mmHg of intra-abdominal pressure in animal models.[3,10,11]

The volume status of the subject determines the magnitude of the effect of intra-abdominal pressure on systemic vascular resistance. Using an intra-abdominal pressure of 20 mmHg in dogs, Kashtan and associates[7] found that cardiac output fell slightly in the presence of normovolemia, decreased significantly with experimental simulation of hypovolemia, and actually increased with experimental simulation of hypervolemia. Others have confirmed the adverse effects of hypovolemia[12] and the beneficial effect of volume loading[13] in the presence of increased intra-abdominal pressure.

Cardiac output is limited by venous return. At low levels of intra-abdominal pressure (less than 10 mmHg), there is augmentation of venous return (and therefore cardiac output), due to 'autotransfusion' from partially emptied abdominal capacitance vessels.[14,15] As intra-abdominal pressures rise above 20 mmHg, venous return and cardiac output tend to decrease (Figure 5.2).[4–6,16]

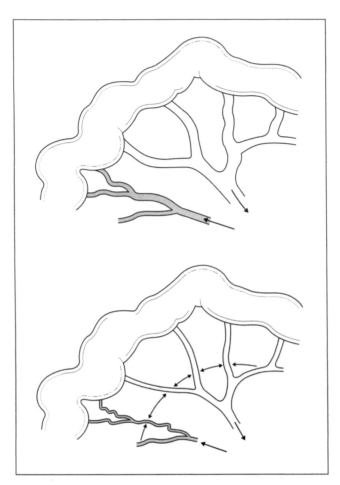

**Figure 5.1**
Sphlanchnic circulation can be markedly restricted.
(Reproduced with permission from Wolf and Stoller ML.[1])

Mean arterial pressure is the product of cardiac output and arterial resistance. At intra-abdominal pressure $\leq 20$ mmHg, there is elevation of mean arterial pressure.[5,8,9,14–18] With intra-abdominal pressure $> 40$ mmHg, arterial pressure falls as cardiac output decreases more than arterial resistance rises.[6,19] Venous pressure is determined, similarly, by the volume of blood collected from the capillaries and the venous resistance. As noted earlier, the venous resistance rises with insufflation.[4,14] It is, however, more difficult to measure and interpret venous pressures during laparoscopy compared with traditional open urologic surgery. The central venous pressure measured by a catheter within the right atrium is the sum of intracardiac (transmural) and intrathoracic (pleural) pressures. The former reflects venous return and is the effective cardiac filling pressure. Intrathoracic pressure, which impedes venous return, rises during laparoscopy.[5,7] It is the increase in this component that is the primary reason the measured central venous pressure rises during laparoscopy. Consequently, the measured central venous pressure is not necessarily a good indicator of cardiac filling unless intrathoracic pressure is taken into account.

The complex effects of increased intra-abdominal pressure on hemodynamics are best summarized by considering again the role of volume status. In general, a small increase in intra-abdominal pressure will increase venous pressure more than it increases resistance, thereby augmenting venous return and cardiac output. As intra-abdominal pressure rises above a certain point, the increase in resistance exceeds the increase in pressure and venous return falls. This transition point occurs at a low intra-abdominal pressure in the hypovolemic state because

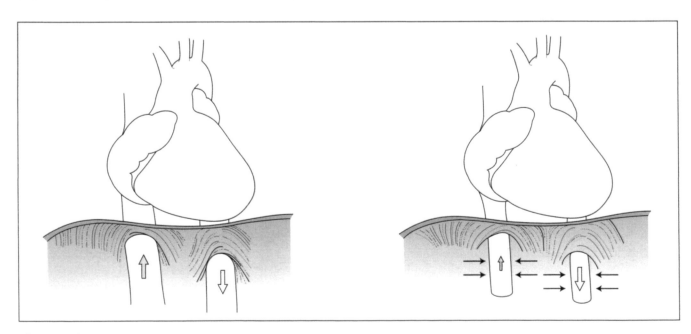

**Figure 5.2**
Reduction of venous return and cardiac output during laparoscopy. (Reproduced with permission from Wolf and Stoller.[1])

vessels collapse easily. In the hypervolemic state, the transition point occurs at a higher intra-abdominal pressure because the full vessels do not collapse as readily; there is less increase in resistance and the pressure increase remains proportional to the elevation of intra-abdominal pressure. In other words, the balance between resistance and pressure changes that determines venous return – and therefore cardiac output – is dependent upon circulating blood volume. Given the avoidance of hypovolemia, maintaining an intra-abdominal pressure less than 20 mmHg should prevent significant hemodynamic alterations in most patients.

## Effects of $CO_2$

The insufflated gas is another determinant of the hemodynamic effects of laparoscopy. The absorption of $CO_2$, the most commonly used gas, has contradictory effects at different sites. The direct effects of $CO_2$ are cardioinhibitory, reducing heart rate, cardiac contractility, and vascular resistance.[20] Stimulation of the sympathetic nervous system by $CO_2$ counteracts these effects, as sympathetic efferents and circulating catecholamines elevate heart rate, cardiac contractility, and vascular resistance. If acidosis develops, parasympathetic stimulation occurs as well.[20] Overall, moderate hypercapnia elevates cardiac output and blood pressure and decreases systemic vascular resistance. The decrease in systemic vascular resistance counteracts the increase created by the mechanical effects of pneumoperitoneum. Insufflation of gases that lack the chemical activity of carbon dioxide results in a lower cardiac output for a given intra-abdominal pressure.[17,18,21–23]

## Effects of positioning

Since laparoscopic retraction can be awkward during laparoscopy, positioning of the patient to use gravity as a retractor is critical. The head-down tilt (Trendelenburg) position during pelvic laparoscopy tends to modestly increase cardiac output.[8,9,24,25] Conversely, the head-up tilt (reverse Trendelenburg) position for upper abdominal laparoscopy is associated with a decrease in cardiac output.[26] The lateral position has minimal effect on hemodynamics unless extreme lateral flexion is applied, which can obstruct the vena cava by impinging on it.[27]

## Integrated cardiovascular response

Table 5.1 delineates the hemodynamic effects of an intra-abdominal pressure of 15 mmHg and moderate hypercapnia. The response of any individual patient may differ, however. Measured central venous pressure, systemic vascular resistance, heart rate, and mean arterial pressure all increase when $CO_2$ is insufflated at 15 mmHg pressure, and the effect on cardiac output in this situation in healthy patients ranges from a decrease of 17–19%,[8,16] to no net change,[4,9] to an increase of 7%.[17] Intra-abdominal pressure less than 5–10 mmHg may increase cardiac output in normovolemic patients by 4–15%,[14,15] while intra-abdominal pressure above 40 mmHg risks marked reduction of cardiac output.[4]

## Retroperitoneal insufflation

Although not as extensively studied as intraperitoneal insufflation, findings suggest that the impact of retroperitoneal insufflation on hemodynamics is less. In two different experimental studies in pigs, extraperitoneal insufflation tended to alter venous pressures and cardiac output in the same direction but with less magnitude compared to intraperitoneal insufflation.[28,29] Giebler and associates did not find any change in cardiac output up to retroperitoneal insufflation pressures of 20 mmHg,[30] and subsequently confirmed the distinction between

| **Table 5.1** *Hemodynamic response to laparoscopy* | | | |
|---|---|---|---|
| | Intra-abdominal pressure of 15 mmHg | Moderate hypercapnia (PaCO$_2$ of 45 mmHg) | Combined |
| Central venous pressure | Increase | Increase | Increase |
| Systemic vascular resistance | Increase | Decrease | Increase |
| Heart rate | Increase | Increase | Increase |
| Mean arterial pressure | Increase | Increase | Increase |
| Cardiac output | Decrease | Increase | Variable |

PaCO$_2$ = arterial partial pressure of carbon dioxide.

intraperitoneal insufflation (decreased venous return) and retroperitoneal insufflation (slightly augmented venous return) with a clinical study using the same testing methodology in both groups.[31] The smaller volume of gas in the latter group may account for some of the difference.

## Physiologic complications

### Tension pneumoperitoneum

When intra-abdominal pressure is excessive ($> 40$ mmHg), the increased vascular resistance becomes overwhelming and tension pneumoperitoneum can occur. Venous return, cardiac output, and blood pressure drop precipitously,[32] which can be fatal.[33] The effect of elevated intra-abdominal pressure is potentiated by hypovolemia,[6,7] so volume status must be optimized before laparoscopy. Parra and associates[34] reported a case of tension pneumoperitoneum during urologic laparoscopy when a malfunctioning insufflator allowed the intra-abdominal pressure to exceed 32 mmHg, resulting in hypotension and bradycardia. Although the procedure was completed following release of the excess pressure and administration of atropine, the patient suffered a cerebrovascular accident that was thought to be due to the intraoperative event. Whenever hemodynamic compromise due to excessive intra-abdominal pressure is suspected, immediate desufflation will quickly improve the situation and the surgeon may be able to complete the procedure at a lower intra-abdominal pressure.[32]

Although brief periods of intra-abdominal pressure above 20 mmHg during laparoscopy are well tolerated by most patients, in general the pressure should be kept below 15–20 mmHg. Even these typically acceptable pressures are no guarantee against problems, as hemodynamic deterioration has been reported at insufflation pressures $\leq 20$ mmHg.[35] Moreover, patients with cardiac disease, either ischemic heart disease or with congestive heart failure, are at greater risk for intraoperative cardiac dysfunction and should be monitored even more closely.[36,37] Laparoscopy can be performed safely in patients with cardiac ejection fractions less than 15% with careful preparation.[38]

### Cardiac dysrhythmias

Cardiac dysrhythmias have been noted during laparoscopy with a frequency of 17–50%.[39,40] Tachycardia and ventricular extrasystoles due to $CO_2$ are usually benign, but fatal dysrhythmias can occur with very high arterial partial pressure of $CO_2$ ($PaCO_2$).[20] Since hypercapnia may also potentiate parasympathetic actions,[20] vagal stimulation by peritoneal manipulation or distention during $CO_2$ laparoscopy can occasionally produce bradydysrhythmias; asystolic arrest during $CO_2$ laparoscopy has been reported.[41,42] Avoidance of hypercapnia will prevent tachydysrhythmias. As vagal reactions may be more profound during laparoscopy under local anesthesia, some recommend premedication with atropine in this setting.[43]

### Fluid overload

The need for intravenous fluid administration is much less during laparoscopy than during open surgery. Not only is the insensible loss of fluid less because there is no body cavity open to air but also urine production is decreased.[44] In one study, urine output during laparoscopy was only 0.03 ml/kg/h, compared to 1.70 ml/kg/h immediately postoperatively, despite an average intravenous intraoperative fluid administration of 13.0 ml/kg/h.[45] An intra-abdominal pressure $< 10$ mmHg caused only mild oliguria, while pressure $> 10$ mmHg produced a 50–100% decrease in urine output in a rodent model.[46] Increased renal vein resistance (with subsequent decreased renal blood flow) and renal parenchymal compression are potential mechanisms.[44,46–50] Pigs exposed to pneumoperitoneum $> 10$ mmHg pressure experienced a 65% fall in urine output, compared to a 29% increase with intra-abdominal pressure $\leq 10$ mmHg.[51] This combination of decreased insensible losses and decreased urine output predisposes to volume overloading during laparoscopy. In Clayman's nephrectomy series, 2 of the first 10 patients developed transient congestive heart failure, possibly due to administration of excessive intravenous fluid and blood products at a time when the decreased urine output during laparoscopy was not yet appreciated.[52] In an effort to prevent this volume overload, however, patients must not be allowed to become hypovolemic, as this will exacerbate the adverse hemodynamic effect of pneumoperitoneum. The volume status of the patient should be optimized prior to insufflation, and then intraoperative fluid administration should be limited to appropriate replacement for blood loss plus a maintenance rate of 5 ml/kg/h.

### Renal failure

Corresponding to the decreased urine output during laparoscopy, there is a reduction in creatinine clearance. During laparoscopic cholecystectomy the creatinine clearance fell in 29 of 48 patients in one study, with the decrease being $> 50\%$ in 8 patients.[53] In a porcine study,[51] the creatinine clearance decreased 18% with intra-abdominal pressures $\leq 10$ mmHg and 53% with pressures

> 10 mmHg. Encouragingly, all renal indices returned almost to baseline within 2 hours of the release of pneumoperitoneum. Moreover, the temporary renal insult does not potentiate the toxicity of nephrotoxic agents such as aminoglycosides[54] and even experiments in a chronic renal insufficiency model failed to reveal anything but a transient effect of pneumoperitoneum.[55] If postoperative renal failure occurs in a laparoscopy patient, then other etiologies should be evaluated before ascribing the event to the pneumoperitoneum. Nonetheless, there has been a single case report of acute renal failure lasting for 2 weeks following laparoscopy in a 67-year-old man with chronic renal insufficiency, renal tubular acidosis, and hypertension.[56]

## Hypertension

Hypertension may accompany hypervolemia during laparoscopy. In addition, hypertension during laparoscopy may be due to hypoxemia, hypercapnia, inadequate anesthesia, or moderately increased intra-abdominal pressure. If hypertension is noted during laparoscopy, the cuff reading should be verified, the intra-abdominal pressure checked, and the adequacy of anesthesia ascertained. If there is doubt as to the accuracy of pulse oximetry and capnography in estimating the arterial partial pressure of oxygen ($PaO_2$) and $PaCO_2$, arterial blood gases should be obtained to evaluate for hypoxemia and hypercapnia.

## Elevated intracranial pressure and cerebral ischemia

In a small animal series, the intracranial pressure rose 5 mmHg in pigs exposed to intra-abdominal pressure of 15 mmHg with $CO_2$ pneumoperitoneum.[57] In 2 myelomeningocele patients with Arnold–Chiari malformations managed with ventriculoperitoneal shunts, the intracerebral pressure increased more than 15 mmHg above baseline during $CO_2$ pneumoperitoneum at $\leq 10$ mmHg intra-abdominal pressure.[58] In another study of 18 patients with ventriculoperitoneal shunts undergoing 19 laparoscopic procedures, there was no trend toward the combined bradycardia and hypertension that would be expected if this intracerebral pressure increase were clinically significant.[59] Cerebral vascular engorgement secondary to restricted venous outflow is the probable mechanism for the increase in intracranial pressure associated with laparoscopy, although in patients with ventriculoperitoneal shunts distal obstruction of the catheter may play a role as well. Patients with head trauma or cerebral mass lesions may suffer from an increase in intra-abdominal pressure during laparoscopy. As the cerebral circulation responds to the increased intracranial volume and pressure with a decrease in blood flow, patients with significant cerebral vascular disease may suffer ischemia.[60]

## Venous thrombosis

The increased abdominal pressure during laparoscopy restricts lower extremity venous return. Mechanical pressure forces blood out of the sphlanchnic circulation into the lower extremities.[61] Femoral vein pressures generally parallel intra-abdominal pressures. Lower extremity venous stasis during transperitoneal laparoscopy can be demonstrated with Doppler flow studies.[62,63] One group evaluated femoral vein flow during intraperitoneal and preperitoneal gas insufflation in the same patients, and found flow to decrease with the former but not the latter.[64] Deep vein thromboses and pulmonary emboli have been reported following laparoscopy.[65–67] It is not known if laparoscopy poses a greater or lesser risk for venous thrombosis than open surgery, although in one study of 61 low-risk laparoscopic patients there were no cases of deep venous thrombosis detected with lower limb venous duplex scans.[63] Prophylaxis against deep venous thrombosis with sequential compression devices makes intuitive sense and has been shown to be effective in reversing the pneumoperitoneum-induced reduction of femoral vein flow during laparoscopy,[68] but the optimal method of prophylaxis in laparoscopy has not been determined.

# Pulmonary, acid–base, and insufflant-related considerations

Investigations of the pulmonary effects of pneumoperitoneum were first directed toward the use of pneumoperitoneum to treat pulmonary tuberculosis and emphysema.[69] These studies focused on the mechanical aspects of pneumoperitoneum. Subsequently, workers have considered the role of gas absorption from pneumoperitoneum. $CO_2$, the most commonly used insufflant, is rapidly absorbed during laparoscopy and consideration of the effects of absorbed $CO_2$ is important in understanding the physiology of laparoscopy.

## Physiology

### Mechanical effect of pneumoperitoneum

Pneumoperitoneum adversely affects pulmonary function. The increased intra-abdominal pressure and volume elevate the diaphragm,[70] reducing both lung capacity and compliance.[15,71] There is worsening of the ventilation/perfusion mismatch.[70]

### Gas absorption

When the peritoneal cavity is filled with gas by insufflation, the total sum of gas movement is directed outwards into the surrounding tissue because the intra-abdominal pressure is above atmospheric pressure.[72] Individual gases move in a direction determined by their partial pressure gradients. The rate of their movement is determined by:

- tissue permeance of the gas
- absorptive capacity of the surrounding tissue
- temperature
- the area of tissue exposed.

The peritoneal cavity is lined by well-vascularized mesothelium with high absorptive capacity. Gases with high tissue permeance are absorbed readily. $CO_2$ has the highest tissue permeance of the gases used for insufflation during laparoscopy (Table 5.2).[73] Insufflated $CO_2$ rapidly diffuses into the bloodstream. The baseline production of $CO_2$ in adults is 150–200 ml/min.[74] The amount of $CO_2$ absorbed from the peritoneal cavity during intraperitoneal $CO_2$ laparoscopy has been estimated to range from 14 to 48 ml/min.[67] Increasing minute ventilation can usually eliminate this excess $CO_2$. When the insufflated gas gains access into the extraperitoneal space or subcutaneous tissues, the surface area exposed for gas absorption increases and a greater amount of $CO_2$ is absorbed.[67,75,76]

### $CO_2$ metabolism and absorption

When $CO_2$ is absorbed or produced by tissue metabolism, it is primarily hydrated to carbonic acid, a reaction catalyzed by carbonic anhydrase. Carbonic acid rapidly ionizes to bicarbonate, which represents 90% of the $CO_2$ in the bloodstream, and hydrogen ions.[74] The hydrogen ions reduce hemoglobin. In the alveolar capillaries the hemoglobin is re-oxidized and the hydrogen ions are released to produce carbonic acid, subsequently forming $CO_2$ and water for expiration. If $CO_2$ elimination cannot keep pace with the sum of metabolic production and absorption of $CO_2$, hypercapnia and respiratory acidosis develop. The absolute rise of $PaCO_2$, which represents the 'rapid' compartment of $CO_2$ storage, is tempered by storage of $CO_2$ in the 'medium' (primarily skeletal muscle) and 'slow' (fat) compartments. These storage sites can hold up to 120 liters of $CO_2$.[74] Therefore, all of the absorbed $CO_2$ is not immediately available for elimination. The situation exists where hypercapnia can develop or persist after the conclusion of an extended laparoscopic procedure.[77]

## Physiologic complications

### Hypercapnia

Hypercapnia (excess of $CO_2$ in the blood) occurs when production and absorption of $CO_2$ exceed its elimination. While moderate hypercapnia is stimulatory to the cardiovascular system overall, if the level of $PaCO_2$ exceeds 60 mmHg the direct cardiodepressive effects predominate. Cardiovascular collapse, severe acidosis, and fatal

**Table 5.2** *Insufflant characteristics*

|  | Solubility[a] | Diffusibility[a] | Tissue Permeance[a] |
|---|---|---|---|
| Nitrogen | 1.0 | 1.0 | 1.0 |
| Helium | 0.7 | 2.7 | 1.3 |
| Oxygen | 1.9 | 0.9 | 1.8 |
| Argon | 2.2 | 0.9 | 2.0 |
| Nitrous oxide | 33.0 | 0.9 | 28.0 |
| Carbon dioxide | 47.0 | 0.9 | 39.0 |

Reproduced with permission from Stoller and Wolf.[73]
[a]Value relative to nitrogen.

dysrhythmias can occur. The respiratory acidosis associated with hypercapnia is responsible for most effects of hypercapnia, but $CO_2$ has direct effects as well. Hypercapnia is related directly to the insufflated $CO_2$, and not to any change in tissue metabolism or pulmonary function. In 3 studies comparing $N_2O$ insufflation to $CO_2$ insufflation in patients under general anesthesia with controlled respiration at a fixed minute ventilation, the average increase in $PaCO_2$ was 0.5 mmHg in the $N_2O$ group and 10.7 mmHg in the $CO_2$ group.[21,78,79] Animal studies have also confirmed that hypercapnia during laparoscopy is due to absorption of $CO_2$ rather than mechanical effects on pulmonary function.[80] The clinical practice during laparoscopy of increasing ventilation rates and tidal volumes in order to increase $CO_2$ elimination is usually but not always effective. Wittgen and associates[81] converted 2 of 30 laparoscopic cholecystectomies to open surgery because of hypercapnia, and conversion to open surgery because of hypercapnia during laparoscopic pelvic lymphadenectomy has been reported.[65,73] Others have described severe cardiovascular depression or cardiac arrest due to hypercapnia during $CO_2$ pneumoperitoneum.[41,42,82]

Clinical studies have suggested that subcutaneous emphysema,[67,76,83] elevated intra-abdominal pressure,[4] extraperitoneal insufflation,[67,75,76] and increased duration of insufflation[22,70,79,84] all increase the rate of $CO_2$ absorption. Other studies have not found extraperitoneal insufflation to be a risk factor.[28,29,85]

Reduction of intra-abdominal pressure is the first maneuver that should be performed when hypercapnia is detected. It allows more effective $CO_2$ elimination by reducing the mechanical interference with ventilation by pneumoperitoneum, and it decreases $CO_2$ absorption. Intra-abdominal pressure should be limited to 20 mmHg. In addition, adjustment of ventilation to keep the partial pressure of end-tidal $CO_2$ ($P(et)CO_2$) between 30 and 40 mmHg is recommended. Finally, alternative gases may be employed for insufflation.

Introduced in 1924 by Zollikofer of Switzerland, $CO_2$ is the most popular gas for insufflation. The advantages of $CO_2$ are its rapid absorption and its inability to support combustion. The rapid absorption of $CO_2$ is beneficial if hypercapnia can be maintained at a low level ($PaCO_2 \leq 45$ mmHg), because its cardiovascular stimulation offsets some of the hemodynamic burden of pneumoperitoneum.[17,18,21–23] At excessive levels, however, hypercapnia can produce dysrhythmias and cardiodepressive acidosis. For this reason, workers have searched for alternative gases for insufflation. Following the first formal reports of the physiologic hazards of $CO_2$ pneumoperitoneum,[86] Alexander and Brown described the use of $N_2O$ for insufflation.[78] $N_2O$ is similar to $CO_2$ in that it is rapidly absorbed (see Table 8.2), but it has few physiologic effects at the blood concentration achieved with intraperitoneal

insufflation and it is less irritating to the peritoneal membrane.[87,88] Unlike $CO_2$, it can support combustion in the abdominal cavity (see Intra-abdominal explosion section below). $N_2O$ is a suitable alternative for intra-abdominal insufflation if electrocautery or laser techniques are not being used.

Other alternative gases include helium (He) and argon (Ar).[23,80] Experiments with He have revealed no cardiopulmonary problems.[80,89] Successful clinical series of laparoscopic cholecystectomy have been performed,[22] and in one case report a laparoscopic nephrectomy associated with extreme hypercapnia was continued safely after switching the insufflatory gas to He.[90] Helium and argon have less chemical activity than $CO_2$ and are absorbed slowly (Table 8.2). Hypercapnia is obviated by the use of He or Ar for insufflation, but the clinical effects of a venous gas embolism may be exacerbated (see Venous gas embolism section below). A practice of switching to He or Ar after initial insufflation with $CO_2$ might be a safe and effective way of preventing hypercapnia.[84,90]

Capnography is used to monitor the $P(et)CO_2$ during operation. The $P(et)CO_2$, being about 3–5 mmHg lower than the $PaCO_2$ during general anesthesia, should be maintained between 30 and 40 mmHg. The difference between $PaCO_2$ and $P(et)CO_2$, the $P(a-et)CO_2$ gradient, is not significantly worsened during short laparoscopic procedures in healthy patients.[71,77,91] Normal pulmonary function is adequate to eliminate the small amount of absorbed $CO_2$ and any increase in $PaCO_2$ is minimal. As $PaCO_2$ rises in patients with pulmonary disease, however, $P(a-et)CO_2$ increases in an unpredictable manner.[81,92] To monitor accurately the $CO_2$ elimination in patients with pulmonary disease, arterial blood gases may be necessary.

## Acidosis

Laparoscopy with $CO_2$ insufflation causes a mild respiratory acidosis due to the absorption of $CO_2$.[6,93] Various investigators have reported coexisting minimal metabolic alkalosis[91] and mild metabolic acidosis.[77,79] Experimentally, the trend towards metabolic acidosis is noted at gas insufflation pressures $\geq 20$ mmHg.[51] Since the metabolic acidosis is not associated with an increased anion gap, the cause is not likely to be lactate acidosis from sphlanchnic hypoperfusion, and may instead be related to retained acids due to the decreased urine output at high intra-abdominal pressures.[51]

## Extraperitoneal gas collections

Gases insufflated into the peritoneal cavity may leak into several extraperitoneal tissue planes or spaces.

Subcutaneous emphysema is the most common site of extraperitoneal gas. Its presence is often attributed to technical causes such as incorrect insufflation needle placement, excessive intra-abdominal pressure, a malfunctioning insufflator, or leakage around a laparoscopic port, but in practice it is sometimes inevitable. Since subcutaneous gas is a risk factor for hypercapnia, its presence should prompt an assessment for hypercapnia and its effects. Gas that is insufflated inadvertently into the preperitoneal space or omentum will interfere with visualization during intraperitoneal laparoscopy and might also increase the risk of hypercapnia. Preperitoneal insufflation is a not an uncommon reason for aborting a laparoscopic procedure.[34]

A deliberate extraperitoneal approach is now being advocated for many laparoscopic procedures. Aside from the surgical implications of this approach, there are some physiologic ones. First, extraperitoneal insufflation may be associated with increased gas absorption,[67,75,76] although not all have found this to be the case.[28,29,85] Secondly, extraperitoneal gas can more easily gain access into the subcutaneous space or thoracic cavity. In one study, subcutaneous emphysema was noted in 91% of patients undergoing laparoscopy with extraperitoneal insufflation and in 53% of patients in whom the insufflation was intraperitoneal. Pneumomediastinum or pneumothorax was noted in 36% of patients undergoing extraperitoneal laparoscopy and in 6% of patients after transperitoneal laparoscopy.[67,76]

Pneumomediastinum and pneumothorax can inhibit cardiac filling and limit lung excursion, and can be fatal.[94] Insufflated gas may get into the thorax through many pathways: persistent fetal connections (pleuroperitoneal, pleuropericardial, and pericardioperitoneal), around great vessels in an extrafascial plane, in between fibers of the diaphragm (extraperitoneal or extrapleural), or dissection of subcutaneous gas from the anterior neck directly into the superior mediastinum (Figure 5.3).[1] Pneumothorax may also occur secondary to barotrauma when the peak airway pressure rises with pneumoperitoneum.[71] Pneumomediastinum is more common than pneumothorax, and when the latter occurs it is almost always accompanied by pneumomediastinum and subcutaneous emphysema.[1,67,76] If $CO_2$ or $N_2O$ has been insufflated, the pneumothorax will usually resolve,[95] but thoracostomy should be performed for a large or symptomatic pneumothorax. Pneumopericardium is occasionally noted after laparoscopy.[96] Subcutaneous gas has been present in all reported cases of pneumopericardium, and in 3 of 4 cases there has been radiographic evidence of pneumomediastinum. The mechanism is most likely entry of mediastinal gas into the pericardial space alongside blood vessels, although persistent embryologic pleuropericardial and pericardioperitoneal connections would also allow gas into the pericardium.

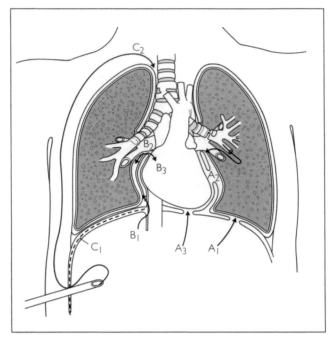

**Figure 5.3**
Possible routes of gas into mediastinum, pericardial sac, or pleural cavity during laparoscopy include the following: persistent fetal connection at the site of pleuroperitoneal membrane (A1, forme fruste of diaphragmatic hernia), pleuropericardial membrane (A2), and pericardioperitoneal canal (A3); rupture of gas through intact membrane at a weak point such as diaphragmatic hiatus (B1), at pulmonary hilum (B2), and pericardial sac alongside blood vessels (B3); gas outside membrane-bound cavities such as pro- or retroperitoneal gas in between fibers of the diaphragm or alongside great vessels (C1) or subcutaneous gas from the anterior neck (C2); gas from the rupture of an airspace (barotrauma) enters the mediastinum or pleural cavity by dissecting along the pulmonary vasculature (D). (Reproduced with permission from Wolf and Stoller.[1])

## Venous gas embolism

A venous gas embolism (VGE) is a gas bubble in the venous system that can pass into the heart and pulmonary circulation. The outflow tract of the right side of the heart can be blocked, producing hypoxemia, hypercapnia, and depressed cardiac output. If the right-heart pressure exceeds that on the left side, a probe patent foramen ovale (present in 20–25% of the population) may open and allow embolization of gas into the arterial system.[5,97,98] The incidence of VGE has been estimated to be between 0.002 and 0.08%,[1] although clinically detectable VGE may occur in as many as 0.59% of laparoscopic cases when careful surveillance is used.[99] Many VGE during laparoscopy have been fatal.[97,98,100] VGE rarely occurs more than a few minutes after initial gas insufflation, but delayed cases have been reported.[97] VGE has been produced experimentally in a bleeding vena cava model, with the riskiest situations appearing to be occlusion of the vena cava distal to the venotomy or following significant blood loss.[101] Clinically, VGE should be suspected when there is hypoxemia, evidence of pulmonary edema, increased airway pressure, hypotension, jugular venous distention, facial plethora, or dysrhythmias. The most useful finding is a sudden fall in $P(et)CO_2$ on capnometry (if the $CO_2$ embolus is large) and an abrupt but transient increase if it is small.[100,102] The auscultation of a mill-wheel murmur and the appearance of a widened QRS complex with right-heart strain patterns on electrocardiography are less sensitive indicators. When these indicators are noted during initial insufflation, VGE should be suspected. Swift response is required, and includes immediate desufflation, rapid ventilation with 100% oxygen, steep head-down tilt with the right side up, and general resuscitative maneuvers.

The type of the gas comprising the embolus is important. Air (~80% nitrogen) is absorbed very slowly in blood. As Table 5.2 indicates, $CO_2$ is 47 times more soluble than nitrogen. Graff and associates[103] found the $LD_{50}$ (lethal dose in 50% of subjects) of $CO_2$ to be 5 times that of air when injected intravenously in dogs. Helium, which has been used as an alternative to $CO_2$ for insufflation in some series,[22,84,90] is even less soluble than nitrogen. In canine experiments, the intravenous injection of He was lethal on 4 of 6 occasions, whereas the same amount of $CO_2$ was followed by hemodynamic recovery in all cases (Figure 8.4).[104] Additionally, argon VGE during laparoscopic use of an argon beam coagulator has been reported.[105] These findings argue against the use of He or Ar for initial insuf-flation, but their use after the pneumoperitoneum has been safely created with $CO_2$ appears safe.[84]

## Hypoxemia

$PaO_2$ may decrease during laparoscopy because of the decreased cardiac output, increased pulmonary shunt, worsened ventilation/perfusion mismatch, decreased alveolar ventilation, and acidosis associated with laparoscopy.[106] Most clinical studies have suggested a slight but clinically insignificant reduction of $PaO_2$ during laparoscopy.[6,71,78,81,93] Corall and associates[107] reported that 2 patients with heavy smoking history experienced a drop in $PaO_2$ to less than 100 mmHg during $N_2O$ laparoscopy, but others have not found $PaO_2$ during laparoscopy to be affected significantly by preoperative pulmonary status.[81] When severe hypoxemia occurs, other complications such as venous gas embolism, pneumothorax, or ventilator malfunction should be considered.

## Hypothermia

Hypothermia may occur during laparoscopy because of the loss of heat to the large volumes of gas exchanged through the patient.[108] Ott found that the core temperature dropped 0.3°C for every 50 liters of $CO_2$ used, and recommended warming the gas prior to insufflation to prevent hypothermia.[109] Others, however, found that heating the gas made no difference in the slight drop in core temperature.[110] Moreover, another study found the core temperature to increase rather than decrease during

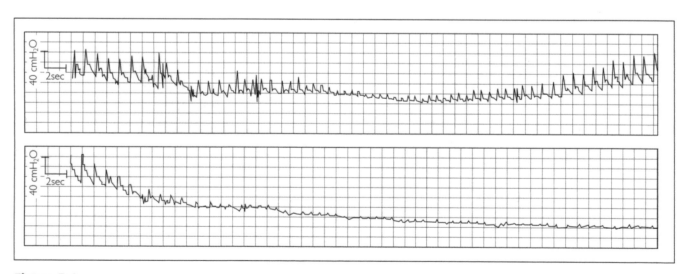

**Figure 5.4**
Arterial tracing after rapid intravenous injection of 7.5 ml/kg $CO_2$ (top) and helium (bottom) in a dog. There is recovery within 1 min after the $CO_2$ injection but complete cardiovascular collapse after helium injection. (Reproduced with permission from Wolf et al.[104])

laparoscopy, even with the use of room temperature gas for insufflation.[111]

## Intra-abdominal explosion

In 1933, Fervers[112] reported an intra-abdominal explosion during laparoscopy with oxygen insufflation, and the use of pure oxygen pneumoperitoneum subsequently has been abandoned. $N_2O$ will support combustion[113] and is explosive in the presence of hydrogen or methane.[114] Although the proper conditions for explosion during laparoscopy are rare,[115] death has occurred due to cardiac rupture from an explosion during $N_2O$ pneumoperitoneum.[116] Neuman and associates[117] found that $N_2O$ content in the peritoneal cavity rose to 36% after 30 min duration of $CO_2$ pneumoperitoneum when the inhaled gas contained 60% $N_2O$. They also reported that 69% hydrogen (the maximum reported content of hydrogen in bowel gas) was combustible in the presence of 29% $N_2O$. Therefore, both inhaled and insufflated $N_2O$ should be avoided when electrocautery or laser might be used. Even without $N_2O$ insufflation, electrocautery injury to the colon can be associated with explosion.[118]

## Summary

The hemodynamic effects of laparoscopy are determined by the intra-abdominal pressure, the type of gas insufflated, and the position of the patient. Cardiovascular complications of laparoscopy include tension pneumoperitoneum, cardiac dysrhythmias, fluid overload, renal failure, hypertension, elevated intracranial pressure, cerebral ischemia, and venous thrombosis. The intraoperative pulmonary stresses of laparoscopy can also be considerable. Pulmonary, acid–base, and insufflant-related complications include hypercapnia, acidosis, extraperitoneal gas collections, venous gas embolism, hypoxemia, hypothermia, and intra-abdominal explosion.

Most patients tolerate laparoscopy well if the intra-abdominal pressure is limited to 20 mmHg, there is adequate (but not excessive) fluid replacement, and $CO_2$ levels are monitored appropriately. Nonetheless, it should be remembered that laparoscopy is in many ways associated with more intraoperative physiologic stress than is open surgery. The unique physiologic stresses of laparoscopy require vigilance on the part of the surgeon and anesthesiologist to prevent, monitor for, and treat the potential physiologic complications of laparoscopy.

## References

1. Wolf JS Jr, Stoller ML. The physiology of laparoscopy: basic principles, complications, and other considerations. J Urol 1994; 152:294–302.
2. Deziel DJ, Millikan KW, Economou SG, et al. Complications of laparoscopic cholestectomy: a national survey of 4,292 hospitals and an analysis of 77,604 cases. Am J Surg 1993; 165:9–14.
3. Caldwell CB, Ricotta JJ. Changes in visceral blood flow with elevated intraabdominal pressure. J Surg Res 1987; 43:14–20.
4. Motew M, Ivankovich AD, Bieniarz J, et al. Cardiovascular effects and acid-base and blood gas changes during laparoscopy. Am J Obstet Gynecol 1973; 115:1002–12.
5. Ivankovich AD, Miletich DJ, Albrecht RF, et al. Cardiovascular effects of intraperitoneal insufflation with carbon dioxide and nitrous oxide in the dog. Anesthesiology 1975; 42:281–7.
6. Diamant M, Benumof JL, Saidman LJ. Hemodynamics of increased intra-abdominal pressure: interaction with hypovolemia and halothane anesthesia. Anesthesiology 1978; 48:23–7.
7. Kashtan J, Green JF, Parsons EQ, Holcroft JW. Hemodynamic effects of increased abdominal pressure. J Surg Res 1981; 30:249–55.
8. Johannsen G, Andersen M, Juhl B. The effect of general anaesthesia on the haemodynamic events during laparoscopy with $CO_2$-insufflation. Acta Anaesthesiol Scand 1989; 33:132–6.
9. Torrielli R, Cesarini M, Winnock S, et al. [Hemodynamic changes during celioscopy: a study carried out using thoracic electric bioimpedance]. Can J Anaesth 1992; 37:46–51.
10. Hashikura Y, Kawasaki K, Munakata Y, et al. Effects of peritoneal insufflation on hepatic and renal blood flow. Surg Endosc 1994; 8:759–61.
11. Eleftheriadis E, Kotzampassi K, Botsios D, Tzartinoglou E, Farmakis H, Dadoukis J. Sphlanchnic ischemia during laparoscopic cholecystectomy. Surg Endosc 1996; 10:324–6.
12. Ho HS, Saunders CJ, Corso FA, Wolfe BM. The effects of $CO_2$ pneumoperitoneum on hemodynamics in hemorrhaged animals. Surgery 1993; 114:381–7.
13. Cullen DJ, Coyle JP, Teplick R, Long MC. Cardiovascular, pulmonary, and renal effects of massively increased intra-abdominal pressure in critically ill patients. Crit Care Med 1989; 17:118–21.
14. Versichelen L, Serreyn R, Rolly G, Vanderkerckhove D. Physiopathologic changes during anesthesia administration for gynecologic laparoscopy. J Reprod Med 1984; 29:697–700.
15. Ekman LG, Abrahamsson J, Biber B, et al. Hemodynamic changes during laparoscopy with positive end-expiratory pressure ventilation. Acta Anaesthesiol Scand 1988; 32:447–53.
16. Lenz RJ, Thomas TA, Wilkins DG. Cardiovascular changes during laparoscopy: studies of stroke volume and cardiac output using impedance cardiography. Anaesthesia 1976; 31:4–12.

17. Marshall RL, Jebson PJR, Davie IT, Scott DB. Circulatory effects of carbon dioxide insufflation of the peritoneal cavity for laparoscopy. Br J Anaesth 1972; 44:680–4.

18. Marshall RL, Jebson PJR, Davie IT, Scott DB. Circulatory effects of peritoneal insufflation with nitrous oxide. Br J Anaesth 1972; 44:1183–7.

19. Richardson JD, Trinkle JK. Hemodynamic and respiratory alterations with increased intra-abdominal pressure. J Surg Res 1976; 20:401–4.

20. Price HL. Effects of carbon dioxide on the cardiovascular system. Anesthesiology 1960; 21:652–63.

21. El-Minawi MF, Wahbi O, El-Bagouri IS, et al. Physiologic changes during $CO_2$ and $N_2O$ pneumoperitoneum in diagnostic laparoscopy. A comparative study. J Reprod Med 1981; 26:338–46.

22. Bongard FS, Pianim NA, Leighton TA, et al. Helium insufflation for laparoscopic operation. Surg Gynecol Obstet 1993; 177:140–6.

23. Eisenhauer DM, Saunders CJ, Ho HS, Wolfe BM. Hemodynamic effects of argon pneumoperitoneum. Surg Endosc 1994; 8:315–21.

24. Sibbald WJ, Paterson NAM, Holliday RL, Baskerville J. The Trendelenburg position: hemodynamic effects in hypotensive and normotensive patients. Crit Care Med 1979; 7:218–24.

25. Reich DL, Konstadt SN, Raissi S, et al. Trendelenburg position and passive leg raising do not significantly improve cardiopulmonary performance in the anesthetized patient with coronary artery disease. Crit Care Med 1989; 17:313–17.

26. Cunningham AJ, Turner J, Rosenbaum S, Rafferty T. Transoesophageal echocardiographic assessment of haemodynamic function during laparoscopic cholecystectomy. Br J Anaesth 1993; 70:621–5.

27. Lawson NW. The lateral decubitus position. In: Martin JT, ed. Positioning in anesthesia and surgery. Philadelphia: WB Saunders, 1987:155–79.

28. Bannenberg JJ, Rademaker BM, Froeling FM, Meijer DW. Hemodynamics during laparoscopic extra- and intraperitoneal insufflation. An experimental study. Surg Endosc 1997; 11:911–14.

29. Giebler RM, Kabatnik M, Stegen BH et al. Retroperitoneal and intraperitoneal $CO_2$ insufflation have markedly different cardiovascular effect. J Surg Res 1997; 68:153–60.

30. Giebler RM, Walz MK, Peitgen K, Scherer RU. Hemodynamic changes after retroperitoneal $CO_2$ insufflation for posterior retroperitoneoscopic adrenalectomy. Anesth Analg 1996; 82:827–31.

31. Giebler RM, Behrends M, Steffens T, et al. Intraperitoneal and retroperitoneal carbon dioxide evoke different effects on caval vein pressure gradients in humans: evidence for the Starling resistor concept of abdominal venous return. Anesthesiology 2000; 92:1568–80.

32. Lee CM. Acute hypotension during laparoscopy: a case report. Anesth Analg 1975; 54:142–3.

33. Arthure H. Laparoscopy hazard. Br Med J 1970; 4:492–3.

34. Parra RO, Hagood PG, Boullier JA, et al. Complications of laparoscopic urological surgery: experience at St. Louis University. J Urol 1994; 151:681–4.

35. Lew JKL, Gin T, Oh TE. Anaesthetic problems during laparoscopic cholecystectomy. Anaesth Intens Care 1992; 20:91–2.

36. Joris JL, Noirot DP, Legrand MJ, et al. Hemodynamic changes during laparoscopic cholecystectomy. Anesthes Analg 1993; 76:1067–71.

37. Safran D, Sgambati S, Orlando R III. Laparoscopy in high-risk cardiac patients. Surg Gynecol Obstetr 1993; 176:548–54.

38. Jones PE, Sayson SC, Koehler DC. Laparoscopic cholecystectomy in a cardiac transplant candidate with an ejection fraction of less than 15%. J Soc Laparoendosc Surg 1998; 2:89–92.

39. Scott DB, Julian DG. Observations on cardiac arrythmias during laparoscopy. Br Med J 1972; 1:411–13.

40. Cimino L, Petitto M, Nardon G, Budillon G. Holter dynamic electrocardiography during laparoscopy. Gastrointest Endosc 1988; 34:72.

41. Shifren JL, Adlestein L, Finkler NJ. Asystolic cardiac arrest: a rare complication of laparoscopy. Obstet Gynecol 1992; 79:840–1.

42. Biswas TK, Pembroke A. Asystolic cardiac arrest during laparoscopic cholecystectomy. Anaesth Intens Care 1994; 22:289–91.

43. Borten M. Choice of anesthesia. In: Laparoscopic complications. Toronto: BC Decker, 1986:173–84.

44. Vukasin A, Lopez M, Shichman S, et al. Oliguria in laparoscopic surgery (abstract #462). J Urol 1994; 151(supplement):343A.

45. Chang DT, Kirsch AJ, Sawczuk IS. Oliguria during laparoscopic surgery. J Endourol 1994; 8:349–52.

46. Kirsch AJ, Hensle TW, Chang DT, et al. Renal effects of $CO_2$ insufflation: oliguria and acute renal dysfunction in a rat pneumoperitoneum model. Urology 1994; 43:453–9.

47. McDougall EM, Monk TG, Hicks M, et al. Effect of pneumoperitoneum on renal function in an animal model (abstract #938). J Urol 1994; 151(supplement):462A.

48. Chiu AW, Azadzoi KM, Hatzichristou DG, et al. Effects of intra-abdominal pressure on renal tissue perfusion during laparoscopy. J Endourol 1994; 8:99–103.

49. Razvi HA, Fields D, Vargas JC, et al. Oliguria during laparoscopic surgery: evidence for direct parenchymal compression as an etiologic factor. J Endourol 1996; 10:1–4.

50. Guler C, Sade M, Kirkali Z. Renal effect of carbon dioxide insufflation in rabbit pneumoperitoneum model. J Endourol 1998; 12:367–70.

51. McDougall EM, Monk TG, Hicks M, et al. The effect of prolonged pneumoperitoneum on renal function in an animal model. J Am Coll Surg 1996; 182:317–28.

52. Clayman RV, Kavoussi LR, Soper NJ, et al. Laparoscopic nephrectomy: review of the initial 10 cases. J Endourol 1992; 6:127–32.

53. Kubota K, Kajiura N, Teruya M, et al. Alterations in respiratory function and hemodynamics during laparoscopic cholecystectomy under pneumoperitoneum. Surg Endosc 1993; 7:500–4.

54. Beduschi R, Beduschi MC, Williams AL, Wolf JS Jr. Pneumoperitoneum does not potentiate the nephrotoxicity of aminoglycosides in rats. Urology 1999; 53:451–4.

55. Cisek LJ, Gobet RM, Peters CA. Pneumoperitoneum produces reversible renal dysfunction in animals with normal and chronically reduced renal function. J Endourol 1998; 12:95–9.

56. Ben-David B, Croitoru M, Gaitini L. Acute renal failure following laparoscopic cholecystectomy: a case report. J Clin Anesth 1999; 11:486–9.

57. Josephs LG, Este-McDonald JR, Birkett DH, Hirsch EF. Diagnostic laparoscopy increases intracranial pressure. J Trauma 1994; 36:815–19.

58. Poppas DP, Peters CA, Bilsky MH, Sosa RE. Intracranial pressure monitoring during laparoscopic surgery in children with ventriculoperitoneal shunts. J Endourol 1994; 8:S93.

59. Jackman SV, Weingart JD, Kinsman SL, Docimo SG. Laparoscopic surgery in patients with ventriculoperitoneal shunts: safety and monitoring. J Urol 2000; 164:1352–4.

60. Prentice JA, Martin JT. The Trendelenburg position. Anesthesiologic considerations. In: Martin JT, ed. Positioning in anesthesia and surgery. Philadelphia: WB Saunders, 1987:127–45.

61. Borten M. Circulatory changes. In: Laparoscopic complications. Toronto: BC Decker, 1986:185–95.

62. Jorgensen JO, Hanel K, Lalak NJ, et al. Thromboembolic complications of laparoscopic cholecystectomy. BMJ 1993; 306:518–19.

63. Wazz G, Branicki F, Taji H, Chishty I. Influence of pneumoperitoneum on the deep venous system during laparoscopy. J Laparoendosc Surg 2000; 4:291–5.

64. Morrison CA, Schreiber MA, Olsen SB, et al. Femoral venous flow dynamics during intraperitoneal and preperitoneal laparoscopic insufflation. Surg Endosc 1998; 12:1213–16.

65. Kavoussi LR, Sosa E, Chandhoke P, et al. Complications of laparoscopic pelvic lymph node dissection. J Urol 1993; 149:322–5.

66. Mayol J, Vincent HE, Sarmiento JM, et al. Pulmonary embolism following laparoscopic cholecystectomy: report of two cases and review of the literature. Surg Endosc 1994; 8:214–17.

67. Wolf JS JR, Clayman RV, Monk TG, et al. Carbon dioxide absorption during laparoscopic pelvic surgery. J Am Coll Surg 1995; 180:555–60.

68. Schwenk W, Bohm B, Fugener A, Muller JM. Intermittent pneumatic sequential compression (ISC) of the lower extremities prevents venous stasis during laparoscopic cholecystectomy. A prospective randomized study. Surg Endosc 1998; 12:7–11.

69. Wright GW, Place R, Princi F. The physiological effects of pneumoperitoneum upon the respiratory apparatus. Am Rev Tuberc 1949; 60:706–14.

70. Hodgson C, McClelland RMA, Newton JR. Some effects of the peritoneal insufflation of carbon dioxide at laparoscopy. Anaesthesia 1970; 25:382–90.

71. Puri GD, Singh H. Ventilatory effects of laparoscopy under general anaesthesia. Br J Anaesth 1992; 68:211–13.

72. Piiper J. Physiological equilibria of gas cavities in the body. In: Fenn WO, Rahn H, ed. Handbook of physiology, Section 3: Respiration. Washington, DC: American Physiological Society, 1965:1205–18.

73. Stoller ML, Wolf JS Jr. Physiological considerations in laparoscopy. In: Das S, Crawford ED, ed. Urologic laparoscopy. Philadelphia: WB Saunders, 1994:17–34.

74. Nunn JF. Carbon dioxide. In: Applied respiratory physiology. London: Butterworths, 1987:207–34.

75. Mullett CE, Viale JP, Sagnard PE, et al. Pulmonary $CO_2$ elimination during surgical procedures using intra- or extraperitoneal $CO_2$ insufflation. Anesth Analg 1993; 76:622–6.

76. Wolf JS Jr, Monk TG, McDougall EM, et al. The extraperitoneal approach and subcutaneous emphysema are associated with greater absorption of carbon dioxide during laparoscopic renal surgery. J Urol 1995; 154:959–64.

77. Liu SY, Leighton T, Davis I, et al. Prospective analysis of cardiopulmonary responses to laparoscopic cholecystectomy. J Laparoendosc Surg 1991; 1:241–6.

78. Alexander GD, Brown EM. Physiologic alterations during laparoscopy. Am J Obstet Gynecol 1969; 105:1078–81.

79. Magno R, Medegård A, Bengtsson R, Tronstad S-E. Acid-base balance during laparoscopy: the effects of intraperitoneal insufflation of carbon dioxide on acid-base balance during controlled ventilation. Acta Obstet Gynecol Scand 1979; 58:81–5.

80. Leighton TA, Liu SY, Bongard FS. Comparative cardiopulmonary effects of carbon dioxide versus helium pneumoperitoneum. Surgery 1993; 113:527–31.

81. Wittgen CM, Andrus CH, Fitzgerald SD, et al. Analysis of the hemodynamic and ventilatory effects of laparoscopic cholecystectomy. Arch Surg 1991; 126:997–1001.

82. Holzman M, Sharp K, Richards W. Hypercarbia during carbon dioxide gas insufflation for therapeutic laparoscopy: a note of caution. Surg Laparosc Endosc 1992; 2:11–14.

83. Sosa RE, Weingram J, Stein B, et al. Hypercarbia in laparoscopic pelvic lymph node dissection. J Urol 1992; 147:A246.

84. Neuberger TJ, Andrus CH, Wittgen CM, et al. Prospective comparison of helium versus carbon dioxide pneumoperitoneum. Gastrointest Endosc 1994; 40:P30.

85. Wright DM, Serpell MG, Baxter JN, et al. Effect of extraperitoneal carbon dioxide insufflation on intra-operative blood gas and hemodynamic changes. Surg Endosc 1995; 9:1169–72.

86. Siegler AM, Berenyi KJ. Laparoscopy in gynecology. Obstet Gynecol 1969; 34:572–7.

87. Sharp JR, Pierson WP, Brady CE III. Comparison of $CO_2$- and $N_2O$-induced discomfort during peritoneoscopy under local anesthesia. Gastroenterology 1982; 82:453–6.

88. Minoli G, Terruzzi V, Spinzi GC, et al. The influence of carbon dioxide and nitrous oxide on pain during laparoscopy: a double-blind, controlled trial. Gastrointest Endosc 1982; 28:173–5.

89. Fitzgerald SD, Andrus CH, Baudendistel LJ, et al. Hypercarbia during carbon dioxide pneumoperitoneum. Am J Surg 1992; 163:186–90.

90. Wolf JS Jr, Clayman RV, McDougall EM, et al. Carbon dioxide and helium insufflation during laparoscopic radical nephrectomy in a patient with severe pulmonary disease. J Urol 1996; 155:2021.

91. Verbessem D, Camu F, Devroey P, Steirteghem AV. Pneumoperitoneum induced pH changes in follicular and Douglas fluids during laparoscopic oocyte retrieval in humans. Human Reprod 1988; 3:751–4.

92. Wahba RWM, Mamazza J. Ventilatory requirements during laparoscopic cholecystectomy. Can J Anaesth 1993; 40:206–10.

93. Kenefick JP, Leader A, Maltby JR, Taylor PJ. Laparoscopy: blood-gas values and minor sequelae associated with three techniques based on isoflurane. Br J Anaesth 1987; 59:189–94.

94. Sivak BJ. Surgical emphysema: report of a case and review. Anesth Analg 1964; 43:415–17.

95. Batra MS, Driscoll JJ, Coburn WA, Marks WM. Evanescent nitrous oxide pneumothorax after laparoscopy. Anesth Analg 1983; 62:1121–3.

96. Pascual JB, Baranda MM, Tarrero MT, et al. Subcutaneous emphysema, pneumomediastinum, bilateral pneumothorax and pneumopericardium after laparoscopy. Endoscopy 1990; 22:59.

97. Root B, Levy MN, Pollack S, et al. Gas embolism death after laparoscopy delayed by 'trapping' in portal circulation. Anesth Analg 1978; 57:232–7.

98. Gomar C, Fernandez C, Villalonga A, Nalda MA. Carbon dioxide embolism during laparoscopy and hysteroscopy. Ann Fr Anesth Reanim 1985; 4:380–2.

99. Hynes SR, Marshall RL. Venous gas embolism during gynaecological laparoscopy. Can J Anaesth 1992; 39:748–9.

100. Beck DH, McQuillan PJ. Fatal carbon dioxide embolism and severe haemorrhage during laparoscopic salpingectomy. Br J Anesth 1994; 72:243–5.

101. O'Sullivan DC, Micali S, Averch TD, et al. Factors involved in gas embolism after laparoscopic injury to inferior vena cava. J Endourol 1998; 12:149–54.

102. Shulman D, Aronson HB. Capnography in the early diagnosis of carbon dioxide embolism during laparoscopy. Can Anaesth Soc J 1984; 31:455–9.

103. Graff TD, Arbegast NR, Phillips OC, et al. Gas embolism: a comparative study of air and carbon dioxide as embolic agents in the systemic venous system. Am J Obstet Gynecol 1959; 78:259–65.

104. Wolf JS Jr, Carrier S, Stoller ML. Gas embolism: helium is more lethal than carbon dioxide. J Laparoendosc Surg 1994; 4:173–7.

105. Mastragelopulos N, Sarkar MR, Kaissling G, et al. [Argon gas embolism in laparoscopic cholecystectomy with the Argon Beam One coagulator]. Chirurg 1992; 63:1053–4.

106. Nunn JF. Oxygen. In: Applied respiratory physiology. London: Butterworths, 1987:235–83.

107. Corall IM, Knights K, Potter D, Strunin L. Arterial oxygen tension during laparoscopy with nitrous oxide in the spontaneously breathing patient. Br J Anaesth 1974; 46:925–8.

108. Ott DE. Laparoscopic hypothermia. J Laparoendosc Surg 1991; 1:127–31.

109. Ott DE. Correction of laparoscopic insufflation hypothermia. J Laparoendosc Surg 1991; 1:183–6.

110. Nelskyla K, Yli-Hankala A, Sjoberg J, et al. Warming of insufflation gas during laparoscopic hysterectomy: effect on body temperature and the autonomic nervous system. Acta Anaesth Scand 1999; 43:974–8.

111. Teichman JMH, Floyd M, Hulbert JC. Does laparoscopy induce operative hypothermia? J Endourol 1994; 8:S92.

112. Fervers C. Die Laparoskopie mit dem Cystoskop. Medizinische Klinik 1933; 29:1042–5.

113. Soderstrom RM. Dangers of nitrous oxide pneumoperitoneum. Am J Obstet Gynecol 1976; 124:668–9.

114. Robinson JS, Thompson JM, Wood AW. Laparoscopy explosion hazards with nitrous oxide. Br Med J 1975; 4:760–1.

115. Vickers MD. Fire and explosions in operating theatres. Br J Anaesth 1978; 50:659–64.

116. El-Kady AA, Abd-el-Razek M. Intraperitoneal explosion during female sterilization by laparoscopic electrocoagulation. A case report. Int J Gynaecol Obstet 1976; 14:487–8.

117. Neuman GG, Sidebotham G, Negoiana E, et al. Laparoscopy explosion hazards with nitrous oxide. Anesthesiology 1993; 78:875–9.

118. Altmore DF, Memeo V. Colonic explosion during diathermy colotomy. Dis Colon Rectum 1993; 36:291–3.

# 6

# Minimally invasive treatment of bladder calculi

David Cuellar, William W Roberts, Steven Docimo

Bladder stones account for only 5% of urinary calculi in the Western world[1] and usually affect adult men with bladder outlet obstruction. In contrast to renal stones, bladder stones are usually composed of uric acid or struvite. Bladder stones in the pediatric population are becoming more frequent as the number of patients undergoing bladder-related surgery (augmentation cystoplasty, exstrophy repair, creation of Mitrofanoff stoma, urinary diversion) increases.

## Incidence

Depending on the type of procedure performed, the incidence of bladder stone formation in children with reconstructed bladders ranges from 5 to 52% (Table 6.1). The incidence with urinary diversions ranges from 3%[7,8] in nonrefluxing colon conduits to as high as 20% in some ileal conduit series[9] and 43% in Kock pouches.[10–13]

## Risk factors

Risk factors for stone formation include mucus production, decrease in urinary citrate levels, chronic bacteriuria (caused by urea-splitting organisms), foreign bodies, and dehydration.[9] Mucus production can act as a nidus for stone formation and harbor urea-splitting organisms while causing poor drainage and stasis. Persistent infection causing alkalinization of the urine combined with chronic hypercalciuria create a suitable environment for stone formation. Conduits and pouches, especially Kock pouches,[10] created with nonabsorbable staples and suture are notoriously associated with stones.

**Table 6.1** *Incidence of bladder calculi*

| Type of bladder | Incidence | Follow-up | Author |
|---|---|---|---|
| Augmentation cystoplasty | 52% | 4 years | Palmer 1993[2] |
| | 10% | 6 years | Kronner 1998[3] |
| | 16% | 4.9 years | Mathoera 2000[4] |
| Exstrophy–epispadias complex | 26% | 6 years | Surer 2003[5] |
| Children on CIC | 7% | 3 years | Barroso 2000[6] |
| no augment. + urethral cath. | 5% | | |
| no augment + Mitrof. cath. | 11% | | |
| augment. and urethral cath. | 8% | | |
| augment. and Mitrof. cath. | 10% | | |

CIC = clean intermittent catheterization; augment. = augmentation cystoplasty; Mitrof. = Mitrofanoff; cath. = catheter.

# Diagnosis

These stones are often found incidentally by plain film, pouchograms or loopograms, ultrasound, computed tomography (CT) scan, or endoscopy. Symptoms that suggest the presence of stones include gross hematuria, recurrent urinary infections, difficulty voiding or catheterizing, increased frequency of catheterization, lower abdominal fullness or discomfort, and incontinence.[14]

# Prevention

There are many strategies for prevention of bladder pouch stones. As with any stone, hydration is important in preventing stone formation. Frequent and complete catheterization/voiding can also help. In those with interposed bowel, daily irrigation of mucus from the bladder can minimize recurrent infection and stone formation. Many of these patients have low urinary citrate levels, raising the possibility that oral citrate repletion may help prevent these stones. Renacidin irrigation has been used to dissolve and prevent bladder stones composed of struvite or phosphate, whereas alkalinization for uric acid stones is also a viable option. Irrigation in a bladder that contains intestine is not generally recommended, however, due to issues related to absorption. When prevention or conservative intervention is not successful, surgical options must be addressed.

# Treatment modalities

The historical treatment for bladder calculi is cystolithotomy. However, technological advances in endoscopic and lithotripsy equipment over the last two decades have made it possible for most bladder calculi in the adult population to be removed via the transurethral approach. Fragmentation can be accomplished with the use of mechanical means, electrohydraulic lithotripsy, ultrasonic lithotripsy, pneumatic lithotripsy (EHL), or holmium–YAG laser lithotripsy. However, the transurethral approach is not always possible in pediatric patients due to the smaller urethral caliber or the presence of a catheterizable stoma. In adult patients, as well, the risk of urethral injury and subsequent stricture is increased when lengthy transurethral procedures are performed for large or numerous calculi. In these patients percutaneous cystolithotomy is a suitable option.

# *The technique of percutaneous cystolithotomy*

The technique of percutaneous cystolithotomy is straightforward and has evolved from previous experience with upper tract percutaneous procedures. A flexible or rigid endoscope is inserted into the bladder through an intact urethra. The pouch is filled with sterile saline and the previous site of a suprapubic tube is identified in those patients with prior bladder reconstruction. The site is transilluminated and examined visually to ensure there is no intervening tissue. Fluoroscopy is seldom required for percutaneous bladder access. A 16- or 18-gauge percutaneous access needle is inserted through the site under direct visualization from the endoscope. A guide wire is passed through the needle before the needle is removed. An 8/10 dilator set or 10F dual-lumen catheter can then be used to introduce a safety wire. This is followed by rigid coaxial dilation of the tract with an Amplatz set or a one-step trocar system under direct visualization. Following dilation, a 26 or 30F access sheath is placed and a nephroscope introduced through the sheath. Improved visualization facilitates fragmentation or intact removal of the stones without risk of urethral injury. Removal of all stones and fragments can be confirmed with a plain abdominal X-ray. A suprapubic catheter is inserted into the bladder through the access sheath, which is subsequently split and pulled back leaving the SP tube in place.

# *Review of results*

Ikari et al reported an 89% success rate using ultrasonic fragmentation through a 26F nephroscope on the percutaneous treatment of bladder stones in 36 patients.[15] The 3 failures were due to inability to fragment the stone with the ultrasonic device. Twenty-two of these patients underwent concomitant TURP (transurethral resection of the prostate) or internal urethrotomy. Wollin et al reported a 100% stone-free rate when performing percutaneous suprapubic cystolithotripsy on 15 adult patients.[16] Patients were considered candidates for this approach if stone size > 3 cm, multiple stones > 1 cm were present, and patient anatomy precluded transurethral access. Using EHL, patients were rendered stone free in one procedure (mean operative time 86 min) and no major complications occurred. Similar success was reported when utilizing this percutaneous approach with an ultrasonic lithotriptor to treat stones of 1.2–3.1 cm in pediatric patients.[17]

Perhaps the greatest indication for percutaneous removal of bladder calculi is found in patients who have undergone urinary diversion. With improved oncologic therapies and procedures, it is now common for patients to live many years with reconstructed urinary systems created from bowel segments. In pediatrics as well, the continued refinement of reconstructive techniques has resulted in greater numbers of patients with augmented bladders and continent pouches. These patients are at greater risk for stone formation, yet standard endoscopic techniques can be limited by altered anatomy and increased risk of damage to surgically created continence mechanisms.

Multiple case reports appeared in the literature in the mid-1990s describing techniques for percutaneous treatment of continent pouch stones.[18–20,21] Franzoni et al presented their experience with percutanous vesicolithotomy in 3 adult patients who had previously undergone continent urinary diversion, bladder neck closure, and appendicovesicostomy.[20] Using intact extraction and ultrasonic lithotripsy, all patients were rendered stone free and discharged the same day. More recently, Cain et al reported on a series of 13 pediatric patients who had developed stones following augmentation cystoplasty. Complete stone removal (intact or with laser or EHL fragmentation) was achieved in 92% without complication. One patient suffered a small bladder perforation and required conversion to open cystolithotomy.[22]

We reviewed our data of 11 pediatric patients undergoing 16 procedures with complete elimination of the entire stone burden in all patients, with one requiring a second-look procedure. The average operative time was 136 min and the average hospital stay was < 1 day with 63% discharged the same day. Minor complications occurred in 5 of the 16 (31%) procedures and included ileus, hypothermia, and extravasation of fluid.[23]

Based upon the available literature, it appears that percutaneous approaches to bladder and urinary pouch calculi result in excellent stone-free outcomes. The few complications that have been reported were easily treated with conversion to traditional open cystolithotomy. Many of these patients have had significant prior reconstructive procedures on the urinary system and within the pelvis, which increases the complexity and the risk of complications when performing open cystolithotomy. With the relatively high rate of stone recurrence in augmented bladders and thus the need for repeated procedures, the importance of decreasing morbidity and hospital stay becomes evident.[24] Minimally invasive percutaneous procedures would therefore seem to be preferable to traditional open approaches. This, however, remains a controversial point.

## Stone recurrence

The data on stone recurrences in these patients are inconclusive, although some feel that intact extraction of stones reduces the stone recurrence rate compared with percutaneous or endoscopic approaches that rely on fragmentation[14] (Table 6.2). A series directly comparing open and

**Table 6.2** *Recurrence rate among stone formers*

| Type of bladder | Recurrence rate | Treatment | Main author |
|---|---|---|---|
| Augmentation cystoplasty | 19% | | Palmer 1993[2] |
| | 44% | | Kronner 1998[3] |
| | 54% | Cystolithalopaxy | |
| | 33% | Open cystolithotomy | |
| Exstrophy–epispadias complex | 38% | | Surer 2003[5] |
| Children on CIC | 32% | | Barroso 2000[6] |
| | 66% | Endoscopically with EHL | |
| | 33% | Open cystolithotomy | |
| Augmentation cystoplasty | 66% | | Docimo 1998[24] |
| | 66% | Open cystolithotomy | |
| | 66% | Percutaneous cystolithotomy | |

CIC = clean intermittent catheterization; EHL = electrohydraulic lithotripsy.

percutaneous techniques, however, found recurrence to be equally common in both groups,[24] suggesting that it is the underlying risk, and not technique, that accounts for high recurrence rates. The bladder stone recurrence rate in our most recent series was 58%, with a mean follow-up of 43 months.[23] Jarrett et al published a modification of the percutaneous approach to address recurrence.[25] They use an entrapment sac which is passed through the access sac. The calculi are then isolated from the remainder of the bladder or pouch inside this sac during fragmentation and removal. This eliminates the need to vigorously irrigate and remove tiny fragments at the end of the case.

# Conclusions

Although not the most frequently encountered, bladder stones and their management do merit discussion, especially when encountered in pediatric patients with reconstructed bladders. Many believe that open cystolithotomy remains the gold standard when addressing these stones with shorter operative times and decreased stone recurrence rates. However, because many of these patients have complex anatomy and have previously been operated on several times, and because they will probably need more bladder stone procedures in the future with high recurrence rates, thought should be given to a minimally invasive percutaneous procedure as described in this chapter.

# References

1. Schwartz BF, Stoller ML. The vesical calculus. Urol Clin North Am 2000; 27(2):333–46

2. Palmer LS, Franco I, Kogan SJ, et al. Urolithiasis in children following augmentation cystoplasty. J Urol 1993; 150:726–9.

3. Kronner KM, Casale AJ, Cain MP, et al. Bladder calculi in the pediatric augmented bladder. J Urol 1998; 160:1096–8.

4. Mathoera RB, Kok DJ, Nijman RJ. Bladder calculi in augmentation cystoplasty in children. Urology 2000; 56:482–7.

5. Surer I, Ferrer FA, Baker LA, Gearhart JP. Continent urinary diversion and the exstrophy-epispadias complex. J Urol 2003; 169:1102–5.

6. Barroso U, Jednak R, Fleming P, et al. Bladder calculi in children who perform clean intermittent catheterization. BJU Int 2000; 85:879–84.

7. Althausen AF, Hagen-Cook K, Hendren HW 3rd. Non-refluxing colon conduit: experience with 70 cases. J Urol 1978; 120:35–9.

8. Hagen-Cook K, Althausen AF. Early observations on 31 adults with non-refluxing colon conduits. J Urol 1979; 121:13–16.

9. McDougal WS. Use of intestinal segments and urinary diversion. In: Walsh PC, Retik AB, Vaughan ED Jr, Wein AJ, eds. Campbell's urology, 7th edn. Philadelphia: WB Saunders, 1998: 3121–61.

10. Arai Y, Kawakita M, Terachi T, et al. Long term follow-up of the Kock and Indiana pouch procedure. J Urol 1993; 150:51–5.

11. Turk TM, Koleski FC, Albala DM. Incidence of urolithiasis in cystectomy patients after intestinal conduit or continent urinary diversion. World J Urol 1999; 17:305–7.

12. Terai A, Ueda T, Kakehi Y, et al. Urinary calculi as a late complication of the Indiana continent urinary diversion: comparison with the Kock pouch procedure. J Urol 1996; 155:69–70.

13. Benson MC, Olsson CA. Continent urinary diversion. In: Walsh PC, Retik AB, Vaughan ED Jr, Wein AJ, eds. Campbell's urology, 7th edn. Philadelphia: WB Saunders, 1998:3190–245.

14. Ginsberg D, Huffman JL, Lieskovsky G, et al. Urinary tract stones: a complication of the Kock pouch continent urinary diversion. J Urol 145: 1991; 956–9.

15. Ikari O, Netto NR, D'Ancona CAL, Palma PCR. Percutaneous treatment of bladder stones. J Urol 1993; 149: 1499–500.

16. Wollin TA, Singal RK, Whelan T, et al. Percutaneous suprapubic cystolithotripsy for treatment of large bladder calculi. J Endourol 1999; 13:739–44.

17. Agrawal MS, Aron M, Goyal J, et al. Percutaneous suprapubic cystolithotripsy for vesical calculi in children. J Endourol 1999; 13:173–5.

18. Hollensbe DW, Foster RS, Brito CG, Kopecky K. Percutaneous access to a continent urinary reservoir for removal of intravesical calculi: a case report. J Urol 1993; 149:1546–7.

19. Seaman EK, Benson MC, Shabsigh R. Percutaneous approach to treatment of Indiana pouch stones. J Urol 1994; 151:690–2.

20. Franzoni DF, Decter RM. Percutaneous vesicolithotomy: an alternative to open bladder surgery in patients with an impassable or surgically ablated urethra. J Urol 1999; 162:777–8.

21. Thomas R, Lee S, Salvatore F, et al. Direct percutaneous pouch cystostomy with endoscopic lithotripsy for calculus in a continent urinary reservoir. J Urol 1993; 150:1235–7.

22. Cain MP, Casale AJ, Kaefer M, et al. Percutaneous cystolithotomy in the pediatric augmented bladder. J Urol 2002; 168:1881–2.

23. Cuellar DC, Docimo SG. Endoscopic treatment of lower urinary tract pathology in the pediatric population. J Endourol, in press.

24. Docimo SG, Orth CR, Schulum PG. Percutaneous cystolithotomy after augmentation cystoplasty: comparison with open procedures. Tech Urol 1998; 4:43–5.

25. Jarrett TW, Pound CR, Kavoussi LR. Stone entrapment during percutaneous removal of infection stones from a continent diversion. J Urol 1999; 162:775–6.

# 7

# Pediatric laparoscopic renal biopsy: techniques and indication

Paolo Caione and Salvatore Micali

## Indications for renal biopsy

The indications for renal biopsy vary according to the ethnic and age characteristics of population studies and geographical location, since these factors influence the incidence of various renal diseases.

Evaluation of a renal biopsy specimen may be useful in establishing the diagnosis, evaluating the acuteness and severity of the disease process, and determining the degree of reversibility. Clinical and laboratory evidence of glomerulonephropathy, either primary or secondary to systemic disease, is one of the most common indications for examination of renal tissue. Biopsies are done to define the prognosis based on the histologic diagnosis in children with nephrotic syndrome, to establish a diagnosis in children with chronic glomerulonephritis, and to determine the nature of disease and the degree of renal injury in patients presenting clinically with acute glomerulonephritis, particularly when it is severe. Percutaneous renal biopsies are often performed by nephrologists for the assessment of pediatric patients with unexplained azotemia, protein-uria, hematuria, or idiopathic nephrotic syndrome resistant to steroids.[1] Moreover, acute nephritis, acute renal failure, chronic renal insufficiency, systemic diseases, and follow-up of disease could be considered clinical indications for renal biopsy. In patients with systemic disorders such as lupus erythematosus or Henoch–Schönlein syndrome, examination of renal tissue may be necessary to document involvement of the kidney and to provide information concerning the histo-logic diagnosis and magnitude of the renal injury. Hypertension without other signs of renal involvement is not an indication for renal biopsy in children. The rate of serious complication of biopsy is increased in hyper-tensive individuals. If renal disease is suspected as the etiology of the hypertension and if a biopsy is to be performed, the hypertension must be well controlled prior to the procedure. Prompt interpretation of biopsy tissue from renal allografts apparently undergoing acute rejection may aid in determining the correct therapy. Biopsy may play a critical role also in the diagnosis of recurrent disease in renal transplants and in determining the presence or absence of cyclosporine toxicity. The use of fine-needle biopsies has been advocated for the latter purpose.

Most authors agree that renal biopsy is of little value in the assessment of children with urinary tract infec-tion. It has been applied only occasionally in the evalua-tion of cystic and dysplastic disorders. It is relatively contraindicated when the presence of an intrarenal neoplasm is suspected because the procedure may lead to intra-abdominal dissemination of the tumor.

Percutaneous needle renal biopsy is the current standard approach, usually performed under ultrasound control. Ultrasonography and radioisotopic scanning could precede biopsy in an attempt to differentiate acute from chronic renal failure and to exclude extrarenal or urologic lesions such as obstruction. Over time, the contraindica-tions of percutaneous needle biopsy of the kidney have decreased with the advent of reliable, minimally invasive imaging techniques and the development of adequate protocols for patient monitoring during the early post-biopsy period.[2] The development of small-caliber biopsy needles has also contributed to the increased safety and reduced morbidity of this technique.

With improvements in safety and reliability, several clinical conditions that were recently considered absolute contraindications for percutaneous biopsy, i.e. solitary kidney and obesity, are now considered relative contraindi-cations.[3] However, there are some pediatric patients in whom a percutaneous approach may be risky, the only remaining option being a renal biopsy under direct visuali-zation. Currently, relative indications for renal biopsy under direct visualization are age less than 7 years old, uncon-trolled hypertension, bleeding disorders, and anticoagulant medications.

# Technical options for renal biopsy

## Percutaneous needle biopsy

The patient can be treated as an outpatient. Ultrasound examination is performed to confirm the normal position of the kidney without anatomical anomalies. Laboratory evaluation must include a complete blood cell count with normal platelet count, partial thromboplastin, pro-thrombin time, fibrinogen level and bleeding time. The biopsy is timed so that an experienced technician or pathologist can attend, to ensure prompt processing of the biopsy tissue.

Food and drink should be withheld for at least 6 hours before biopsy. The child should be sedated, but awake, so if possible he can cooperate during the procedure. The patient lies in the prone position with a rolled sheet under the abdomen and draped in a sterile fashion. The left kidney is usually preferred, but either side can be chosen for biopsy. Then, the lower pole of the kidney is marked on the skin with a pen after localization by ultrasound. Local anesthetic is infiltrated first in the skin, and then in deeper tissues, taking care not to enter the kidney. A small incision is made through the skin. A disposable core tissue biopsy needle (16-gauge) mounted on a biopsy gun (Bard Magnum, CR Bard, Inc., Covington, Georgia) is preferred for biopsy in larger children (over 5 years old) because of its ease of use and sharp cutting edge. The biopsy needle can now be inserted into the desired position. When the kidney capsule is punctured, a loss of resistance can be felt. The needle will move with inspiration when the child is ask to breathe, confirming that it is within the renal parenchyma. The entire needle with tissue sample is then removed. Usually, two cores of tissue are necessary for optimal evaluation. If tissue cannot be obtained after several passes, the biopsy should be attempted another way. The child is kept supine in bed for 24 hours, urine is observed for gross hematuria and the hematocrit should be rechecked at 4 and 24 hours after the biopsy. The child may be discharged the next day if no complications arise.

## Retroperitoneoscopic renal biopsy

Following the administration of adequate general endotracheal anesthesia, a transurethral Foley catheter and a nasogastric tube are placed. The patient is placed in the full flank position and secured to the operating table (Figure 7.1). A two-port technique is used via a retroperitoneal route: a 10 mm laparoscopic port is placed between the iliac crest and the 12th rib, in the posterior axillary line. A 5 mm port is inserted at the same level on the anterior axillary line (Figure 7.2). In all children the first trocar is positioned under direct vision using the Visiport (AutoSuture, US Surgical Corporation, Norwalk, Connecticut). This device allows the surgeon to incise and advance the cannula through each tissue layer under direct vision until the retroperitoneal space is reached. Insufflation with $CO_2$ at 15 mmHg is started. The laparoscope is then used to bluntly dissect the retroperitoneal space and mobilize the lateral peritoneum from the anterior abdominal wall (Figure 7.3). The 5 mm port is also inserted under direct vision (Figure 7.4). Finally, the $CO_2$ insufflation pressure is turned down to 8–10 mmHg. Minimal dissection is required in order to expose the lower pole of the kidney (Figure 7.5). Short 5 mm laparoscopic cut biopsy forceps are used to grasp two superficial cortical biopsy specimens (Figures 7.6 and 7.7). The biopsy site is fulgurated with monopolar or bipolar electrocautery, and a sheet of oxidized cellulose (Surgicel, Johnson & Johnson, Arlington, Texas) is applied. Upon conclusion, the gas is evacuated and the skin is closed with absorbable sutures. Time required is usually 20–40 min. Blood loss tends to be minimal. The retroperitoneoscopic procedure may be performed on an outpatient basis or the patient may spend the night in hospital. Patients are allowed to return to their usual activities within a few days.

## Traditional open renal biopsy

This technique today is rarely used because minimally invasive techniques are preferred in almost all the pediatric hospitals, either with percutaneous needle or laparoscopic procedures.

Open biopsy is performed under general anesthesia. The kidney can be directly visualized even through a small muscle-splitting lumbotomy incision. One advantage of the open approach is that a larger sample may be obtained via wedge biopsy than can be obtained with the laparoscopic biopsy forceps.

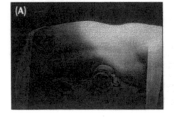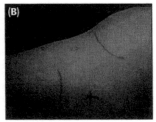

**Figure 7.1**
(A) Patient position for retroperitoneal open renal biopsy or laparoscopic biopsy. (B) Trocar positions are underlined.

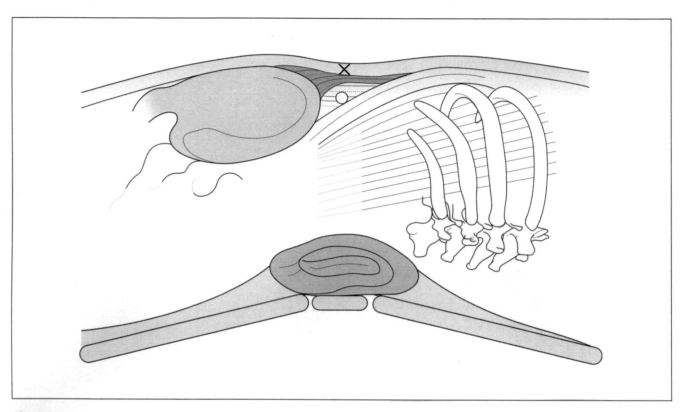

**Figure 7.2**
Anatomic landmarks for retroperitoneal laparoscopy: 12th rib, iliac crest. Trocar positioning for minor renal operative procedures through retroperitoneal laparoscopic access: X = 10 mm port, O = 5 mm port.

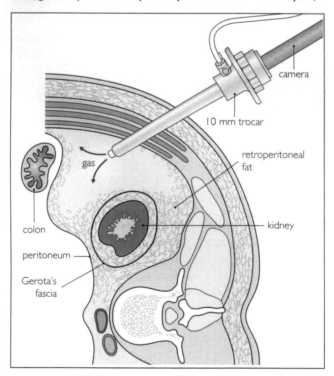

**Figure 7.3**
After retroperitoneal access is obtained, blunt dissection is used to mobilize the lateral peritoneum from the anterior abdominal wall.

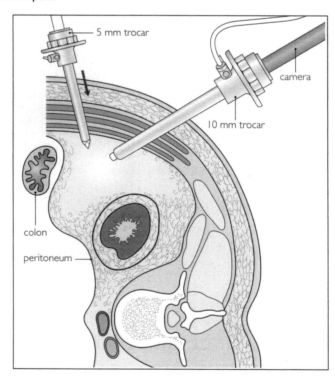

**Figure 7.4**
After the development of the retroperitoneal space, a 5 mm trocar is placed at the anterior axillary line. Care must be taken to prevent entry into the peritoneal cavity.

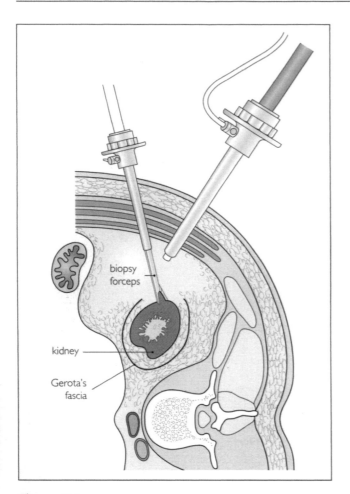

**Figure 7.5**
After localization of the kidney, Gerota's fascia is incised and the renal parenchyma is exposed.

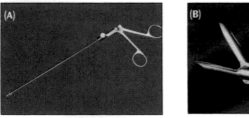 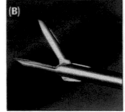

**Figure 7.6**
Pediatric biopsy forceps (A) and particular of the jaws for renal biopsy (B).

# Clinical considerations, complications, and results

Histologic evaluation of renal tissue is often necessary in the evaluation and management of several renal diseases. Pathologic diagnosis often provides useful information in determining prognosis and guiding treatment.[1,4,5] Several methods to sample renal tissue are available, including

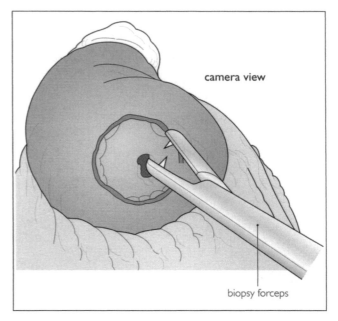

**Figure 7.7**
Renal core biopsies are obtained via a 5 mm laparoscopic cut biopsy forceps.

blind and image-guided percutaneous needle biopsy or aspiration and open or laparoscopic approaches. Percutaneous needle biopsy is the most common method of sampling renal tissue in adults and pediatric patients, because it is minimally invasive and can be performed under local anesthesia with minimal morbidity.[3] Unfortunately, as many as 5–20% of percutaneous needle biopsies yield inadequate renal tissue for diagnosis[6] and significant complications such as hemorrhage and even renal loss have been reported.[7–9] Moreover, in children younger than 7 years of age who do not cooperate adequately during the procedure, the percutaneous approach may be hazardous even under local anesthesia.

In addition, our experience in children indicates contraindications to percutaneous renal biopsy, such as uncontrolled hypertension, bleeding disorders, anatomic abnormalities, solitary kidney, and anticoagulant medication.[1,7,10] In these patients, a renal biopsy under direct vision may be preferred (Table 7.1).

The development of laparoscopic renal biopsy now provides a minimally invasive alternative to open renal biopsy. General anesthesia is required as in the open technique, but the kidney is better identified with the optical magnification of the laparoscopic lens. Only two ports are required for the retroperitoneal procedure. During our retroperitoneoscopic procedure, a nephrologist is present in the operating room, and a preliminary macroscopic examination of the kidney, including site, size, color, and bleeding intensity is performed. Moreover, biopsy and hemostasis are achieved under direct vision in a controlled minimally invasive fashion.[11–14]

**Table 7.1**  *Indications for pursuing a laparoscopic approach in 20 consecutive patients[19]*

| Patient No. | Age (years old) | Contraindications for percutaneous biopsy |
|---|---|---|
| 1 | 10 | Uncontrolled hypertension |
| 2 | 4 | Uncontrolled hypertension, age |
| 3 | 4 | Age |
| 4 | 7 | Age, parents' request |
| 5 | 7 | Age |
| 6 | 4 | Uncontrolled hypertension, age |
| 7 | 11 | Uncontrolled hypertension |
| 8 | 17 | Anticlotting medications |
| 9 | 14 | Uncontrolled hypertension |
| 10 | 2 | Age |
| 11 | 16 | Uncontrolled hypertension |
| 12 | 11 | Medullary cystic disease |
| 13 | 12 | Uncooperative patient |
| 14 | 5 | Age |
| 15 | 11 | Parents' request |
| 16 | 9 | Unsuccessful previous needle biopsy |
| 17 | 14 | Uncontrolled hypertension |
| 18 | 18 | Parents request |
| 19 | 4 | Age |
| 20 | 5 | Age |

**Table 7.2**  *Hystopathologic diagnosis in the 20 retroperitoneal laparoscopic renal biopsies[19]*

| Patient No. | Age (years old) | Pathologic diagnosis |
|---|---|---|
| 1 | 10 | Proliferative glomerulonephritis, Henoch-Schönlein syndrome |
| 2 | 4 | Proliferative glomerulonephritis |
| 3 | 4 | Proliferative glomerulonephritis |
| 4 | 7 | Alport's syndrome |
| 5 | 7 | Proliferative glomerulonephritis |
| 6 | 4 | Thrombotic microangiopathy |
| 7 | 11 | Proliferative glomerulonephritis |
| 8 | 17 | Proliferative lupus glomerulonephritis |
| 9 | 14 | Proliferative lupus glomerulonephritis |
| 10 | 2 | Proliferative glomerulonephritis, Henoch-Schönlein syndrome |
| 11 | 16 | Proliferative glomerulonephritis |
| 12 | 11 | Medullary cystic disease |
| 13 | 12 | IgA nephropathy |
| 14 | 5 | Alport's syndrome |
| 15 | 11 | Alport's syndrome |
| 16 | 9 | IgA nephropathy |
| 17 | 14 | Mesangial proliferative glomerulonephritis |
| 18 | 18 | IgA nephropathy |
| 19 | 4 | Focal segmental glomerulosclerosis |
| 20 | 5 | Henoch-Schönlein syndrome |

Using an entirely retroperitoneal approach, we were able to obtain sufficient renal tissue for the histopathologic diagnosis in 20 children (Table 7.2). No bleeding complications or hematuria occurred in any of our patients, and none of them required blood transfusion. The high success rate and lack of bleeding complications in our experience is equal to that reported in large open renal biopsy series.[6,15,16] In contrast, the incidence of bleeding complications was found to be 5.0% in a contemporary percutaneous renal biopsy series.[9] We feel that our technique potentially reduces the risk of hemorrhage, hematuria, and the development of secondary arteriovenous fistulas as compared with the percutaneous needle approach. Two primary advantages are noted: hemostasis is achieved and confirmed under direct vision and the cup biopsy forceps yields generous and superficial cortical specimens, without injuring the underlying central vessels or the collecting system. Biopsy needles, which can potentially reach collecting system and/or large segmental vessels, are avoided.

Squadrito and Coletta[17] were the first to report laparoscopic renal biopsy in a human patient via a transperitoneal approach. Gaur[18] popularized the retroperitoneoscopic approach and reported the use of a balloon to develop the retroperitoneal space. Gaur et al.[11] first reported a series of 17 patients in whom retroperitoneoscopic renal biopsy was performed. The authors reported two complications in their series. When deep cup biopsies were performed, hemostasis was achieved through an enlarged incision in one case. Another patient developed gross hematuria, which resolved spontaneously in 2 days. We prefer the retroperitoneal approach for renal biopsy because there is less risk of injuring intraperitoneal viscera or causing a postoperative ileus.[19] According to our experiences, we have modified the Gaur technique by entering the retroperitoneum using the Visiport device through a standard 1 cm incision, rather than performing a larger cutdown. We rapidly develop the retroperitoneal space with a blunt technique, using the laparoscope rather than a balloon.[20] We find that the retroperitoneal space in children is smaller than in adults, and the peritoneum is thin and easily entered. Therefore, the Visiport device enables us to see the peritoneum and preserve its integrity safely. In addition, our technique uses only two ports as compared to the three commonly required for other techniques.

In small children we recommend the use of short pediatric instruments (dolphin forceps, scissors, and biopsy forceps). At the end of the procedure, the insufflation pressure is gradually decreased, and the biopsy site is observed and any bleeding is controlled.[21]

# Conclusion

Laparoscopic renal biopsy is a safe, reliable, and minimally invasive alternative to open renal biopsy. With experience and a systematic, anatomic approach, retroperitoneoscopic renal biopsy can be efficiently performed in pediatric patients older than 6 months of age.

# References

1. Gault MH, Muehrcke RC. Renal biopsy: current views and controversy. Nephron 1983; 34:1–34.

2. Donovan KL, Thomas, DM, Wheeler DC, et al. Experience with a new method for percutaneous renal biopsy. Nephrol Dial Transplant 1991; 6(10):731–3.

3. Schow DA, Vinson RK, Morrisean PM. Percutaneous renal biopsy of the solitary kidney: a contraindication? J Urol 1992; 147:1235–7.

4. Morel-Maroger L. The value of renal biopsy. Am J Kidney Dis 1982; 1:244–8.

5. Manoligod JR, Pirani CL. Renal biopsy in 1985. Sem Neph 1985; 5:237–9.

6. Nomoto Y, Tomino Y, Endoh M, et al. Modified open renal biopsy: results in 934 patients. Nephron 1987; 45:224–8.

7. Diaz-Buxo JA, Donadio JV Jr. Complications of percutaneous renal biopsy: an analysis of 1,000 consecutive cases. Clin Nephrol 1975; 4(6):223–6.

8. Rosenbaum R, Hoffsten PE, Stanley RJ, et al. Use of computerized tomography to diagnose complications of percutaneous renal biopsy. Kidney Int 1978; 14(1):87–92.

9. Wickre CG, Golper TA. Complications of percutaneous needle biopsy of the kidney. Am J Nephrol 1982; 2:173–8.

10. Healey DE, Newman RC, Cohen MS et al. Laparoscopically assisted percutaneous renal biopsy. J Urol 1993; 150:1218–21.

11. Gaur DD, Agarwal DK, Khochikar MV, et al. Laparoscopic renal biopsy via retroperitoneal approach. J Urol 1994; 151: 925–6.

12. Keizur JJ, Tashima M, Das S. Retroperitoneal laparoscopic renal biopsy. Surg Laparosc Endosc 1993; 3:60–2.

13. Chen RN, Moore RG, Micali S, et al. Retroperitoneoscopic renal biopsy in extremely obese patients. Urology 1997; 50(2):195–8.

14. Gimenez LF, Micali S, Chen RN, et al. Laparoscopic renal biopsy. Kidney Int 1998; 54:525–9.

15. Patil J, Bailey GL, Mahoney EF. Open-renal biopsy in uremic patient. Urology 1974; 3:293–6.

16. Bolton WK, Vaughan ED. A comparative study of open surgical and percutaneous renal biopsies. J Urol 1977; 117:696–8.

17. Squadrito JF Jr, Coletta AV. Laparoscopic renal exploration and biopsy. J Laparoendosc. Surg 1991; 1:235–9.

18. Gaur DD. Laparoscopic operative retroperitoneoscopy: use of a new device. J Urol 1992; 148:1137–9.

19. Caione P, Micali S, Rinaldi S, et al. Retroperitoneal laparoscopy for renal biopsy in children. J Urol 2000; 164:1080–3.

20. Micali S, Caione P, Virgili G, et al. Retroperitoneal laparoscopic access in children using direct vision technique. J Urol 2001; 165:1229–32.

21. Micali S, Caione P. Retroperitoneal access. In: Caione P, Micali S, Kavoussi LR, eds. Retroperitoneoscopy and Extraperitoneal Laparoscopy in Pediatric and Adult Urology. Milan: Springer, 2003: 31–7.

# 8

# Minimally invasive approaches to the ureteropelvic junction and upper ureter

Craig A Peters

## Pathologic anatomy of the ureter

The basis for nearly all pathologic conditions of the ureter in children is abnormal ureteral development, which follows fairly consistent patterns. The ureteral pathology itself is rarely the problem, but the effects on urinary transit and renal function are the principal concerns. Understanding the patterns of abnormal ureteral development is essential to selection and application of appropriate therapeutic interventions.

## Embryology

The ureter develops in conjunction with the kidney in a mutually inductive process. Recent evidence has suggested that the metanephric blastema, the precursor for the ultimate kidney, may actively induce ureteral budding,[1] in contrast to separate ureteral budding with subsequent induction of the metanephric mesenchyme by the ureteral bud. This would suggest that any renal mesenchyme abnormalities might then induce ureteral budding anomalies, such as reflux or ectopia. There is clearly an association between the two, and this was best described by the Mackie–Stephens theory: progressively more anomalous and ectopic ureteral budding leads to increasing degrees of renal dysplasia. While this theory has provided an explanation for many patterns of anomalous development, it does not explain all, and exceptions can be found. It does not permit a simplistic approach to these anomalies either, and their features must be carefully evaluated to develop an appropriate treatment plan for each child.

The molecular signals mediating ureterorenal development are now being elucidated and include a variety of signaling molecules (Pax2),[2] Foxc (transcription factor),[1] Wnt-6,[3] Tmp21-I (a protein traffic regulator),[4] Vitamin A

(with Ret, a signaling molecule),[5] glial-derived neurotrophic factor (GDNF),[2] endostatin (an angiogenesis inhibitor),[6] matrix metalloproteinases,[7] and components of the angiotensin system.[8] The regulation of branching morphogenesis is a critical element in normal ureterorenal embryogenesis and has been the subject of much investigation relevant to normal ureteral development.[9,10] Several excellent reviews of the current focus of research on ureterorenal development have been published.[11–13]

During ureteral development there is good evidence that the ureter passes through a stage in which the initially tubular structure condenses into a solid cord.[14] This feature of development has been highly quoted and the evidence is fairly strong. It is observed in both human and animal embryonic specimens. The importance of this stage is that many obstructive conditions are considered due to incomplete subsequent recanalization. The specific causes for this are unknown, as is the process of recanalization. Presumably it is mediated by increased growth of the peripheral aspects of the ureter. This may relate to the process of muscular ingrowth into the ureter from the surrounding mesenchyme.[15] The driving factors in these processes are still undefined, but their elucidation may provide useful insight into pathological processes.

Development of the ureteropelvic junction (UPJ) itself, the site of the vast majority of ureteral obstructions is relatively undefined.

The response of the ureter to anomalous development is important to consider as well, since it may determine the efficacy of various treatment modalities. Obstruction and reflux are the most common patterns of pathology for the ureter and each induces similar, but likely, functionally distinct responses. These responses are probably very similar to those of the renal pelvis as well. In general, any process that induces dilation of the ureter is characterized by increased amounts of ureteral smooth muscle with increased interstitial connective tissue.[16] The underlying mechanisms of these pathologic responses, which may be compensatory, but nonetheless pathologic, are being investigated. There seem to be increased expression of smooth muscle, suggesting dysregulation of ureteral smooth muscle cell (SMC) growth factors.[17] Increased extracellular matrix (ECM) may be the product of altered balance between connective tissue synthesis and breakdown.[18] Breakdown may itself be the product of imbalance between degradation and natural inhibition of degradation. These processes are seen in the bladder as well. Recognizing the patterns of these processes and their driving forces may permit more specific therapy for the abnormal ureter. It is also important to recognize that treatments directed at the ureter are dealing with abnormal tissue that may be fibrotic and poorly compliant. This will clearly affect healing and remodeling, and may well explain some failures of therapy. Precise definition of those aspects, however, is still lacking.

As the ureter develops, it is involved in a delicate two-way dance with the developing kidney and their respective fates are intertwined. Mutual coinduction is probably the most appropriate description of this process. Clearly, then, the abnormal ureter may be associated with an abnormal kidney. This is not, however, certain, and detailed evaluation is still needed. It should also not be assumed that abnormalities of kidney function associated with an abnormal ureter are immutable and fixed. This is particularly true in the setting of apparent obstruction, in which the abnormal ureter, with deranged function, may cause worsening of renal function that may already be less than normal.

## Pathologic patterns

The most common abnormality of the ureter is ureteropelvic junction obstruction (UPJO). Because this is a spectrum of disorders, precise definition of the incidence is difficult to establish. In prenatal detection, the incidence is between 0.1 and 2.0% of cases, depending upon the threshold for 'hydronephrosis'. Thomas reports in-utero dilation to have an incidence of 1 in 60 pregnancies with 1 in 500 having a significant urologic problem, half of which were UPJ abnormalities.[19] There is a male predominance (2:1) of these conditions, which also occur more often on the left side (2:1). The clinical and functional significance of any given UPJO is very controversial. Prenatal ultrasound has shown many patients with an apparent UPJO that may resolve spontaneously, challenging the accuracy of other series. The controversy of the functional significance of any of these conditions remains unsettled. Treatment options must therefore be viewed in the context that no gold standard exists for defining a 'significant' or 'surgical' UPJO. Within the group of UPJOs are those crossed by a lower pole renal vessel, usually an artery,

which produces a mechanical fixation point of the ureter, about which it will kink. This may produce intermittent obstruction, with attendant acute symptoms, so-called Dietl's crisis.[20]

# Pathophysiology of ureteral anomalies

The most significant ureteral anomalies produce obstruction, and the response of the developing or juvenile kidney is the key deleterious effect. The spectrum of severity in ureteral obstruction is paralleled by the spectrum of response of the kidney. Precise detection of where in the spectrum a particular patient's condition may fall remains an ongoing challenge and is controversial. This is particularly true of patients whose obstruction has been detected by prenatal ultrasound and who are usually symptom-free. It is clear that some UPJOs produce an ongoing loss of renal function, with the further risk of infection, pain, or stone formation. Others, however, and a large number, are less severe and appear to resolve spontaneously when followed nonsurgically. Distinguishing the two may be difficult, and there is a broad gray area in which the distinction is unclear. The response of the prenatal kidney is complex, yet viewed broadly it reflects the altered growth and differentiation of various components of renal function.[21] There are injury responses such as fibrosis that are also important and play a significant role in the functional response to obstruction. These responses should ultimately permit more accurate determination of the severity of the obstruction from a renal standpoint and allow clinical decisions that reflect more than simple appearance. The functional effects at the ureteral level are still important and are clearly the foundation of the renal response.

The function of the ureter is to transmit urine from the kidney to the bladder at low pressure, and be able to do this efficiently at differing rates of urine production. This is mediated through a peristaltic action of the ureter in which a regular progression of smooth muscle contractions and relaxations travels from the calyces through the renal pelvis to the ureter. These form discrete boluses of urine, which are trapped by the contracting ureter above and propel the urine downward. Disturbances in this mechanism result from three sources.

**1. Mechanical obstructive effect such that the rate of urine passage at the pressure generated from above is much lower than the urine output.** While the ureter may still be patent, it is limited in its volume capacity. To some extent, this effect can be overcome by increased pressure, but clearly this can be limited and may have negative hydrostatic effects on the kidney. Of course, this is what will ultimately lead to the indication of obstruction, hydronephrosis, as the system attempts to maintain normal function in the face of reduced volume capacity. Above the point of hold-up, several things may happen and these include the second cause of disturbed urine transmission.

**2. With increasing pressures, the system tends to dilate and this reduces wall tension according to Laplace's law.**  This will serve, presumably to protect the tissues from pathologic tension/pressure, particularly the renal parenchyma, but in so doing, it will reduce the ability to transmit the peristaltic wave. This is due to the inability to coapt or come together with the peristaltic wave. This, then, permits regurgitation of urine backward, much the same as in valvular regurgitation of the heart. As the dilation progresses, transport efficiency declines and the system is in a decompensated mode.

**3. The third means by which urine transport is impaired in the ureter is by way of disordered ureteral peristalsis.**  This results in lack of propagation or discoordinated propagation of the peristaltic wave. It is presumed that developmental anomalies of the ureter can lead to segmental maldevelopment, where the contraction wave is not conducted appropriately. Histologic examinations of resected UPJ segments show various patterns of disordered smooth muscle organization, increased connective tissue, and narrowing.[22–26] These areas may not be able to propagate the ureteral contraction appropriately. Similarly, surgical division of the ureter can also be seen to disrupt propagation, but this can heal.[27–29] Persistent apparent obstruction following surgery may be explained by failure to re-establish appropriate cell-to-cell interactions that seem to be the basis for peristaltic propagation.

Disordered urine transport has been used as the basis for several diagnostic studies of ureteral pathology, including the pressure perfusion test (Whitaker test) and the MAG3 diuretic renogram. Interpretation of the results of these tests remains controversial. Clearly, a better understanding of how the ureter fails to transmit urine in pathologic states, as well as the effect of that failure on renal function, are the keys to diagnosing significant obstruction and may yield insights into more specific therapies.

## Ureteral healing

Ureteral healing is an important aspect to be considered in treatment modalities, and our understanding is approaching the point where we may be able to enhance healing and identify patients at risk for complications of healing. Early studies of the ureter have indicated that smooth muscle regrowth is rapid and occurs from the outside inward.[28,29] This allows circumferential reconstitution of the ureter within days and subsequent muscularization shortly thereafter. This experimental observation supports the empiric observation that was the basis for the Davis intubated ureterotomy, in which a narrow ureter could be longitudinally incised, stented, and would regenerate the ureteral wall and demonstrate appropriate peristalsis with healing. This is the basis for modern endopyelotomy. Dismembering the ureter was initially considered to be doomed to failure, due to interruption of peristaltic transmission. Experimental studies in the 1950s showed that peristalsis would regenerate within 4 weeks, indicating reconstitution of the cell–cell junctions transmitting the peristaltic wave.[30] These processes do not always succeed and there is still more to be learned about ureteral healing. Several model systems have been developed and may provide insight into the healing of the ureter and ways in which it may be enhanced.[31,32]

# Clinical presentation and evaluation of ureteral anomalies

## Ureteropelvic junction obstruction

The classic presentation of UPJO is episodic flank pain with nausea and vomiting, often triggered by a fluid load. This pattern may be readily mistaken for gastrointestinal conditions and many patients have undergone unrevealing gastrointestinal investigations until a dilated kidney is noted by chance. The pattern of intermittent severe pain that totally resolves and often occurs at night should at least initiate a cursory consideration for renal pathology using ultrasound. Occasionally, this will be normal when no symptoms are present, and if the pattern is suggestive, those patients are best approached by obtaining an emergency ultrasound during an attack of colic. While this may be cumbersome, it may be the only way to confirm the diagnosis. In some of these cases, stimulating a high urine output with diuretic will trigger an attack. This can be done with furosemide and ultrasound or with a diuretic renogram. Occasionally, a crossing lower pole vessel may be identified sonographically, but this is difficult and not a universal ultrasonic finding.

Currently, the most common pediatric presentation of UPJO is through prenatal detection of hydronephrosis. This group of patients poses the greatest challenge, as they are generally asymptomatic and present with a wide spectrum of severity. Significant controversy has evolved in the last 15 years as to which patients need to undergo any corrective intervention, and the concern for selecting patients in whom the apparent obstruction is severe enough to risk affecting renal function and who will not resolve spontaneously has become a major challenge.[33,34] This chapter cannot hope to cover or resolve this controversy, but the basic approach to these patients can be presented in the context of choosing therapy using minimally invasive techniques. Of course, as those minimally invasive techniques evolve, the therapeutic balance between the risk and impact of intervention and observation will also change, and may facilitate decision making.

In children with prenatally detected hydronephrosis, the initial level of decision-making is to decide who should have testing. This remains to be definitively defined, as it depends largely upon the level of certainty that one desires and the level of risk reduction sought: it is difficult, if not impossible, to quantitate and generalize. For practical purposes, functional testing beyond ultrasonography is recommended for those with some likelihood of requiring surgical intervention. These are the patients with generalized caliectasis of the affected kidney. A diuretic renogram is then recommended to assess both relative function by uptake and drainage of the affected kidney. The interpretation of these data remain controversial, but in the setting of a kidney with normal uptake and drainage that is not markedly abnormal, observational management is reasonable.[35] The thresholds for intervention are fluid, and largely dependent upon the individual's as well as the parents' level of comfort. Intravenous pyelography (IVP) is an option if there is question about the anatomic basis for obstruction or if there is discordance between the ultrasound and radionuclide images. Many of these patients may be followed expectantly, although the burden of follow-up must be communicated to the parents. The decision as to how long to monitor these patients when the hydronephrosis does not resolve is difficult.

## Ureteral polyps

A rare etiology of apparent UPJO is a ureteral polyp(s) at the UPJ.[36,37] These are considered to be both congenital and acquired, and their pathogenesis is poorly defined. They may be intermittent in their obstruction, or produce a constant degree of obstruction, leading to hydronephrosis. They are not usually visualized on ultrasound but may be seen on retrograde pyelography or IVP. Surgical management is not different from conventional UPJO and the affected segment, which should contain the pedicle of the polyp, is resected and a spatulated anastomosis performed. Endoscopic resection is a reported option, limited only by ureteral size.[38] Histologically, these polyps show a transitional cell surface and an edematous

core with a vascular stalk. They may be multilobulated. No difference in postoperative follow-up is needed.

## Megaureter (obstructive)

Recognition of the obstructed megaureter is the essential part of therapy. The dilated ureter may be missed on ultrasound imaging. The best image to exclude a dilated ureter is the bladder view, in which the dilated distal ureter is usually noted. Determining if the ureterovesical junction obstruction (UVJO) is functionally significant is more difficult, as many will resolve spontaneously.[39] Those presenting with symptoms in later life are more likely to benefit from intervention. Prenatally detected UVJO rarely undergoes surgical intervention today, but those with extreme dilation and reduced function are likely to benefit from surgical therapy.

## Goals of therapy and clinical decision making

It should always be kept in mind that the goal of therapy of the dilated renal pelvis is to protect renal function and reduce the risk of complications due to stasis. The judgment as to which patient is at what level of risk for functional loss or complications is fraught with uncertainty, and remains controversial. While it may not be settled in this review, the basic principle to be followed might be that if renal function is already impaired, it is at higher risk to continue to do so, and that if a process has not improved in a reasonable waiting period (e.g. 2 years) it might be unlikely to do so. If the degree of dilation is of a similar nature as those associated with decreased function (severe by whatever scale), even if function is preserved, intervention seems reasonable.

If early surgery is not deemed to be appropriate, a monitoring program needs to be adopted to prevent unrecognized functional decline. The specifics of this are also poorly defined. Annual or every 2-year functional studies would seem a minimum of security. All of this is predicated on the notion that if functional decline is noted, intervention at the time of detection will permit return to prior function. This is not the universal experience in observational studies and some recognition of this risk is essential.[34,40]

In those patients in whom surgical repair is deemed appropriate, the options available should be discussed with the family in a realistic context. In part, this is age-dependent in that some of the minimally invasive procedures have little track record in infants. None have the degree of certainty of open surgical repair, which remains the gold standard of therapy, but there is ongoing development of less-invasive modalities.

# Ureteropelvic junction obstruction

## Endopyelotomy

### Antegrade direct vision

Endopyelotomy in children may be performed using an antegrade or retrograde approach, and in smaller children the antegrade technique is the most reasonable. There are several reports of this method in primary UPJO,[41–43] and the original reports were related to secondary obstructions.[44] In the dilated pelvis, access is not difficult, although it is important to access from the mid pole of the kidney rather than the lower pole to facilitate direct access to the UPJ. A guide wire is passed down the ureter, which may be difficult, but this is essential, as stenting after the incision is necessary. Incision may be performed using either a hot or cold knife. With small numbers in each category the potential success rate is about 82% ($n = 11$) for retrograde, 69% ($n = 48$) for antegrade, and 84% ($n = 32$) for secondary endopyelotomy in pediatric series (Figure 8.1) This compares to a general average of about 80–85% success in adult series. Risk factors identified for failure include the presence of a crossing vessel, as indicated by lower success rates in symptomatic patients.[45]

The basic principle of this approach, of course, is based upon the Davis intubated ureterotomy, in which the incised and stented ureter will tubularize itself, including musculature within several weeks, and regain peristaltic function. Today, this concept is well used in the Snodgrass tubularized incised plate hypospadias repair. The critical

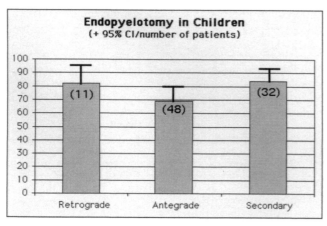

**Figure 8.1**
Endopyelotomy in children.

parameters that mediate ureteral healing in this context remain unknown, although a recent study suggested that the cytokine transforming growth factor $\beta_1$ (TGF-$\beta_1$) may play an important role in healing.[46] The importance of developing this understanding would be in the ability to manipulate these healing programs to increase efficacy. The basic principles tell us that to be successful the incision should be complete, through the entire wall of the ureter, which is usually signaled by visualization of retroperitoneal fat.

Duration of stenting usually generates debate and there are no clear data in children undergoing endopyelotomy. A reasonable compromise would be between 2 and 4 weeks.[47] Leaving a stent for 6 weeks is difficult if it is external.

### Retrograde incision/balloon dilation

Retrograde endopyelotomy in children is largely limited by the size of the patient. Current technology permits ureteral access in almost any child, but the manipulative instruments are limited. There is no Accusize-type system that could be passed into a child younger than 6 or 8 years old without predilation. No custom-built incising instruments are available to date. Direct vision incision requires access to the proximal ureter and this can be performed, and often is facilitated with prestenting. The cold knife instrument is larger than most ureters of children under 6 years old could usually tolerate. Smaller incising systems may be put together, but none of these have any background of use. The Accusize is the most established instrument for this purpose, using complete radiographic control, and yet can realistically be used only in adolescents.[48,49]

## Balloon rupture

A limited series of infants with UPJO were presented in whom balloon rupture of the UPJ was presented, suggesting that this might be a viable option for early obstruction.[50,51] This method has not been reported elsewhere and the follow-up period is short. The concept is probably similar to the intubated ureterotomy in that the rupture produces a single line of rupture in the ureter; however, the uncontrolled and traumatic nature of the procedure seems counterintuitive for pediatric use. At present it remains a procedure that is yet to be proven with long-term outcomes studies.

## Percutaneous pyeloplasty

A recent report in adults has presented a method combining endopyelotomy and laparoscopic pyeloplasty.[52]

This method is based upon percutaneous access and incision of the UPJ. A Heineke–Mikulicz closure of the longitudinal incision is performed to open the narrow UPJ. The closure is performed using a device that permits placement of two or three sutures to allow transverse closure and knot tying that is performed extracorporeally. There are no reports in children as yet, and the bulk of the instruments and lack of precision of suture closure seem at odds with standard pediatric practice, yet the concept is novel and intriguing.

# Laparoscopic pyeloplasty

Laparoscopic pyeloplasty has been performed and reported in several dozen children and has shown itself to be technically feasible and effective. The precise parameters of its utility and generalizability remain to be defined. With new robotic technology, it may become more readily applied by a wider spectrum of urologic surgeons.

## Dismembered pyeloplasty

The standard procedure used in lap pyeloplasty is a dismembered method, based upon the Anderson–Hynes approach that is the standard of open surgery. Lap pyeloplasty was first reported in 1993[53,54] and in young children in 1995,[55] yet there have been a limited number of reports since then, in contrast to large numbers in the adult literature.[56–59] Success rates seem to be acceptable and close to or equal to open surgical outcomes, yet the procedure has clearly not taken hold. The success depends upon delicate suturing and this seems to be the limiting feature. Unless one has the chance to perform numerous laparoscopic procedures and to develop the skills of intracorporeal suturing, embarking on a lap pyeloplasty in a child is a challenging undertaking. The reported series that include both transperitoneal and extraperitoneal approaches indicate that the procedure can be effective with steadily improving surgical times and excellent outcomes.[56–59] Hospital stay seems shorter, but this is difficult to ascertain as many of the series are from countries where surgical stay is distinctly different than in the United States. It may be very difficult to prove that this approach is 'better' than open surgery. The impact of the postoperative recovery and the scar is difficult to assess in children. These are difficult parameters to assess in an adult, and even more so in a child. It is also a challenge to know how a family will interpret the impact of a permanent large scar in contrast to small laparoscopic incisions.

In a comparison of open and laparoscopic pyeloplasty,[13] school age and adolescent patients underwent laparoscopic pyeloplasty (mean age 15 years old) and 11 open pyeloplasty (mean age 9 years old). All patients had successful repair of UPJO at greater than 12 months follow-up. Mean perioperative narcotic use was similar between the groups. However, both hospital stay (2.6 days vs. 5.6 days) and operating room time (3.68 hours vs. 4.19 hours) were shorter for laparoscopic vs open pyeloplasty.[59] Although open pyeloplasty times in this range are unlikely to be the norm, the study demonstrates the potential for equivalent outcomes without a burden of increased operative times.

Both transperitoneal and retroperitoneal approaches have been used for lap pyeloplasty in children. The relative merits and challenges of each are shown in Table 8.1. It is intuitively more appealing to approach the kidney from the retroperitoneum, but it is difficult to demonstrate that this is 'better'.[58,62]

Transperitoneal lap pyeloplasty is performed with the patient on the operative table, having a wedge support under the affected side of the patient. The table is tilted to lower this side and allow transperitoneal access of the camera and working instruments. Once these instruments are in place, the table is turned to raise the affected kidney. The pelvis may be readily visible through the peritoneum, in which case a transmesenteric approach may be used. Alternatively, the colon is reflected medially to expose the kidney and pelvis. The ureter is dissected free of attachments. This is done carefully to avoid devascularizing the ureter. Once the renal pelvis is defined, the UPJ can be identified and a traction suture placed at the most dependent portion of the pelvis. A hitch stitch is often helpful in lifting the renal pelvis, after being passed through the anterior abdominal wall. After ureteral spatulation, the anastomosis is begun at the vertex of the spatulation to the most dependent portion of the renal pelvis. A running monofilament suture is used for the closure, usually 5–0 or 6–0, with the back side being closed first followed by the anterior. Placement of a stent is optional, but for conventional laparoscopic pyeloplasty, it has been our preference. In that case, no drain is used.

**Table 8.1** *Comparison of Transperitoneal and Retroperitoneal Laparoscopic Pyeloplasty*

| Transperitoneal | Retroperitoneal |
|---|---|
| Greater working area | Direct access to UPJ |
| Transmesenteric direct access to UPJ possible | Avoid direct contact with intraperitoneal contents |
| Port placement and access more rapid | More readily drained post-op |
| Direct visualization of intraperitoneal contents | Any urine leak contained |
| Best approach for initial learning | |

Retroperitoneal pyeloplasty is usually performed in the lateral position; however it can be performed in the prone position, providing direct access to the renal pelvis, but offering a more limited working space. The procedure is otherwise identical to transperitoneal repair.

With the emergence of clinically useful robotic devices to assist in laparoscopic surgery, laparoscopic pyeloplasty in children can become more widely performed. By providing enhanced vision, including magnified three-dimensional images, full range of motion manipulating devices at the ends of laparoscopic instrument arms and a very natural feel for the operator, pyeloplasty even in the small child can be readily accomplished. This has largely been performed transperitoneally due to the larger size of the instruments, but as these are being scaled down, retroperitoneal access in small children will be feasible. The exposure and operative steps are essentially identical to conventional laparoscopic pyeloplasty (Figures 8.2 and 8.3) Early experience has shown excellent results with improving efficiency.[62]

## Fenger-plasty

An alternative, nondismembered, method of correcting UPJ obstruction has been described based upon the Heineke-Mikulicz principle,[63] which involves a longitudinal incision through the stenotic segment of the ureter that is closed simply in a transverse direction. This is obviously well suited to laparoscopic methods as it has a limited amount of suturing. The clinical data on its efficacy are limited, however. A few reports of its use in laparoscopic applications have been presented.[56,64,65] To date, the data are not very convincing that this is a broadly

useful method of correcting pediatric UPJO. One concern is the means by which the complex anatomy often seen in children is handled. Many children, as noted above, have a tortuous UPJ that is not readily amenable to a simple longitudinal incision. If the operator is not comfortable with alternative means of pyeloplasty, how would such a case be handled intraoperatively as the anatomy is unknown until the UPJ is exposed? Similarly, with a crossing vessel that necessitates transposition of the ureter, this approach is of no value. Since the identification of a crossing vessel preoperatively is imperfect, the utility of this method is limited.

## Ureteral polyps

Endourologic management of ureteral polyps has been described in one child.[38] At the time of a laparoscopic pyeloplasty, the polyps could be readily removed and would not pose any problem with repair, just as with open pyeloplasty. In the less complex techniques, it would be important to recognize the possibility of polyps and be able to recognize them if present. In general, simple resection is adequate and no formal change in the reconstruction is needed. It would seem reasonable to proceed with a formal repair of the UPJ in any event, as there is some suggestion that the polyp is a secondary process to obstruction in a peristalsing lumen. Whether that is a universal observation is uncertain, but it would seem the safest approach to assume an obstruction complicated by polyp, and thereby to repair both, than assume the polyp as the only factor in the obstruction and risk the need for reoperation.

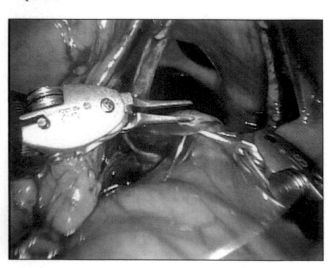

**Figure 8.3**
Robotic pyeloplasty using the daVinci surgical robot. A 5-0 absorbable suture is being passed through the posterior aspect of the renal pelvis for the beginning of the anastomosis. The exposure is transperitoneal.

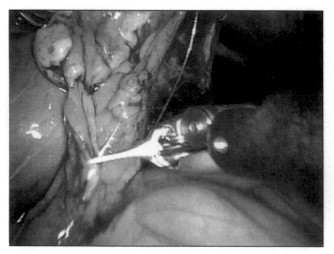

**Figure 8.2**
Robotic pyeloplasty using the daVinci surgical robot. The ureter has been spatulated and the vertex suture is being placed.

# Secondary ureteropelvic junction obstruction

## Strategies

While identification of the patient with a failed pyeloplasty may be very obvious, at times this may be as challenging as with the initial diagnosis in the asymptomatic patient. If pain, persistent leakage or marked increase in hydronephrosis occurs, some early intervention is needed. More often, there is very slow improvement in the degree of dilation, or lack of improvement in the washout parameters on diuretic renography. In the asymptomatic patient one must factor in the degree of initial dilation, the age of the patient, and the nature of the obstruction. The most rapid improvement in dilation is seen in the young patient with moderately severe dilation, especially associated with a crossing vessel, while the most delay is seen in the older child with massive dilation and an intrinsic narrowing. We usually perform a postoperative ultrasound at 1 month and, as long as the degree of dilation is no more than preoperative, that is considered a satisfactory result. If there is more dilation or symptoms develop, a functional study such as an IVP or diuretic renogram is performed to make sure there is not a high-grade obstruction.

In the setting of a symptomatic patient or in whom there is clearly severe ongoing obstruction; an early intervention as described below is performed. If the results are ambiguous, a further period of observation is appropriate, as it is well known from the days of routine nephrostomy use in pyeloplasty that delayed opening of the UPJ after successful repair is frequent, and not of great risk. This might be a follow-up ultrasound or repeat functional study. Invasive evaluation such as retrograde pyelography or percutaneous antegrade studies are reserved for patients warranting intervention.

## Therapeutic options and decision making

If it is determined that the result of the pyeloplasty is inadequate, intervention is appropriate and can be either retrograde stenting or antegrade drainage and possible stenting. Very early stenting is difficult and risks disruption of a repair that is only transiently obstructed. Therefore, an antegrade approach is preferred, usually with a temporary nephrostomy for drainage. Passage of contrast by the repair is assessed after the period of drainage, as the repair may open spontaneously after taking the pressure off. If still closed, an antegrade stent may be placed for passive dilation.

For persistent UPJO more than 3 months postoperative, retrograde assessment, dilation, and stenting are reasonable options. There are no good data in children regarding optimal timing or duration of such stenting maneuvers. Dilation is best achieved using a small, 8F, dilating balloon (Microvasive, Watertown, Massachusetts), followed by stenting with a 5–6F double-J stent, or a nephroureteral stent if approached antegrade. The limitation of the double-J stenting approach is that access to the ureter is lost with testing patency, unless an antegrade nephrostomy is left in place. Parallel nephrostomy and ureteral stenting can be used, but this is cumbersome. A nephroureteral stent (e.g. Salle stent; Cook, Spencer, Indiana), replaced by a simple nephrostomy, may also be used. With this arrangement, the patency of the anastomosis may be tested and assured prior to removing a drainage tube. It is best to clamp the nephrostomy temporarily to ensure asymptomatic adequate drainage.

Endopyelotomy for persistent UPJO has been described and has its proponents. The usual approach is through retrograde incising balloon (Accusize, Applied Medical), although the large size (10F deflated, 24F inflated) of the instrument limits its utility to teens. Stenting for 2–4 weeks after is recommended. There are limited follow-up data and our institutional experience is less than enthusiastic. Open repair after endopyelotomy is often challenging, due to the inflammatory effects of the obligate extravasation induced.

Direct vision endopyelotomy is also an option from an antegrade approach, but again there are few data and limited experience. These approaches are generally worth an attempt after careful discussion with parents who are already frustrated. In many cases a more definitive approach of reoperative open or laparoscopic pyeloplasty is most advisable. The anticipated success rate is probably in the 85% range for open reoperative pyeloplasty, but there are very few reports, and none for pediatric redo laparoscopic pyeloplasty.

# References

1. Kume T, Deng K, Hogan BL. Murine forkhead/winged helix genes Foxc1 (Mf1) and Foxc2 (Mfh1) are required for the early organogenesis of the kidney and urinary tract. Development 2000; 127(7):1387–95.

2. Brophy PD, Ostrom L, Lang KM, Dressler GR. Regulation of ureteric bud outgrowth by Pax2-dependent activation of the glial derived neurotrophic factor gene. Development 2001; 128(23):4747–56.

3. Itaranta P, Lin Y, Perasaari J, et al. Wnt-6 is expressed in the ureter bud and induces kidney tubule development in vitro. Genesis 2002; 32(4):259–68.

4. Baker LA, Gomez RA. Tmp21-I, a vesicular trafficking protein, is differentially expressed during induction of the ureter and metanephros. J Urol 2000; 164(2):562–6.

5. Batourina E, Choi C, Paragas N, et al. Distal ureter morphogenesis depends on epithelial cell remodeling mediated by vitamin A and Ret. Nat Genet 2002; 32(1):109–15.

6. Karihaloo A, Karumanchi SA, Barasch J, et al. Endostatin regulates branching morphogenesis of renal epithelial cells and ureteric bud. Proc Natl Acad Sci USA 2001; 98(22):12509–14.

7. Pohl M, Sakurai H, Bush KT, Nigam SK. Matrix metalloproteinases and their inhibitors regulate in vitro ureteric bud branching morphogenesis. Am J Physiol Renal Physiol 2000; 279(5):F891–900.

8. Oshima K, Miyazaki Y, Brock JW 3rd, et al. Angiotensin type II receptor expression and ureteral budding. J Urol 2001; 166(5):1848–52.

9. Zent R, Bush KT, Pohl ML, et al. Involvement of laminin binding integrins and laminin-5 in branching morphogenesis of the ureteric bud during kidney development. Dev Biol 2001;238(2):289–302.

10. Sakurai H, Bush KT, Nigam SK. Identification of pleiotrophin as a mesenchymal factor involved in ureteric bud branching morphogenesis. Development 2001; 128(17):3283–93.

11. Pohl M, Bhatnagar V, Mendoza SA, Nigam SK. Toward an etiological classification of developmental disorders of the kidney and upper urinary tract. Kidney Int 2002; 61(1):10–19.

12. Baker LA, Gomez RA. Embryonic development of the ureter. Semin Nephrol 1998; 18(6):569–84.

13. Ichikawa I, Kuwayama F, Pope JC, et al. Paradigm shift from classic anatomic theories to contemporary cell biological views of CAKUT. Kidney Int 2002; 61(3):889–98.

14. Alcaraz A, Vinaixa F, Tejedo-Mateu A, et al. Obstruction and recanalization of the ureter during embryonic development. J Urol 1991; 145(2):410–16.

15. Baker LA, Gomez RA. Embryonic development of the ureter and bladder: acquisition of smooth muscle. J Urol 1998; 160(2):545–50.

16. Santis WF, Sullivan MP, Gobet R, et al. Characterization of ureteral dysfunction in an experimental model of congenital bladder outlet obstruction. J Urol 2000; 163(3):980–4.

17. Stehr M, Adam RM, Khoury J, et al. Platelet derived growth factor-BB is a potent mitogen for rat ureteral and human bladder smooth muscle cells: dependence in lipid rafts for cell signaling. J Urol 2003; 169(3):1165–70.

18. Peters CA, Freeman MR, Fernandez CA, et al. Dysregulated proteolytic balance as the basis of excess extracellular matrix in fibrotic disease. Am J Physiol 1997; 272(6 Pt 2):R1960–5.

19. Thomas DF. Fetal uropathy. Br J Urol 1990; 66(3):225–31.

20. Dietl. J, Wandernde nieren and deren einklemmung. Wien Med Wochenschr 1864; 14:153–66.

21. Peters CA. Urinary tract obstruction in children. J Urol 1995; 154:1874–84.

22. Hanna MK, Jeffs RD, Sturgess JM, Baskin M. Ureteral structure and ultrastructure. Part II: Congenital ureteropelvic junction obstruction and primary obstructive megaureter. J Urol 1976; 116:725–30.

23. Hanna MK, Jeffs RD, Sturgess JM, Barkin M. Ureteral structure and ultrastructure. Part I. The normal human ureter. J Urol 1976; 116(6):718–24.

24. Hanna MK, Jeffs RD, Sturgess JM, Barkin M. Ureteral structure and ultrastructure. Part IV. The dilated ureter, clinicopathological correlation. J Urol 1977; 117(1):28–32.

25. Hanna MK, Jeffs RD, Sturgess JM, Barkin M. Ureteral structure and ultrastructure. Part III. The congenitally dilated ureter (megaureter). J Urol 1977; 117(1):24–7.

26. Zhang PL, Peters CA, Rosen S. Ureteropelvic junction obstruction: morphological and clinical studies. Pediatr Nephrol 2000; 14(8–9):820–6.

27. Oppenheimer R, Hinman F. Ureteral regeneration: contracture vs. hyperplasia of smooth muscle. J Urol 1955; 74:476.

28. Weaver R. Ureteral regeneration: experimental and clinical II. J Urol 1957; 77:164–72.

29. Weaver R, Henderson J. Ureteral regeneration: experimental and clinical. J Urol 1954; 71:274–86.

30. Butcher H, Sleator W. The effect of ureteral anastomosis upon conduction of peristaltic waves: an electro-urographic study. J Urol 1956; 75:650–8.

31. Wolf JS Jr, Soble JJ, Ratliff TL, Clayman RV. Ureteral cell cultures II: collagen production and response to pharmacologic agents. J Urol 1996; 156(6):2067–72.

32. Wolf JS Jr, Soble JJ, Ratliff TL, Clayman RV. Ureteral cell cultures. I. Characterization and cellular interactions. J Urol 1996; 156(3):1198–203.

33. Hanna MK. Antenatal hydronephrosis and ureteropelvic junction obstruction: the case for early intervention [editorial]. Urology 2000; 55(5):612–5.

34. Koff SA. Postnatal management of antenatal hydronephrosis using an observational approach. Urology 2000; 55(5):609–11.

35. Ulman I, Jayanthi VR, Koff SA. The long-term followup of newborns with severe unilateral hydronephrosis initially treated nonoperatively. J Urol 2000; 164(3 Pt 2):1101–5.

36. Cooper CS, Hawtrey CE. Fibroepithelial polyp of the ureter. Urology 1997; 50(2):280–1.

37. Karaca I, Sencan A, Mir E, et al. Ureteral fibroepithelial polyps in children. Pediatr Surg Int 1997; 12(8):603–4.

38. Faerber GJ, Ahmed MM, Marcovich R, et al. Contemporary diagnosis and treatment of fibroepithelial ureteral polyp. J Endourol 1997; 11(5):349–51.

39. McLellan DL, Retik AB, Bauer SB, et al. Rate and predictors of spontaneous resolution of prenatally diagnosed primary nonrefluxing megaureter. J Urol 2002; 168(5):2177–80; discussion 2180.

40. Ransley PG, Dhillon HK, Gordon I, et al. The postnatal management of hydronephrosis diagnosed by prenatal ultrasound. J Urol 1990; 144:584–7; discussion 593–4.

41. Tan HL, Najmaldin A, Webb DR. Endopyelotomy for pelviureteric junction obstruction in children. Eur Urol 1993; 24(1):84–8.

42. Schenkman EM, Tarry WF. Comparison of percutaneous endopyelotomy with open pyeloplasty for pediatric ureteropelvic junction obstruction. J Urol 1998; 159(3):1013–15.

43. Rodrigues Netto N Jr, Ikari O, Esteves SC, D'Ancona CA. Antegrade endopyelotomy for pelvi-ureteric junction obstruction in children. Br J Urol 1996; 78(4):607–12.

44. Kavoussi LR, Meretyk S, Dierks SM, et al. Endopyelotomy for secondary ureteropelvic junction obstruction in children. J Urol 1991; 145(2):345–9.

45. Nicholls G, Hrouda D, Kellett MJ, Duffy PG. Endopyelotomy in the symptomatic older child. BJU Int 2001; 87(6):525–7.

46. Jabbour ME, Goldfischer ER, Anderson AE, et al. Failed endopyelotomy: low expression of TGF beta regardless of the presence or absence of crossing vessels. J Endourol 1999; 13(4):295–8.

47. Kumar R, Kapoor R, Mandhani A, et al. Optimum duration of splinting after endopyelotomy. J Endourol 1999; 13(2):89–92.

48. Bolton DM, Bogaert GA, Mevorach RA, et al. Pediatric ureteropelvic junction obstruction treated with retrograde endopyelotomy. Urology 1994; 44(4):609–13.

49. Gerber GS, Kim J, Nold S, Cromie WJ. Retrograde ureteroscopic endopyelotomy for the treatment of primary and secondary ureteropelvic junction obstruction in children. Tech Urol 2000; 6(1):46–9.

50. Tan HL, Roberts JP, Grattan-Smith D. Retrograde balloon dilation of ureteropelvic obstructions in infants and children: early results. Urology 1995; 46(1):89–91.

51. Wilkinson AG, Azmy A. Balloon dilatation of the pelvi-ureteric junction in children: early experience and pitfalls. Pediatr Radiol 1996; 26(12):882–6.

52. Desai MM, Gill IS, Carvalhal EF, et al. Percutaneous endopyeloplasty: a novel technique. J Endourol 2002; 16(7):431–43.

53. Kavoussi LR, Peters CA. Laparoscopic pyeloplasty. J Urol 1993; 150(6):1891–4.

54. Schuessler WW, Grune MT, Tecuanhuey LV, Preminger GM. Laparoscopic dismembered pyeloplasty. J Urol 1993; 150:1795–9.

55. Peters CA, Schlussel RN, Retik AB. Pediatric laparoscopic dismembered pyeloplasty. J Urol 1995; 153(6):1962–5.

56. Janetschek G, Peschel R, Altarac S, Bartsch G. Laparoscopic and retroperitoneoscopic repair of ureteropelvic junction obstruction. Urology 1996; 47(3):311–16.

57. Tan HL, Roberts JP. Laparoscopic dismembered pyeloplasty in children: preliminary results. Br J Urol 1996; 77(6):909–13.

58. Yeung CK, Tam YH, Sihoe JD, et al. Retroperitoneoscopic dismembered pyeloplasty for pelvi-ureteric junction obstruction in infants and children. BJU Int 2001; 87(6):509–13.

59. Schier F. Laparoscopic Anderson–Hynes pyeloplasty in children [see comments]. Pediatr Surg Int 1998; 13(7):497–500.

60. Pulagiri AV, Moore RG, Steinhardt G, Pugach J. Pediatric/adolescent laparoscopic vs open dismembered pyeloplasty: preliminary results on postoperative morbidity. J Endourol 1999; 13(1):24.

61. Pulagiri AV, Pattaras JG, Pugach JL, et al. Pediatric/adolescent laparoscopic vs open dismembered pyeloplasty: results on postoperative morbidity. J Urol 2000; 163(4):81.

62. El-Ghoneimi A, Valla JS, Steyaert H, Aigrain Y. Laparoscopic renal surgery via a retroperitoneal approach in children. J Urol 1998; 160(3 Pt 2):1138–41.

63. Fenger C. Konservative operation für renale retention infolge von strikturen oder klappenbildung am ureter. Langenbecks Arch Chir 1900; 52:528.

64. Soulie M, Salomon L, Patard JJ, et al. Extraperitoneal laparoscopic pyeloplasty: a multicenter study of 55 procedures. J Urol 2001; 166(1):48–50.

65. Ben Slama MR, Salomon L, Hoznek A, et al. Extraperitoneal laparoscopic repair of ureteropelvic junction obstruction: initial experience in 15 cases. Urology 2000; 56(1):45–8.

# 9

# Anomalies of the lower ureter: minimally invasive treatment options

Lars Cisek

The ureter is the conduit for urine in its path to the bladder. Consequently, ureteral anomalies are poised to disrupt this transit and therefore compromise renal function. This chapter will focus on problems of the ureter itself leaving abnormalities of the proximal junction (UPJ) and distal anomalies such as reflux to other chapters of the book.

## Ureteral stricture, valves, and folds

This category represents a rare cause of functionally significant ureteral obstruction in children. Congenital ureteral strictures represent a fixed anatomic narrowing of the ureter;[1,2] this may occasionally present with multiple lesions in the same ureter. Further, dilation of the segment between narrowed regions may occur. Ureteral valves represent a transverse fold of mucosa containing muscle,[3,4] and are obstructive entities. More common are mucosal folds, although these are seldom the source of true obstruction.[4,5] These lesions represent redundancy of the mucosa, which most often resolves spontaneously over time. This later lesion can be seen in IVPs distorting the ureteral contrast column; the critical feature is the absence of obstruction. It is important to note that folds and valves may be the result of tortuosity of the ureter proximal to an obstruction, and may themselves not be obstructive.[6]

In cases with functionally significant obstructions, presentation may be through incidental finding, infection, flank pain, hypertension, or the finding of (prenatal) hydronephrosis and associated proximal ureterectasis. Ultrasonography will demonstrate proximal dilation (of both the ureter and kidney) without distal ureteral dilation. Evaluation of the function of the affected renal unit may show reduced functional contribution. In flow-dependent nuclear imaging, the dilated proximal ureter may be seen, and the clearance ($T_{1/2}$) will be prolonged. Similarly, an anatomic study such as an IVP will demonstrate proximal dilation, define the location of the narrowing, and facilitate operative planning. The need for intervention is based on findings of obstruction coupled with symptoms – e.g. urinary tract infection (UTI), pain – or evidence of functional impairment of the kidney in obstructed but otherwise asymptomatic cases.

Therapeutic options are analogous to the treatment of acquired strictures. Options include balloon dilation, 'endopyelotomy' methods, laparoscopic or open uretero-ureterostomy, transuretero-ureterostomy, psoas hitch with reimplant, or nephrectomy. Nephrectomy is appropriate in cases of minimal renal function in the affected side. In patients with short lesions (< 2 cm) or greater than 25% renal function, endoscopic means may be considered[7] if appropriately sized instruments are available. One caution in considering these techniques in children is that the often generous 'cushion' of retroperitoneal fat that isolates the ureter from adjacent structures (bowel, vessels) in adults provides a far smaller margin of safety for most children. The size of instrumentation is the other significant limiting factor; at present, common commercial ureteroscopes are in the 7F range and the smallest currently available cutting balloon is 10F (Applied Medical – Acusize). Biliary sphincterotomes without balloons could be considered and are available to 3.5F. Of note, a ureteral valve is a pathology conceptually best addressed by incision. In this entity, the mucosal flap/fold is the issue and intraureteric mucosal and muscle incision alone should repair this. At present, there are essentially no available data in children to guide the urologist in the success rate for minimally invasive approaches for these problems. All recommendations are derived by analogy from adults.

'Endopyelotomy' methods demonstrate success rates in the 55–85% range for strictures shorter than 2 cm in adults.[8–10] Laparoscopic series are rare in the literature, although Nezhat et al[11] reported a 77% success rate with ureteroureterostomy in a group of 9 patients with iatrogenic injuries.

## Acusize or balloon dilation ureteral stricture or valve method

- Equipment: fluoroscopy, cystoscope, acucize balloon, guide wires, contrast media, appropriate length double J stent.
- Preoperative: urine culture and treatment of any current UTI. Magnesium citrate or bisacodyl bowel preparation 1 day preoperatively for improved radiologic visualization. Antibiotic prophylaxis.
- Position for fluoroscopy.
- Cystoscopy with retrograde pyelogram, define site(s) of obstruction.
- Place wire past obstruction.
- Place balloon/acusize catheter over the working wire.
- Advance to the position of the ureteral narrowing, following the bracketing markers on the balloon to center on the site of the obstruction.
- Inflate, cutting current with orientation based on location (proximal to iliac vessels – posteriolateral; vessel – anterior; distal to iliac vessels – posterior).
- Contrast injection looking for exstravasation if cutting for stricture. Note: for a ureteral valve, full-thickness incision is not required.
- Place stent for 4 weeks. (If valve may stent for 1 week only.)
- Remove stent and confirm patency with retrograde pyelogram/balloon calibration.
- Follow up with renal ultrasonography (RUS) at 1 month if clinically well. Failure of hydronephrosis to improve should prompt reinvestigation.

## Endoscopic incision method

- Equipment: Fluoroscopy, cystoscope, guide wires, ureteroscope, holmium laser source and fiber, contrast media, double J stent.
- Preoperative: urine culture and treatment of any current UTI. Magnesium citrate or bisacodyl bowel preparation 1 day preoperatively for improved radiologic visualization. Antibiotic prophylaxis.
- Position for fluoroscopy.
- Cystoscopy with retrograde pyelogram to define anatomy.
- Place wire/safety wire.
- Dilate ureteral orifice if needed. Note it may be necessary to 'pre-stent' smaller patients to gain access to the

ureter without unnecessary trauma. This should be short duration only to preserve proximal dilation so as to be able to clearly identify the location of narrowing.
- Advance ureteroscope to region of narrowing.
- Visualize obstructing region.
- Incise with holmium laser to visualize fat in the retroperitoneum. Note: for a ureteral valve, full-thickness incision is not required (proximal to iliac vessels – posteriolateral; vessel – anterior; distal to iliac vessels – posterior).
- Place stent for 4 weeks. (If valve may stent for 1 week only.)
- Remove with retrograde pyelogram/balloon calibration.
- Follow up with RUS at 1 month if clinically well. Failure of hydronephrosis to improve should prompt reinvestigation.

## Laparoscopic ureteroureterotomy method

- Equipment: fluoroscopy, cystoscope, guide wire, contrast media, ureteral occlusion balloon catheter, double J stent, 3 laparoscopy ports (3–5 mm format; typically, short length preferred), 5 mm Babcock, 3 mm needle driver, 3 mm scissor, 3 mm grasper, scissor, and dissector, 6-0 absorbable suture on BV-1 or TF needle, a bipolar cautery or harmonic scalpel will be useful. We prefer the use of Koh (Stortz) instruments for fine suturing tasks as these instruments will handle 6-0 and 7-0 suture and fine needles well.
- Preoperative: magnesium citrate or bisacodyl bowel preparation 1 day preoperatively.
- Position for fluoroscopy.
- Cystoscopy with retrograde pyelogram to define anatomy.
- Place occlusion balloon above stricture and inflate. With balloon inflated, confirm a 'snag' at the region of identified stricture. Fix position thoroughly by securing to Foley catheter at bladder neck.
- Position patient with a 30° roll, contralateral side down. Secure to table to allow full range of motion. Maintain capacity for fluoroscopy and dye injection to confirm location of pathology, if needed. Catheter should be accessible from field to manipulate.
- Access abdomen.
- Port placement based on site of stricture. Port sites can be either 3 – 3 mm, mixed size 3 mm and 5, or 3–5 mm. We prefer one 5 mm (which allows the use of a 5 mm Babcock to handle the ureter) and two 3 mm ports.
- The ureter can usually be easily observed in children directly through the retroperitoneum and mesentery

and the site of the balloon localized visually. Expose the ureter, limiting the mobilization of the ureter to preserve blood supply. Confirm site of stricture via a balloon tug. Repeat retrograde pyelogram via wire port if needed. In some cases it may be necessary to reflect the colon.

- Place marking suture(s) to define position and manipulate the ureter; avoid the balloon.
- Ureterotomy at the site of narrowing. Identify the valve or stricture. If a true stricture, remove involved segment. If a valve is present, opening the ureter through the region of the valve is the critical feature, with incision, although the valve with Heineke–Mikulicz closure is sufficient.
- Reattach or close the ureter using intracorporeal 6-0 Monocryl or PDS (on BV-1 needles) interrupted sutures. Rotation of the ureter by 120° or less is of no apparent consequence.
- A stent is typically used. Place wire from below, following back wall closure. The wire may be introduced via an occlusion balloon wire port.
- A drain may also be placed. At minimum, either a drain or a stent is required. If a drain is chosen, a 3 mm port can be placed posteriorly and advanced to the peritoneum. Once the peritoneum tents, the trocar is removed and the port advanced through the retroperitoneum to the region of the anastomosis. A 7F round JP drain can be introduced via one of the other port sites, grasped and delivered through skin using this port site.
- Close the retroperitoneum if windowed or reaffix colon if reflected.
- Remove ports under direct vision. In children, it is our practice to close all ports where the fascia can be seen regardless of size. We close the fascia of all port sites 5 mm or greater.
- Follow up with RUS at 1 month if clinically well. Failure of hydronephrosis to improve should prompt reinvestigation.

# Ureterocele

A ureterocele is a submucosal cystic dilation of the terminal segment of the ureter. There are several classifications for ureteroceles:[12,13]

- Intravesical or extravesical – located within or distal to the bladder, respectively.
- Solitary system or duplex – associated with a single renal collecting system or the upper pole of a duplex system, respectively.
- Orthotopic or ectopic – insertion of the ureter into the bladder in the normal or distal (i.e. medial and inferior) position. The orthotopic ureterocele is usually found associated with a single renal unit with one collecting system and is more common in adults.
- Cecoureteroceles are elongated beyond the ureterocele orifice by tunneling under the trigone and the urethra.[13] These may commonly be obstructive at the bladder neck.

With the increasing use of prenatal ultrasound, many ureteroceles are now detected as prenatal hydronephrosis.[14] The findings include hydronephrosis and a fluid-filled structure within the bladder. The most common clinical presentation of a ureterocele postnatally is a UTI with sepsis in the first few months of life.[15,16] Patients may also present with hematuria, purulent urine, pyelonephritis, or abdominal pain.[17] Urinary incontinence or retention may also be seen if the ureterocele causes an obstruction at the level of the bladder.

## Evaluation

Ultrasonography noninvasively depicts anatomic changes in the kidney and bladder. Imaging should be performed with the bladder empty and filled to eliminate nonvisualization of ureteroceles due to either compression of the bladder or the ureterocele. Sonography is the most sensitive test and often the only radiologic evaluation required for the diagnosis of ureteroceles. A ureterocele is seen as a fluid-filled cystic intravesical mass. It is also known as a 'cyst within a cyst.' Ureteroceles may be missed if the patient's bladder is empty or fully distended, if the ureteroceles are small, or if the patient's body habitus precludes proper examination. Ultrasonography also defines the degree of hydronephrosis, and it possibly depicts renal dysplasia or cortical thinning. With their distinct split renal pelves, duplex renal systems may also be identified on the initial ultrasonographic examination.[18] The finding of upper pole hydronephrosis and a dilated ureter should prompt careful inspection of the bladder for a ureterocele.[19]

Because of the association with reflux (vesicoureteral reflux is present in about 50% of ipsilateral lower pole moieties in duplex systems and 10–25% of contralateral moieties in single and duplex systems,[14,20] a voiding cystourethrogram (VCUG) is necessary. The presence of reflux will favor bladder level management of the ureterocele. Early imaging prior to complete opacification of the bladder with contrast material may show the ureterocele as a filling defect. VCUG defines the degree of vesicoureteral reflux in both ipsilateral and contralateral systems and also possible inferior displacement of the lower pole to a large obstructed upper pole. The drooping lily sign is a classic description of moderate-to-high-grade reflux into a displaced lower pole.

In addition, VCUG may be performed to evaluate the size, position, tension, degree of detrusor backing, and compressibility of ureteroceles. Eversion of ureteroceles on VCUGs may be seen as protrusions outside the urethral or vesical wall.[21]

A functional study (DMSA or MAG3) is indicated in those cases with significant obstructive components in the upper pole moiety associated with the ureterocele, as minimal function favors excision of the affected kidney and ureter.[22]

Treatment options must be individualized, based on the unique anatomy, pathophysiology, and renal function found in the patient with a ureterocele. Treatment often involves surgical intervention. The anatomy of the urinary tract must be delineated as clearly as possible prior to surgical intervention. Ipsilateral and contralateral renal function must be assessed. The four goals of intervention are:

1. control and elimination of infection
2. minimization of vesicoureteral reflux and bladder outlet obstruction
3. maintenance of urinary continence mechanisms
4. preservation of renal function.

## Medical therapy

Mere observation is rarely a good option in symptomatic ureteroceles. Antibiotics should be instituted during the initial diagnostic evaluation and during surgical intervention for both pediatric and adult ureteroceles. In infants with symptomatic ureteroceles, antibiotics should be used to treat UTIs. Following therapy, antibiotic prophylaxis is instituted, and may be used to delay surgical intervention until the bladder matures. Small asymptomatic ureteroceles may be observed with careful serial physical and ultrasonographic examinations.

## Surgical therapy

Surgical options include endoscopic ureterocele incision, and, depending on renal function, percutaneous diversion, ureteropyelostomy, partial or total nephroureterectomy, or complete reconstruction. At present, minimally invasive approaches that aim to address the problem at the 'lower tract' level are limited. In complete reconstruction, the approach is often a combined approach with minimally invasive upper tract surgery coupled with open bladder level reconstruction.

Indications for surgical treatment for both pediatric and adult ureteroceles depend on the site of the uretero-cele, the clinical situation, associated renal anomalies, and the size of the ureterocele. Common indications are reflux, infection, obstruction (both of the associated renal moiety and potentially bladder outlet), and impairment of continence. The surgical approach is individualized, and is based upon the following: age of the patient, size and location of the ureterocele, renal function, presence and degree of vesicoureteral reflux, and comorbid conditions (risk of anesthesia).[23]

Surgical therapy for both pediatric and adult uretero-celes may include endoscopic incision or transurethral unroofing of the ureterocele in the adult patient, upper pole heminephrectomy and partial ureterectomy with ureterocele decompression, ureteropyelostomy, excision of ureterocele and ureteral reimplantation, and nephro-ureterectomy. There is a significant debate as to whether management should be 'lower tract' or 'upper tract' based. In general, the moiety associated with the ureterocele is not a significant contributor to renal function, and the approach should eliminate problems with obstruction while correcting any concurrent issues (reflux).

A useful guide to therapy proposed by Churchill et al[24] can be used to guide therapeutic considerations in children:

1. *Upper pole nonfunction*
   - One renal unit in jeopardy – only the upper pole drained by the ureterocele is affected (other renal units normal, may have grade I–II vesicoureteral reflux): perform upper pole heminephrectomy.
   - Entire ipsilateral renal unit or all renal units in jeopardy – ipsilateral and/or contralateral renal units affected by hydronephrosis or high-grade vesicoureteral reflux: perform upper pole nephroureterectomy, ureterocele excision with ureteral reimplantation.
2. *Indeterminate function*
   - Perform endoscopic incision and reassessment of function.
3. *Upper pole function present*
   - One renal unit in jeopardy: perform uretero-pyelostomy and ureterocele drainage.
   - Entire ipsilateral renal unit or all renal units in jeopardy: perform ureteropyelostomy, ureterocele excision, and ureteral reimplantation.

*Note:* the endoscopic incision is also considered first in infants who are medically unstable because of sepsis or coexistent medical conditions.

## Endoscopic incision

Endoscopic incision is the least invasive method for decompressing the ureterocele. It is an ideal method for dealing with a neonate with ureterocele-induced obstructive uropathy and sepsis. Other indications are a single-system intravesical ureterocele with obstruction or a duplex-system ureterocele with indeterminate function of the affected renal moiety. In the endoscopic approach, a small endoscopic incision is made inferiorly and medially on the anterior wall of the ureterocele above its base at the bladder neck.[25–27] This minimally invasive method is associated with low morbidity rates and represents an effective method of decompression in infants. The incision is designed to effect drainage without loss of a 'flap valve' function and resultant creation of reflux. The endoscopic approach is highly successful for small, single-system intravesical ureteroceles.[27] With this procedure, the reported incidence of iatrogenic reflux and incontinence ($< 10\%$) is low, and secondary procedures are often not needed (10–15%).[25,26] The endoscopic approach represents a good first-line method for the acute management of symptomatic ureteroceles. In particular, as regards an infected renal unit, it serves as the method of first choice to relieve the obstruction.

In addition to its therapeutic value, this technique may be employed when the contribution of the associated renal moiety to overall renal function is uncertain. Improvement in renal function after an incision indicates that reconstruction is favorable, if necessary, and poor function indicates that excision of the upper pole moiety is preferable. This procedure allows palliative decompression in children at high risk (secondary to concurrent medical illness), so that definitive reconstruction can be delayed until an adequate healing period has occurred. This decompression may allow the ureter to reduce in size, facilitating reconstruction. This approach is seldom definitive in those patients with reflux, who will likely require lower tract reconstruction.[28]

## Transurethral unroofing

Transurethral unroofing of a ureterocele reliably achieves decompression and allows effective treatment of infection in symptomatic ureteroceles, but invariably results in reflux into the affected moiety. The potential for vesicoureteral reflux limits the use of endoscopic unroofing in children to infection control.

## Upper pole heminephrectomy and ureterectomy

Upper pole heminephrectomy and partial ureterectomy with ureterocele decompression involves removal of the upper pole of the kidney, as well as the affected proximal ureter to a position as distal as is reasonable. The remaining distal ureterocele is not excised but rather is decompressed. This is approached as definitive treatment in patients with an obstructed ectopic ureterocele and a dysplastic upper pole, but without associated vesicoureteral reflux. If reflux is present preoperatively, the distal ureter should be ligated rather than allowing it to remain decompressed. Nephroureterectomy is performed in patients with single-system ureterocele and a nonfunctioning kidney.

This operation has been noted to cause spontaneous resolution of ipsilateral vesicoureteral reflux and contralateral reflux and/or obstruction. Upper pole heminephrectomy and partial ureterectomy with ureterocele decompression has been reported to cause spontaneous resolution of grade I and II vesicoureteral reflux in 60% of cases, while higher grades of reflux necessitated bladder reconstruction in 96% of cases. While upper pole heminephrectomy provides effective decompression, the likelihood of subsequent bladder surgery may be significant, especially if reflux is already present.[29–33]

Factors that may predict the likelihood of future surgical intervention include high-grade reflux (grades III, IV, V) and poor detrusor backing behind the remaining ureterocele.[32,33] Therefore, upper pole heminephrectomy is an excellent first-line procedure for the child with a ureterocele that affects only the ipsilateral upper pole. It is a good choice in the child with a ureterocele with only ipsilateral renal involvement (which may include upper pole obstruction and lower pole reflux, for example). In any case, the patient and family should be counseled about the potential need for further surgical procedures.

This upper tract approach is ideally suited to a laparoscopic approach, as access to the kidney and ease of defining the associated vascular anatomy is excellent. It also allows access to the entire upper pole ureter, facilitating removal.[34–37]

## Ureteropyelostomy

Ureteropyelostomy joins the upper pole ureter to the lower pole renal pelvis. This is preferred if the affected renal unit demonstrates significant function and no reflux or obstruction is present. Alternatively, a high ureteroureterostomy will achieve similar ends. This bypasses the obstructing distal problem, and is an option if upper pole function is significant. This upper tract solution can also be effected efficiently through a laparoscopic approach, although no reports of ureteropyelostomy or ureteroureterostomy have yet been made for this indication.

## Excision of the ureterocele and ureteral reimplantation

Excision and ureteral reimplantation is the primary procedure of choice if the patient has significant vesicoureteral reflux in the lower pole moiety and a well-functioning upper pole moiety and/or significant contralateral vesicoureteral reflux. Both ipsilateral ureters may be reimplanted within a common sheath or via uretero-ureterostomy. Note the common sheath reimplantation has a distinct disadvantage of reimplanting a very dilated distal upper pole ureter into the small bladder. The decision whether to taper the ureters must be made on an individual basis. This operation is commonly delayed until the child is older (approximately 2 years old); however, the operation should be performed before the child is toilet trained, since it has a significant potential to be disruptive to or alter urinary continence.

In the pediatric population, the excision and reimplantation procedure is commonly employed as a secondary procedure (after previous heminephrectomy or endoscopic incision of a ureterocele) because of UTI, voiding disturbance, persistent vesicoureteral reflux, or obstruction. Significant vesicoureteral reflux on initial VCUG usually indicates that lower tract reconstruction will be necessary. Of note, if this procedure is selected as the first-line treatment in the appropriate patient, the rate of secondary surgery is low.

A lower tract reconstruction approach has not yet been reported using laparoscopic techniques.

## Total reconstruction

The traditional method of correcting an ectopic ureterocele in a duplex system has been to perform a total reconstruction. This involved surgery at both the bladder and renal level. The bladder surgery required excision of a ureterocele, reconstruction of the detrusor, and reimplantation of the ipsilateral ureter. This was followed by a flank incision and upper pole heminephrectomy.[38] Since most ureteroceles typically present in young children (often < 1 year old), total reconstruction is technically challenging, and complications were common. This lends itself well to a combined approach where the upper tract surgery is done laparoscopically and the ureter and upper pole moiety are placed in the pelvis for removal through a conventional Pfannenstiel incision used to effect the lower tract reconstruction.

**Preoperative details.** The goals of the preoperative evaluation of the ureterocele are as follows:

- detailed delineation of upper and lower urinary tract anatomy
- estimation of differential function of all renal moieties
- determination of the presence of obstruction (anatomic or functional) or vesicoureteral reflux.

## Endoscopic incision of the ureterocele

This is the least invasive technique. The patient is placed in the lithotomy position. Cystoscopy is performed, and any issues related to the location of the ureteral orifice or anatomy can be resolved concurrently. Incision of the ureterocele is performed via the pediatric resectoscope or a cystoscope using a small Bugbee electrode (3F) and a cutting current. Create a small puncture at the lowest point (most distal edge) just above the base of the ureterocele. The endpoint of the incision is observation of a clear jet of urine from the ureterocele or ability to visualize the urothelium on the inside of the ureterocele. A retrograde can be performed if any question remains.

Note the ability to visualize the ureterocele is dependent on the degree of bladder filling as the ureterocele will efface as the bladder fills. The procedure is best done at minimum bladder filling to allow visualization of the bladder and ureterocele.

**Postoperative details.**   A dose of intravenous antibiotics is given perioperatively unless concurrent infection is present, in which case ongoing therapy is employed. Prophylaxis is used following discharge until reflux status is confirmed.

**Follow-up care.**   Follow-up care consists of serial monitoring of renal function, periodic evaluation of voiding symptoms and bladder function, and interval radiologic studies to assess renal growth, hydroureteronephrosis, and vesicoureteral reflux. A typical schedule in the absence of infection or other problems is an ultrasound at 2–4 weeks and VCUG and ultrasound at 3–6 months postoperatively. If reflux is absent, prophylaxis can be discontinued.

## Laparoscopic nephroureterectomy

This procedure is employed for a single-system ureterocele associated with nonfunction of the renal unit.

**Equipment.**   Laparoscopic 'cart', Visiport (USSC, Norway, Connecticut), harmonic scalpel, 5 mm clip applier, 10 mm entrapment sac (often not required), grasper, dissector, scissors.

**Operative steps.**   For prone retroperitoneoscopic nephrectomy:

1. Patient positioned prone and secured, with support at iliac crests and axilla.
2. Confirm lack of pressure or limitation of forward fall of abdomen.
3. Visiport access, costovertebral angle inferior to 12th rib and lateral to sacrospinalis.

4. Gentle pressure on Visiport to keep against sacrospinalis, orientation of blade in sagittal plane.
5. No muscles traversed, incise fascia of erector muscle, sacrospinalis medial, open fat lateral.
6. Come to lumbodorsal fascia, incise, quadratus lumborum in front of lens, drift Visiport laterally slightly, incise.
7. Once retroperitoneal fat seen, orient scope towards psoas, pointing to pelvis, initial dissection of space.
8. If balloon desired, place and inflate (5 min for minor vessel tamponade).
9. Fully free space with 10 mm lens, identify peritoneum and psoas.
10. Increase pressure to 15 mmHg.
11. Place two 5 mm working ports, incise skin 3–7 mm stab wound: one 1–2 cm above iliac lateral to sacrospinalis; one 1–2 cm above iliac at posterior axillary line, avoid transgressing the peritoneum which has been actively reflected as far anteriorly as possible.
12. Suture secure all ports.
13. Reduce pressure to working level.
14. Grasper/dissector and scissors to working ports.
15. Dissection anterior to ('below') 10 mm port lower pole of the kidney located here.
16. Dissect lower pole free, move superiorly to free posterior aspect of kidney.
17. Find ureter by dissection medially from the lower pole.
18. Follow ureter superiorly to hilum.
19. Additional dissection of kidney will tend to allow kidney to fall laterally.
20. Free hilum, identify artery and vein, dissect artery free.
21. Suction aspirate to keep field highly visible.
22. Clip renal artery, proximal and distal.
23. Observe kidney to loss of perfusion, identify additional arteries as needed.
24. Divide arteries which have been clipped.
25. Dissect renal veins, apply clips, proximal and distal.
26. Divide veins.
27. Mobilize, free kidney from attachments anteriorly, maintain caution for missed or upper pole vessels.
28. Once fully mobile, dissect ureter distally as far as possible (to level of vas in males, to bladder in females), once secure end length, may divide proximally prior to continued distal dissection/ligation.
29. Divide ureter, electrocautery for nonrefluxing, EndoLoop for refluxing units.
30. Irrigate field.
31. Reduce pressure, confirm hemostasis.
32. Switch to 2–5 mm lens.
33. Return to normal working pressure.
34. Specimen extraction, via 10 mm port site: direct for small specimen, small extension of incision or entrapment sac for larger specimen.
35. Remove kidney.
36. Reduce pressure to reconfirm hemostasis.
37. Insufflate.
38. Remove ports.
39. Remove two 5 mm ports, direct vision closure of 10 mm port.
40. Suture incisions and close with benzoin and Steri-Strip.

**Postoperative details.** Only single-dose perioperative intravenous antibiotics are used unless a concurrent infection is suspected, in which case a longer course is used.

**Follow-up care.** In the absence of contralateral reflux/anomoly, follow-up is restricted to the immediate postoperative period. Late complications are unusual, and the procedure is typically definitive.

# Upper pole heminephrectomy, partial ureterectomy with ureterocele decompression

Partial nephrectomy to remove a dysfunctional upper pole segment is similar to that noted above, and consists of identification of the upper and lower pole vessels and ureter. Once the structures are sorted to upper or lower pole, division of the vessels to the dysfunctional segment, and division of the renal cortex along the line of demarcation identified following ligation of the associated vessels is performed.

The procedure follows the same approach as nephrectomy, except that identification of upper and lower segments and their vascular supply is critical. A harmonic scalpel is an excellent device to divide the parenchyma while avoiding hemorrhage. Typically, if the upper pole vasculature is divided prior to incising the renal parenchyma, no significant bleeding is encountered.

In mobilizing the ureter, care must be taken to avoid stripping the blood supply to the lower pole ureter. Dissection should take place directly on the surface of the upper pole ureter. Injury to the upper pole ureter is inconsequential. The ureter is mobilized distally as far as possible, then divided, as noted for nephrectomy. This can usually be done at a position at the level of the trigone. If difficulty separating the ureters due to an adherent common sheath or common wall is encountered, it is best to terminate distal dissection and divide the ureter.

**Postoperative details.** Intravenous antibiotics are continued until the patient is discharged from the hospital. Prophylaxis is used following discharge until reflux status is confirmed. Urethral catheters are removed when urine is clear. It is not uncommon for a fever to be present postoperatively and speculation as to the possibility of a portion of devitalized upper pole tissue as the genesis of the trouble can be entertained. If the fever is high grade or protracted, evaluation with computed tomography (CT) or ultrasound is indicated.

**Follow-up care.**   Follow-up care consists of serial monitoring of renal function, periodic evaluation of voiding symptoms and bladder function, and interval radiologic studies to assess renal growth, hydroureteronephrosis, and vesicoureteral reflux. A typical schedule in the absence of infection or other problems is an ultrasound at 1 month and VCUG and ultrasound at 3–6 months postoperatively. If reflux is absent, prophylaxis can be discontinued. Issues under evaluation are resolution or development of ipsilateral reflux and evidence of unimpaired drainage from the lower pole system.

## Ureteropyelostomy

In this procedure we anastomose the upper pole ureter to the lower pole renal pelvis in a fashion analogous to a pyeloplasty. This is typically approached in transperitoneal fashion to afford a larger working environment for intracorporeal suturing. A stent is typically placed, and this can be placed cystoscopically at the start of the procedure or percutaneously after the pelvis is opened. This procedure at present is currently best restricted to children > 15 kg because of working space limitations in smaller children.

**Operative steps.**   For laparoscopic ureteropyelotomy:

1. Patient positioned supine and secured, 30° wedge under ipsilateral side or full flank position.
2. Roll table 30° away from surgeon to 'flatten' patient.
3. Obtain access to peritoneal cavity.
4. Increase pressure to 15–20 mmHg.
5. Transilluminate abdominal wall for vessels.
6. Place working ports, incise skin 7 mm incisions, ipsilateral mid-upper abdomen at the paramedian position, ipsilateral mid-lower abdomen lateral to the rectus.
7. Suture secure all ports.
8. Reduce pressure to working levels.
9. Roll table 30° towards surgeon.
10. Grasper/dissector and scissors to working ports.
11. Divide ipsilateral line of Toldt, reflect colon medially. A mesenteric window may be used if the region of the UPJ can be visualized.
12. Expose kidney, freeing medially at the lower pole to begin exposure of hilum.
13. Attention towards lower pole to identify ureters, dissect ureters free. Follow this superiorly to the lower pole renal pelvis.
14. May place two 5 mm addition working ports: anterior to mid axillary line for additional working points.

15. Anterior-lateral traction on ureter to better expose hilum.
16. Free hilum, to expose the lower pole pelvis and UPJ.
17. Suction aspirate to keep field highly visible.
18. Place a hitch stitch in the pelvis to lift and secure the pelvis towards the midpoint of the lower two ports. These ports are the working ports for suturing.
19. Open the renal pelvis above the UPJ.
20. Incise and divide the upper pole ureter at a position lined up with the pelvic incision.
21. Spatulate the upper pole ureter over a matching length to the pelvis incision.
22. A single suture is placed in the crotch of the ureter spatulation to the dependent portion of the pelvis and tied. The suture is left with a tag to identify this position.
23. The back wall is sutured with a running stitch, and tied at the superior apex.
24. A ureteral stent is introduced if it was not previously placed by use of a 2 mm trocar placed at the subcostal margin in the midclavicular line. The stent is advanced down the trocar directly into the ureter.
25. The upper loop of the stent is placed in the renal pelvis of the upper pole moiety.
26. The front wall of the new UPJ is closed with a running suture.
27. Reduce pressure to confirm hemostasis.
28. Return to working pressure.
29. A drain may be placed if desired.
30. Reduce pressure, reconfirm hemostasis.
31. Insufflate.
32. Secure fascia as appropriate: 10 mm sites in adults are best closed using direct vision closure, 5 mm ports do not require closure. In children, 5 mm ports should be closed.
33. Remove ports.
34. Suture incisions and close with benzoin and Steri-Strip.

**Postoperative details.**   Intravenous antibiotics are continued until the patient is discharged from the hospital. Prophylaxis is used following discharge until reflux status is confirmed. Urethral catheters are removed when urine is clear. If an internal stent has been placed, it is removed 3–6 weeks after surgery. A postoperative ultrasound is obtained 1 month following the removal of the stent.

**Follow-up care.**   Follow-up care consists of serial monitoring of renal function, periodic evaluation of voiding symptoms and bladder function, and interval radiologic studies to assess renal growth, hydroureteronephrosis, and vesicoureteral reflux. A typical schedule in the absence of infection or other problems is an ultrasound at 1 month and VCUG and ultrasound at 3–6 months postoperatively. If reflux is absent, prophylaxis can be discontinued.

# References

1. Allen TD. Congenital ureteral strictures. J Urol 1970; 104:196–204.

2. Cussen LJ. The morphology of congenital dilatation of the ureter: intrinsic ureteral lesions. Aust NZ J Surg 1971; 41:185–94.

3. Dajani AM, Dejani YF, Dahabrah S. Congenital ureteric valves – a cause of urinary obstruction. Br J Urol 1982; 54:98–102.

4. Wall B, Wachter H. Congenital ureteral valve: its role as a primary obstructive lesion. Classification of the literature and report of an authentic case. J Urol 1952; 68:684.

5. Kirks DR, Currarino G, Weinberg AG. Transverse folds in the proximal ureter: a normal variant in infants. AJR Am J Roentgenol 1978; 130:463–4.

6. Sant GR, Barbalias GA, Klauber GT. Congenital ureteral valves – an abnormality of ureteral embryogenesis? J Urol 1985; 133:427–31.

7. Wolf JS Jr, Elashry OM, Clayman RV. Long-term results of endoureterotomy for benign ureteral and ureteroenteric strictures. J Urol 1997; 158:759–64.

8. Conlin M, Bagley D. Incisional treatment of ureteral strictures. In: Smith A, Badlani G, Bagley D (eds), Smith's textbook of endourology. St. Louis: K Berger, 1996: 497.

9. Meretyk S, Albala DM, Clayman RV, et al. Endoureterotomy for treatment of ureteral strictures. J Urol 1992; 147:1502–6.

10. Yamada S, Ono Y, Ohshima S, Miyake K. Transurethral ureteroscopic ureterotomy assisted by a prior balloon dilation for relieving ureteral strictures. J Urol 1995; 153:1418–21.

11. Nezhat CH, Nezhat F, Seidman D, Nezhat C. Laparoscopic ureteroureterostomy: a prospective follow-up of 9 patients. Prim Care Update Ob Gyns 1998; 5:200.

12. Glassberg KI, Braren V, Duckett JW, et al. Suggested terminology for duplex systems, ectopic ureters and ureteroceles. J Urol 1984; 132:1153–4.

13. Stephens D. Caecoureterocele and concepts on the embryology and aetiology of ureteroceles. Aust NZ J Surg 1971; 40:239–48.

14. Pfister C, Ravasse P, Barret E, et al. The value of endoscopic treatment for ureteroceles during the neonatal period. J Urol 1998; 159:1006–9.

15. Coplen DE, Duckett JW. The modern approach to ureteroceles. J Urol 1995; 153:166–71.

16. Monfort G, Guys JM, Coquet M, et al. Surgical management of duplex ureteroceles. J Pediatr Surg 1992; 27:634–8.

17. Glazier DB, Packer MG. Infected obstructive ureterocele. Urology 1997; 50:972–3.

18. Cremin BJ. A review of the ultrasonic appearances of posterior urethral valve and ureteroceles. Pediatr Radiol 1986; 16:357–64.

19. Athey PA, Carpenter RJ, Hadlock FP, et al. Ultrasonic demonstration of ectopic ureterocele. Pediatrics 1983; 71:568–71.

20. Caldamone A, Duckett J. Update on ureteroceles in children. AUA Update Series 1984; 3.

21. Bellah RD, Long FR, Canning DA. Ureterocele eversion with vesicoureteral reflux in duplex kidneys: findings at voiding cystourethrography. AJR Am J Roentgenol 1995; 165:409–13.

22. Arap S, Nahas WC, Alonso G, et al. Assessment of hydroureteronephrosis by renographic evaluation under diuretic stimulus. Urol Int 1984; 39:170–4.

23. Decter RM, Roth DR, Gonzales ET. Individualized treatment of ureteroceles. J Urol 1989; 142:535–7; discussion 542–3.

24. Churchill BM, Sheldon CA, McLorie GA. The ectopic ureterocele: a proposed practical classification based on renal unit jeopardy. J Pediatr Surg 1992; 27:497–500.

25. Blyth B, Passerini-Glazel G, Camuffo C, et al. Endoscopic incision of ureteroceles: intravesical versus ectopic. J Urol 1993; 149:556–9; discussion 560.

26. Hagg MJ, Mourachov PV, Snyder HM, et al. The modern endoscopic approach to ureterocele. J Urol 2000; 163:940–3.

27. Rich MA, Keating MA, Snyder HM 3rd, Duckett JW. Low transurethral incision of single system intravesical ureteroceles in children. J Urol 1990; 144:120–1.

28. Husmann D, Strand B, Ewalt D, et al. Management of ectopic ureterocele associated with renal duplication: a comparison of partial nephrectomy and endoscopic decompression. J Urol 1999; 162:1406–9.

29. Caldamone AA, Snyder HM 3rd, Duckett JW. Ureteroceles in children: followup of management with upper tract approach. J Urol 1984; 131:1130–2.

30. Mandell J, Colodny AH, Lebowitz R, et al. Ureteroceles in infants and children. J Urol 1980; 123:921–6.

31. Reitelman C, Perlmutter AD. Management of obstructing ectopic ureteroceles. Urol Clin North Am 1990; 17:317–28.

32. Scherz HC, Kaplan GW, Packer MG, Brock WA. Ectopic ureteroceles: surgical management with preservation of continence – review of 60 cases. J Urol 1989; 142:538–41; discussion 542–3.

33. Shekarriz B, Upadhyay J, Fleming P, et al. Long-term outcome based on the initial surgical approach to ureterocele. J Urol 1999; 162:1072–6.

34. Janetschek G, Seibold J, Radmayr C, Bartsch G. Laparoscopic heminephroureterectomy in pediatric patients. J Urol 1997; 158:1928–30.

35. Jordan GH, Winslow BH. Laparoendoscopic upper pole partial nephrectomy with ureterectomy. J Urol 1993; 150:940–3.

36. Miyazato M, Hatano T, Miyazato T, et al. Retroperitoneoscopic heminephrectomy of the right upper collecting system emptying into an ectopic ureterocele in a 5-year-old girl: a case report. Hinyokika Kiyo 2000; 46:413–16.

37. Valla JS, Breaud J, Carfagna L, et al. Treatment of ureterocele on duplex ureter: upper pole nephrectomy by retroperitoneoscopy in children based on a series of 24 cases. Eur Urol 2003; 43:426–9.

38. Hendren WH, Mitchell ME. Surgical correction of ureteroceles. J Urol 1979; 121:590–7.

# 10

# Renal dysplasia and cystic disease options

Alaa El-Ghoneimi

Renal dysplasia is a common kidney disorder. It is frequently associated with congenital obstructive uropathy that leads to renal failure in children.[1]

Despite the frequent occurrence of renal dysplasia in association with obstructive uropathy, its pathogenesis remains unknown. Abnormal metanephric differentiation in cases of renal dysplasia results in abnormal renal organization and poor development of renal elements. This abnormal differentiation may be secondary to a disturbance in the inductive interaction between the ureteric bud and the metanephric mesenchyma. It has also been suggested that renal dysplasia is not an end-stage phenomenon, but rather involves the abnormal expression of genes normally found in the cascade of renal differentiation, leading to malformed kidney. Various growth and transcription factors, including human growth factor, platelet-derived growth factor, fibroblast growth factor, keratinocyte growth factor, transforming growth factor, glial cell line-derived neurotrophic factor and their receptors are dysregulated in renal dysplasia.[2–4] This dysregulation may provide a continuous signal for proliferation, which may explain persistent dysplastic tubules in the postnatal period.[3]

Renal dysplasia is a histologic term defining a malformed part or the whole kidney and the presence of primitive ducts lined with undifferentiated columnar epithelium and surrounded by undifferentiated fibromuscular collar with sometimes a metaplastic element such as cartilage.

Classically, kidney malformations including dysplasia are classified based on histology. Recent advances in molecular biology and genetics have led Woolf and Winyard to suggest a more straightforward classification to describe kidney malformations. The abnormalities can be divided into groups based on the underlying cell biology, such as aberrant early development or defects in terminal maturation.[5,6] The aberrant early development group includes dysplastic kidneys, whether large multicystic dysplastic kidneys (MCDKs) or small organs with a combination of hypoplasia/dysplasia and some obstructed kidneys.

Defects in terminal maturation are observed in polycystic kidney disease (PKD). Initial nephron and collecting duct malformation is unremarkable in these kidneys, but there is later cystic dilation of these structures, causing secondary loss of adjacent normal structures. The commonest types are the autosomal dominant and autosomal recessive PKD. Cyst decortication is sometimes indicated in adults and the laparoscopic techniques has been thoroughly described in cases of complicated cysts of PKD.[7,8] This category of renal diseases is usually not associated with obstructive uropathy and is mainly managed by nephrologists for the development of renal failure and hypertension; their description is beyond the field of this chapter.

Dysplastic kidneys can be any size, ranging between massive kidneys with multiple large cysts up to 9 cm, which are commonly termed MCDKs, to normal or small kidneys, with or without cysts. Dysplasia can be unilateral, bilateral, or segmental, affecting only part of the kidney. Unilateral incidence is 1 in 3000–5000 births, compared to 1 in 10,000 for bilateral dysplasia.[5,9] MCDK can be familial, but is most commonly a sporadic anomaly. The mode of familial transmission can be an autosomal dominant inheritance with variable expressivity and reduced penetrance. Belk et al[9] did not find any significant renal anomalies in any of the 94 first-degree relatives of the MCDK index cases; therefore, formal screening of relatives is not recommended.

## Diagnosis

Commonly, dysplasia is applied to the bright echogenic appearance secondary to the lack of normal renal parenchyma and structurally abnormal kidney. Meanwhile, this ultrasonographic appearance is not pathognomonic to histologically defined dysplasia.[10] The current classic presentation of MCDK is the prenatal sonographic diagnosis. The typical sonographic appearance is a multiloculated abdominal mass consisting of multiple thin-walled cysts, which do not appear to connect (Figure 10.1). To be differentiated from hydronephrosis, no renal pelvis or parenchyma can be demonstrated in MCDK. Other sonographic patterns are circumferential cysts in kidneys of more normal size, particularly in bilateral cases associated with lower urinary tract obstruction. The amniotic fluid volume is usually normal in unilateral cases in contrast with bilateral cases, where oligo- or anhydramnios is the most common associated findings.[11] Small hypo/dysplastic kidneys are difficult to detect prenatally and in unilateral cases their postnatal follow-up is difficult because of their small size. These small kidneys are commonly misdiagnosed as renal agenesis.[9,12] Even with evident prenatal diagnosis, a postnatal work-up is needed to confirm the diagnosis and search for associated anomalies. A thorough clinical examination will complete the full fetal sonographic examination for other structural abnormalities, including heart, spine, extremities, face, and umbilical cord, as up to 35% may have extrarenal anomalies.[13,14] These are more likely to occur with bilateral than unilateral MCDK. Risks of chromosomal defects are low if there is isolated renal dysplasia.[11] Lazebnik et al[13] have found in a study of 102 cases with MCDK, 10 (9.8%) had an abnormal karyotype, but in all cases there were extrarenal anomalies present. Associated anomalies of kidneys contralateral to dysplastic kidneys are either structural (duplex system, pelviureteric obstruction, or ectopic) or affected by vesicoureteric reflux. The frequency of such anomalies is between 20 and 50%, according to published series.[11,15–17] Vesicoureteric reflux on the same side as the MCDK was reported in 17% of cases.[18]

Renal dysplasia frequently develops in conjunction with lower urinary tract malformation. Experimental urinary tract obstruction in animal models during development has generated dysplastic changes in renal structures.[19,20] The lower urinary tract should be assessed in cases of presumed renal dysplasia.

Our current postnatal work-up for prenatally detected MCDK includes a routine detailed ultrasound, voiding cystourethrography, and renal isotope scan. If the diagnosis is unclear, a Uro-MRI to differentiate MCDK from obstructive uropathy (Figure 10.2) or duplex system is performed.

# Natural history and prognosis of dysplastic kidneys

The prognosis of dysplastic kidneys depends mainly on whether the anomaly is unilateral or bilateral. Bilateral cases have poor prognosis and the fetus often has anhydramnios; death occurs in the neonatal period secondary to pulmonary hypoplasia. Other less severe forms of bilateral cases may survive the early childhood period and develop terminal renal failure later in life.[11,16]

The prognosis of patients with unilateral dysplasia with a normal contralateral kidney is much better. The majority of dysplastic kidneys involute[9] without causing any problems. The natural history is usually towards spontaneous regression of the cysts. Recently, Oliveira et al[21] found partial involution in 68%, complete involution in 21%, and an increase in unit size in 11%. The mean age at complete or partial involution of the lesion was 18 months. In unilateral cases, there is often a compensatory hypertrophy of the contralateral kidney.[22]

It was originally suggested that dysplastic kidneys be removed to avoid rare complications such as hypertension,

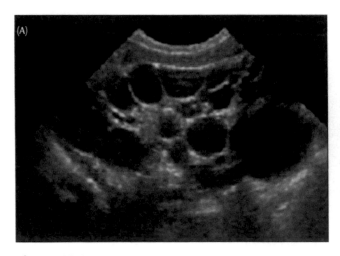
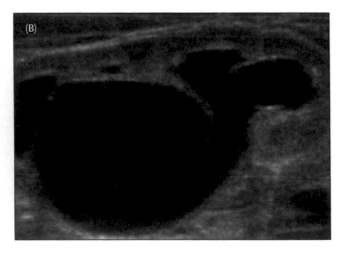

**Figure 10.1**
Sonographic diagnosis of multicystic dysplastic kidney (MCDK). Typical sonographic appearance of MCDK, a multiloculated retroperitoneal mass consisting of multiple thin-walled cysts, which do not appear to connect. To be differentiated from hydronephrosis (B), no renal pelvis or parenchyma can be demonstrated in MCDK (A). The cysts are distributed randomly and the kidney is enlarged with irregular outline.

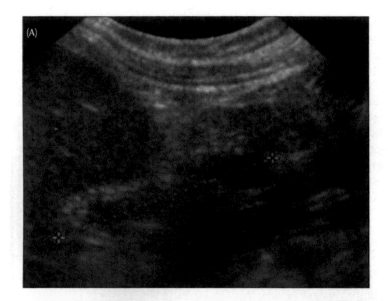

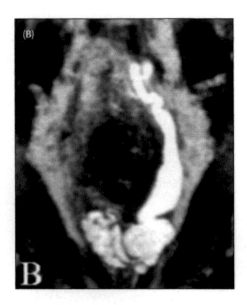

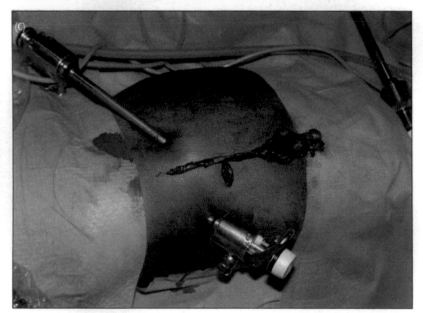

**Figure 10.2**
Magnetic resonance imaging (MRI) diagnosis of associated uropathy to a dysplastic nonfunctioning kidney. The sonographic appearance of an echogenic small nondifferentiated kidney (A). The MRI showed a small left kidney with ectopic implantation in the seminal vesicle (B). The anatomy of the entire left urinary tract can be detailed before surgery. The DMSA renal scan showed no function and a retroperitoneal left nephroureterectomy was done at 10 months of age (C).

tumors, and infections. However, the risk of these complications appears to be very low now that an elective nephrectomy is no longer routinely performed in most of centers. The likelihood of developing such complications is higher in cases associated with contralateral anomalies.[17] Patients with bilateral disease or associated genitourinary (GU) anomalies had a higher incidence of urinary tract infection (UTI) and progression to renal failure. Complex MCDK was associated with a worse outcome (50% chronic renal insufficiency or failure). Even the risk for chronic renal failure is very high: up to 22% with obstruction and 14% with contralateral reflux.[22]

Rare complications have been reported. Pain associated with MCDK was reported as the only symptom in older patients (mean age of 40 years old) with resolution after nephrectomy.[23] Exceptionally huge cysts may need percutaneous decompression to relieve the respiratory distress in infants.[24] Infection was suggested as a complication of MCDK, but any true association is not well documented. The reported cases were mostly associated with other urinary tract anomalies such as reflux or contralateral obstruction. In the registry of the American Academy of Pediatrics (AAP) for MCDK, 16 of the 608 nonoperated MCDK were associated with UTI.[25] Association between MCDK and hypertension was found in less than 1% in the published long-term series;[25] meanwhile, sporadic reports have demostrated resolution of hypertension after nephrectomy.[26] Seeman et al[27] monitored blood pressure in children with unilateral MCDK and found anomalies only in children who had ultrasonographic and/or laboratory signs of contralateral kidney abnormalities.

There is ongoing controversy concerning the management of MCDK, particularly with regard to the potential for malignant transformation. Well-documented sporadic cases of malignancy with MCDK have been reported. The tumor may be Wilms' tumor, renal cell carcinoma, or mesothelioma.[28,29] Age is variable and can even be detected as early as 3 months. The discovery of the renal tumor on the initial ultrasound is more toward an association than the new development of tumor in the natural history of the disease. Even though this association or the malignant degeneration is exceptional, a careful initial ultrasound examination is mandatory and any equivocal diagnosis with suspicious nature of the cysts should lead to surgical removal of the kidney. These sporadic reported cases may lend support to the surgical management of MCDK, particularly as nephrectomy can now be performed in a day surgery setting with minimal morbidity.[26]

Few authors still advocate surgical removal of MCDK to avoid multiple and inadequate evaluations of those children with a single functioning renal unit.[16,26] Perez et al[30] have shown that early nephrectomy is more cost-effective than observation in neonates with MCDK only when observation involves screening with ultrasonography every 3 months until the child is 8 years old.

Controversy exists as to whether any screening program is necessary. When screening is instituted, options include monthly parental abdominal palpation vs serial renal ultrasound. The frequency is variable according to authors, between every 3 and 12 months until age 5–8 years old. The aim of this screening is dual: to screen for early stage tumors and to follow up contralateral renal growth.

# Management of solitary renal cyst

Other cystic diseases of the kidney are very uncommon in children. A single renal cyst is unusual, and even with otherwise normal-appearing kidneys, the diagnosis of PKD should always be suspected. Ultrasonography remains the modality primarily used for their evaluation. In general, computed tomography (CT) and magnetic resonance imaging (MRI) are limited to cases in which the ultrasonographic appearances are confusing or complications such as cyst rupture, hemorrhage, or neoplasia are suspected.[31] Once cystic lesions have been diagnosed by ultrasonography, a careful examination should rule out the group of cystic renal tumors that includes cystic Wilms' tumor and multilocular cystic nephroma. The multilocular cystic nephroma is a benign cystic tumor of the kidney occurring primarily in infant boys between 3 months and 4 years of age and in middle-aged women.[32] The tumor appears as a complex multicystic mass with thin septa separating the cysts.

The fetal simple renal cyst represents a distinct entity within the spectrum of cystic kidney disease. A fetal simple renal cyst can be identified by ultrasonography in early pregnancy.[33] In the absence of associated anatomic or chromosomal abnormalities, the majority of cysts will resolve during pregnancy without any sequelae.

Congenital calyceal cyst is another exceptional congenital anomaly that is also referred to as a calyceal diverticulum. The cysts are typically located more centrally adjacent to the collecting system. They may communicate with the collecting system and facilitate their diagnosis with the presence of contrast product in the cystic cavity on CT, but the communication may be stenotic and the diagnosis becomes less evident.[34]

Indications for surgical removal of solitary renal cysts in children are exceptional, as the natural history is spontaneous resolution and complicated cysts are seen more often in adults than in children. Laparoscopic unroofing of a solitary cyst in adults has been successful and is recommended in case of recurrence after percutaneous ultrasound-guided needle aspiration.[7,35] Few cases of cyst removal have been reported in children through a retroperitoneal laparoscopic approach. The access is the same as for nephrectomy and removal of the cyst can be achieved completely in a reasonable operative time not exceeding 1 hour.[36,37]

# Laparoscopic nephrectomy

The first laparoscopic nephrectomy in adults was reported in 1991 by Clayman et al.[38] One-year later Ehrlich et al[39] reported their first series of pediatric cases. Since then many authors have reported successful results of nephrectomy and nephroureterectomy in pediatrics, all advocating the transperitoneal approach.[40,41] Roberts suggested the retroperitoneal approach to the kidney in 1976,[42] reporting his experience with retroperitoneal endoscopy with gas insufflation in animals. Retroperitoneal operative laparoscopy was described for the first time by Gaur in 1992[43] and then by others in adult and pediatric urology.[44–46] Despite the expanding application of retroperitoneal laparoscopic renal surgery in adults,[47,48] this technique was adapted later by pediatric urologists and is progressively expanding in different centers.[36,46,49–51] We previously reported that the retroperitoneal approach is a well-adapted laparoscopic technique for renal surgery in children and is comparable to that of conventional renal surgery.[36,52]

Guilloneau et al[45] reported in a retrospective study of adults and children that retroperitoneal and transperitoneal approaches were equivalent in terms of morbidity and postoperative stay, but operating time was shorter with the retroperitoneal approach.

Effects of retroperitoneal $CO_2$ insufflation have been studied in animals and in children.[52,53] We have demonstrated a significant increase in systolic blood pressure and end-tidal carbon dioxide, while there was no modification of the other hemodynamic or ventilatory parameters. These changes do not need any special modification of the ventilatory parameters, whereas caution is required in hypertensive patients.

## Indications and contraindications

Currently, malignant renal tumors in children are not considered for laparoscopy. The most common renal tumor in children is nephroblastoma. These tumors are of large size, frequently extending outside the kidney, and with high risk of rupture during dissection. In adults, radical nephrectomy for renal cancer less than 5 cm in size can be safely achieved by a laparoscopic approach.[47]

Indications for nephrectomy in children are mainly for nonfunctioning kidneys secondary to obstructive uropathy or reflux. Although laparoscopic nephrectomy for MCDK is an easy and safe procedure, the indications for nephrectomy are still debatable. The acceptable indications for these cases are the increase in size of cysts or the rare complications of hypertension or infection.

Nephrectomy may be indicated for children with end-stage renal disease before transplantation when the primary renal disease is associated with hypertension, severe nephrotic syndrome, or severe uremic hemolytic syndrome.[52] In such cases, during open surgery, a large incision is necessary to control the renal pedicle in optimal conditions and to extract a large kidney, so here we find the ultimate advantage of laparoscopic procedures. Laparoscopic bilateral nephrectomy has been performed in adults.[54] In our experience, synchronous bilateral nephrectomy was performed in 10 children, and technically the procedure was performed as 2 unilateral cases, as position and draping were changed between the two procedures.

## Patient and preoperative preparation

The surgery is thoroughly explained to the child (adapted to his age) and to his parents. The possibility of conversion to open surgery has to be mentioned in the consent, along with the possible operative incidents.

Patient preparation is not different from the conventional surgery preparation. Personally we do not prescribe any specific diet measures before surgery. We follow the usual recommendations for general anesthesia preparations. The child is on a strict diet for a period between 4 and 8 hours, depending on his age, and premedicated before going to the operating theater. Some surgeons recommend a fluid diet and enema on the night preceding surgery.[55]

An indwelling bladder catheter is recommended in the case of high-grade reflux or each time that ureterectomy is indicated to facilitate the dissection of the ureter as close as possible to its junction with the bladder. Usually it is recommended in the transperitoneal approach to avoid bladder injury during trocar insertion. A preoperative catheter is also needed when urine output monitoring is mandatory for the anesthesia management in certain associated cardiac or renal diseases.

A nasogastric tube is placed after the endotracheal general anesthesia. Noninvasive hemodynamic and ventilatory monitoring is needed during the laparoscopic nephrectomy in either transperitoneal or retroperitoneal approach.

## Recommended equipment and instruments

Standard laparoscopic instruments are suitable for nephrectomy without special instruments or equipments. The usual laparoscopic equipment is necessary: monitor, insufflator, cold light source, and camera.

For any laparoscopic renal surgery, we recommend the following instruments.

### Conventional surgical instruments for access

1. Sterile marker to identify the major landmarks and optimal trocars placement.
2. Stab scalpel, No. 11, to achieve stab incision adapted for trocar insertion.
3. Blunt dissection scissors, helpful for muscle dissociation.
4. Needle driver.
5. Nontoothed forceps.
6. Nonresorbable monofilament suture with tapered needle for the purse-string suture.
7. Two artery forceps.
8. Pair of retractors, narrow and long blades.
9. Sutures necessary for wound closure.
10. Drains, at surgeon's convenience, with or without suction.
11. A complete conventional open surgery set, to be available in the operating room in case of conversion to open surgery.

### Laparoscopic instruments

The choice of single-use or reusable instruments depends usually on the surgeon's convenience and the economic impact. Currently, most of the instruments are available in the two categories. It is convenient to harmonize the type of instruments for all the surgeons and the different departments of surgery working together in the same operating theater. The laparoscopic instruments are the same for general pediatric surgery, and a common pool of instruments can be of great help, especially in the initial phase during the learning curve. Personally, we mostly use reusable instruments, and for few unavailable instruments, we use the single-use ones. Anyway, a full set of single-use instruments is necessary as back-up to reusable instruments:

1. Laparoscope: 5 mm 0° is the standard laparoscope for pediatric nephrectomy.
2. Trocars: 4 trocars of 5 mm; one of them should be blunt for the placement of the first trocar. Self-retaining trocars are interesting, especially in young children, to avoid the slipping of the trocars outside the abdominal wall.
3. Atraumatic grasping forceps.
4. Curved dissecting forceps for vascular dissection.
5. Scissors.
6. Monopolar diathermy.
7. Bipolar diathermy or harmonic scalpel.
8. Needle driver.
9. Toothed grasping forceps for organ retrieval.
10. Resorbable ligature for endocorporeal vascular or ureteral ligation when needed. A readymade laparoscopic loop suture can be used for ureteral ligature.
11. Resorbable suture, with round 3/8 curved needle, for transfixing ligature when needed or repair of vascular tear.
12. Vascular clips, reusable or single use.
13. Laparoscopic bag for organ retrieval; the currently available bags are at least 10 mm diameter and if the kidney is of big size, the first trocar and the laparoscope should be of 10 mm from the beginning to avoid trocar replacement at organ retrieval.
14. Irrigation–suction device.

# Renal access

The kidney can be accessed by a retroperitoneal or transperitoneal approach.

## Retroperitoneal access

**Lateral approach.** The patient is placed lateral, with sufficient flexion of the operating table so as to expose the area of trocars placement, between the last rib and the iliac crest (Figure 10.3). Retroperitoneal access is achieved

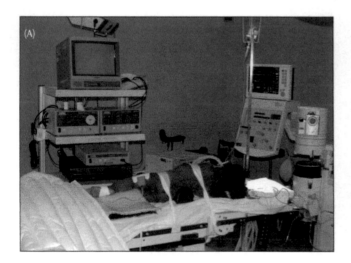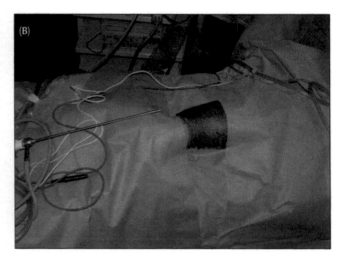

**Figure 10.3**
Patient positioning for left retroperitoneal laparoscopic nephrectomy. (A) The patient is placed lateral, with sufficient flexion of the operating table so as to expose the area of trocars placement, between the last rib and the iliac crest; for younger children, as shown, a lumbar support is sufficient for the exposure. The child is wrapped by two adhesive bands, one on the greater trocanter level and a second on the chest, to keep the child at a perpendicular angle with the table. The surgeon, assistant, and scrub nurse are all on the back side of the child. The front side of the child is left free for the monitor, which is placed cranial while doing the kidney dissection and caudal to proceed for the distal ureterectomy. (B) Drapping is planned with fixation of all the connections with the monitor and insufflator towards the bottom and the head of the child leaving the exposed area free for instruments movement without difficulty.

through the first incision, 10–15 mm in length, and one fingerwidth from the lower border of the tip of the 12th rib (Figure 10.4). The use of narrow retractors with long blades allows a deep dissection with short incision. The Gerota's fascia is approached by a muscle-splitting blunt dissection; it is then opened under direct vision and the first blunt trocar (5 or 10 mm) is introduced directly inside the opened Gerota's fascia. A working space is created by gas insufflation dissection, and the first trocar is fixed with a purse-string suture that is applied around the deep fascia to ensure an airtight seal and to allow traction on the main trocar if needed to increase the working space. A second trocar (3 or 5 mm) is inserted posteriorly in front of the lumbosacral muscle. A third trocar (3 or 5 mm) is inserted in the anterior axillary line, a fingerwidth from the top of the iliac crest. To avoid transperitoneal insertion of this trocar, the working space is fully developed and the deep surface of the anterior wall muscles is identified before the trocar insertion. Insufflation pressure does not exceed 12 mmHg, and the $CO_2$ flow rate is progressively increased from 1 to 3 l/min. Access to the retroperitoneum and creation of the working space are the keys of success in the retroperitoneal renal surgery. Age is not a limiting factor for this approach. Young children have less fat and the access is easier; our youngest child was 6 weeks old.

**Prone posterior approach.** The access begins with an incision in the costovertebral angle at the edge of the paraspinous muscles. The secondary trocars are placed just above the iliac crest – one medially at the edge of the paraspinous muscles and one laterally at the posterior clavicular line.[55] In a randomized prospective study on 36 complete and 19 partial nephrectomies, Borzi[56] compared the lateral to the posterior retroperitoneal approach in children. There was no significant difference in the operative time. Our preference goes to the lateral approach: it permits any type of renal surgery at any age with good exposure to the distal ureter.

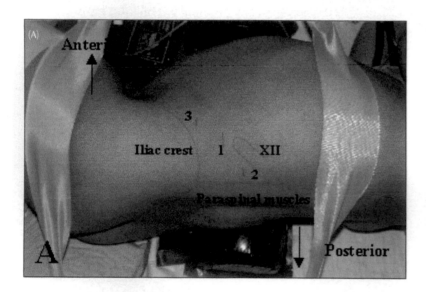

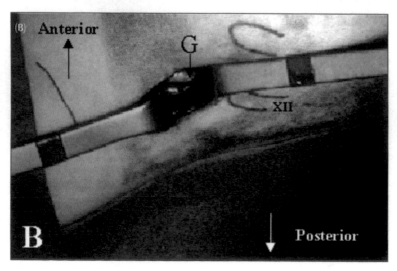

**Figure 10.4**

Trocars placement and retroperitoneal access for nephrectomy. (A) Area of trocars placement, between the last rib and the iliac crest. Retroperitoneal access is achieved through the first incision (1), 10–15 mm in length, and one fingerwidth from the lower border of the tip of the 12th rib. A second trocar (2) is inserted posteriorly in the costovertebral angle. A third trocar (3) is inserted in the anterior axillary line, a fingerwidth from the top of the iliac crest. (B) The Gerota's fascia (G) is approached by a muscle-splitting blunt dissection; it is then opened under direct vision and the first blunt trocar is introduced directly inside the opened Gerota's fascia to start insufflation. The use of narrow retractors with long blades allows a deep dissection with short incision.

**Other techniques to access the retroperitoneal space.**
Since the description by Gaur,[43] balloon dissection has
been the method applied by most urologists.
Disadvantages of balloon dissection are the cost of the
disposable material and the possible complications with
rupture of the balloon.[57] On the other hand, balloon
dissection allows the creation of a working space without
opening Gerota's fascia, which is important for radical
nephrectomy of malignant tumors in adults.

Micali et al[37] reported the use of the Visiport visual
trocar to access directly to the retroperitoneal space. The
advantage of this method is the possibility of using a small
incision for the first trocar, which is interesting in the
reconstructive surgery but not in ablative surgery, as the
first incision is needed for organ retrieval.

## Transperitoneal access

Several options exist in terms of patient positioning. The
most frequently described is the flank position.[55] The
pneumoperitonium is created through an open umbilical
approach. The child is positioned with the surgeon
standing in front of the abdomen (opposite side of
nephrectomy). The most frequent configuration has been
with the umbilical port and two ipsilateral ports in the
midclavicular line above and below the umbilicus. A
fourth trocar may be placed in the midaxillary line for
exposure to retract the liver or spleen if needed. The
kidney is exposed by medial mobilization of the colon.

## *Nephrectomy by lateral retroperitoneal approach*

The landmarks of the retroperitoneal space are first identified in order to be oriented with the retroperitoneal
exposure. The psoas muscle is the posterior landmark and
should remain in the bottom of the screen. The kidney
remains attached anteriorly to the peritoneum, and should
remain upward on the screen. The renal pedicle is
identified and approached posteriorly (Figure 10.5), and
dissected close to the junction with the aorta and inferior
vena cava (IVC), to avoid multiple ligations of branches of
the renal vessels. On the left side, the vein is ligated distal
to the genital and adrenal branches. On the right side, the
vein is short and a careful dissection at its junction with the
vena cava will avoid the confusion with dissecting the vena
cava. After dissecting the renal artery then the vein, the
vessels are clipped, ligated, or coagulated. The choice of
method depends on the vessel diameter and the surgeon
experience. In general, small arteries of MCDK can be
coagulated by bipolar cautery, while the most common
method is to double ligate the artery proximally by two
clips and distally by one. The vein is generally clipped in
the same way: if the diameter is bigger than the length of
the clip, the vein is first ligated by resorbable intracorporeal knot, then clipped. The use of staples, as described in
adult nephrectomy, requires a 12 mm port and is not
needed in pediatric patients. The ureter is then identified
and dissected as far as necessary. In the absence of reflux,

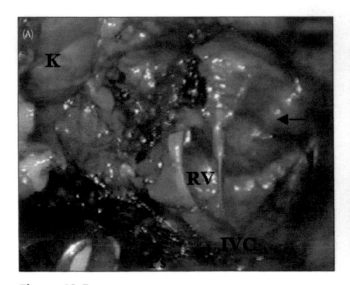
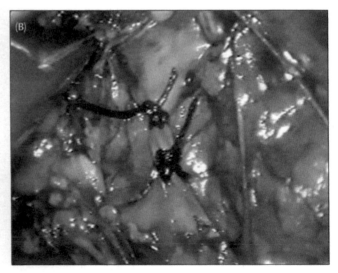

**Figure 10.5**
Retroperitoneal exposure and ligature of the renal pedicle. (A) The landmarks of the retroperitoneal space are first identified in order
to be oriented with the retroperitoneal exposure. The psoas muscle (Ps) is the posterior landmark and should remain in the bottom
of the screen. The kidney (K) remains attached anteriorly to the peritoneum, and should remain upward on the screen. The renal
pedicle is identified and approached posteriorly. In this picture the artery is already ligated and sectioned and dissected close to the
junction with the aorta and vena cava. On the right side, the renal vein (RV) is short and a careful dissection at its junction with the
inferior vena cava (IVC) will allow a safe exposure of its full length. Intestinal loops are visible behind the peritoneum and very close
to the pedicle; monopolar cautery should be avoided in this area. (B) Ligature of the renal vein with intracorporeal knots.

the ureter is coagulated and sectioned at the level of the lumbar ureter (especially in pretransplant nephrectomy, the native ureter might be used for the transplantation). In the presence of reflux, the dissection is distally followed, the vas deferens is identified in males, and the ureter is ligated as close as possible to the ureterovesical junction. During this distal dissection, the surgeon moves towards the head of the child, and the screen goes towards the feet of the child. In the beginning of our experience, we were using a fourth trocar to dissect and ligate the distal ureter.[36] Currently, we use an endoloop or, if the ureter is large, a transparietal suture to fix the ureter to the abdominal wall to facilitate its distal dissection and ligation. As the peritoneum is very close to the ureter in this distal part, its dissection is left to the end of the procedure to avoid any peritoneal tear.

The last part of dissection is the anterior surface of the kidney. The kidney is dissected from the peritoneum very close to its capsule in the cleavage plane of areolar tissue. Usually no hemostasis is necessary in this plane, whereas, in inflammatory adherent kidneys, a sharp dissection with bipolar coagulation may be necessary. In the rare cases of xanthogranulomotous pyelonephritis, we perform the dissection of the adherent kidney through the subcapsular plane to avoid injury to intraperitoneal structures.

## Kidney retrieval

The kidney is usually retrieved through the initial incision (Figure 10.2). A 5 mm telescope is inserted through the accessory port, and a toothed grasping forceps is introduced through the 10 mm port to extract the kidney. The kidney is grasped at one of the poles, and pulled in this axis, to pull on its smallest diameter. In most cases, the kidney can be divided under vision during extraction through the muscle wall. In cases of severe pyelocalyceal dilatation or MCDK, direct evacuation by puncture helps in organ retrieval. An extraction bag is used for infected or large kidneys, and the kidney is morcellated inside the bag (Figure 10.6). Our current preference is for routinely using the bag for extraction to avoid extending the incision and the spillover of the parenchyma in the retroperitoneum, which might produce more postoperative inflammation. This is particularly important in the pretransplant group, where we have to minimize all the factors that might increase the postoperative retroperitoneal adhesions. In our experience these adhesions can render the vascular dissection during transplantation more difficult. If nephrectomy is associated to other lower urinary tract procedures, nephrectomy is performed first and the kidney is placed near to the bladder without transecting the ureter. Retrieval is carried out through the Pfannenstiel incision.

## Postoperative care

Postoperative care after transperitoneal laparoscopy is identical to any transperitoneal laparoscopic surgery in children.

The retroperitoneal nephrectomy does not require specific postoperative care. The nasogastric tube is removed at the end of the surgery. Analgesics are given according to the child's comfort and adapted pain scores. In few cases, especially after a difficult procedure or perioperative bleeding, postoperative ileus may develop, requiring special measures of gastric suction and fasting until the intestinal movements are reestablished. In the case of postoperative abdominal distention or discomfort, repeated abdominal examination is mandatory and completed by imaging if needed to exclude any intraperitoneal organ injury. Even in the retroperitoneal approach, the surgeon should keep in mind the possibility of such complications, especially if monopolar diathermy was used, with the possible injury of adjacent intraperitoneal organs.

## Results

In the exclusively pediatric laparoscopic nephrectomy series, results are consistent with the feasibility of the procedure and a very low rate of conversion to open surgery ranging from 0 to 3%.[36,51,58–60]

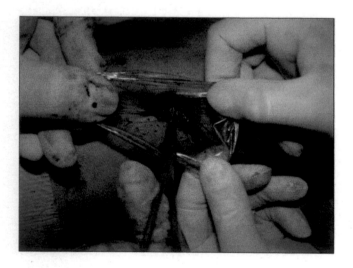

**Figure 10.6**
Kidney retrieval after retroperitoneal nephrectomy. The endobag is introduced through the first trocar and the kidney is placed inside the bag. Morcellation of the kidney by an artery forceps under direct vision allows kidney retrieval without the need to extend the incision.

The operative time is variable in the different series, according to the approach, indications, and the experience of the surgeon. In the retroperitoneal series, the mean operative time for nephrectomy or nephroureterectomy ranges from 47 to 110 min,[36,51,56] with longer time observed in the pretransplant group of children, with a mean operative time of 2 hours.[52] In the transperitoneal pediatric nephrectomy series, the mean operative time is relatively longer, at around 160 min.[59,60] As each group of surgeons does one of the two approaches, it is difficult to take into consideration this difference of operative time as comparison between the two approaches.

Pain and discomfort evaluation is a delicate procedure and should not be considered in nonrandomized series. To our knowledge, such a study on laparoscopic nephrectomy has yet to be published. The general impression of different authors is towards less consumption of analgesics, especially opiates, in the laparoscopic group. The shorter post-operative hospital stay may suggest that children are more comfortable and discharged earlier; here again, prudence is required in the analysis of retrospective nonrandomized series.

The hospital stay after laparoscopic nephrectomy depends on the indications. Most of the children operated on for urologic indications are discharged less than 24 hours after surgery.[36,51,60] Meanwhile, for pretransplant nephrectomy, the hospital stay is longer, with a mean of 4 days.

Although there is no comparative study on the cosmetic results of the treatments, it is obvious that the cosmetic results are excellent after laparoscopic nephrectomy, especially if the 3 or 5 mm trocar is used and the kidney retrieval is done through a laparoscopic bag when needed without extension of the incision.

## Laparoscopic versus open nephrectomy

To our knowledge, no prospective randomized study has proved the advantages of the laparoscopic approach over open surgery. We have retrospectively studied a comparable group of children who underwent pretransplant nephrectomy in our department before beginning our experience with retroperitoneal laparoscopic nephrectomy.[52] In this specific group of patients with end-stage renal disease, the hospital stay was significantly shorter after laparoscopic vs open nephrectomy (5.2 vs 8.4 days). Even when the operating time for laparoscopic vs open nephrectomy was longer (120 vs 104 minutes), the difference was not statistically significant. Hamilton et al[58] found comparable results on transperitoneal laparoscopic nephrectomy with significant decrease in hospital stay after laparoscopic compared with open nephrectomy (22.5

vs 41.3 hours). Operative time was significantly longer in the laparoscopic group (175.6 vs 120.2 min). Other studies on mixed groups of adults and children had comparable results, with a significantly briefer postoperative course in the laparoscopic group.[61]

## Common and unusual intraoperative problems and how to identify them

Complications of abdominal laparoscopy for urologic procedures, such as bowel and great vessel injury, have been documented in the adult and pediatric populations.[62–64] In a multicentered survey of 5400 pediatric urologic laparoscopic procedures, Peters[62] showed that the clearest predictor of complication rate was laparoscopic experience. Soulie et al[64] have reported a decrease of complication rate from 9% for the first 100 to 4% for the subsequent 250 procedures. Most intraoperative complications (2.6%) were vascular and visceral injuries, whereas postoperative complications (2.8%) were predominantly thromboembolism and wound infection at trocar sites. Complications of retroperitoneal renal surgery are rare and mainly vascular or colonic injury. Kumar et al[65] reported a major complication rate of 3.5% of 316 patients (aged 4–88 years) who underwent retroperitoneoscopic urologic surgery. Vascular injuries occurred in 7 patients, 5 of whom required immediate conversion to open surgery. Four patients (1.2%) had other major complications, including colonic injury, retroperitoneal collections, and incisional hernia.

In our experience with 65 retroperitoneal nephrectomy cases, we had one vascular tear, during a teaching session, at the origin of a lumbar vein, in a case of xanthogranulomatous pyelonephritis. A clip without the need to convert to open surgery successfully closed the tear. In retroperitoneal procedures, traction on the kidney towards the top of the screen stretches renal vessels, reducing bleeding while evaluating the feasibility of the hemostasis by laparoscopic measures. The only postoperative complication we experienced was a postoperative hematoma after pretransplant bilateral nephrectomy; this hematoma was drained percutaneously. In the pretransplant kidney, we recommend an indwelling drainage tube for 24 hours.

The most common incident of the retroperitoneal approach is the pneumoperitonium secondary to peritoneal tear.[36,65] This incident occurred in nearly 30% of our cases in the early experience, but then could be avoided by careful preparation of the retroperitoneal space for insertion of the anterior working ports. When this occurs at the beginning of the procedure, the retroperitoneal working space is reduced by the effect of the pneumoperitoneum.

This can be managed either by laparoscopic suturing of the tear or, if this is not possible, by inserting a Veress needle in the peritoneal cavity to evacuate the gas during the procedure. If the tear occurs after the ligature of the renal vessels, during dissection of the anterior surface of the kidney or the ureter, the procedure can usually be accomplished without special management of the pneumoperitoneum.

# Conclusion

Minimally invasive procedures emphasize our goals of improving patient comfort and safety while adapting the laparoscopic procedures as closely as possible to conventional surgical techniques with respect to the operative time, cost, and surgical principles.

Indications of laparoscopy in pediatric urology are expanding with more centers being involved in the evolution of the different procedures. To avoid a discouraging learning curve, we recommend pediatric urologists acquire their experience in a progressive pattern. Nephrectomy for MCDK or hydronephrosis is a relatively safe and easy procedure for getting the surgeon to use the laparoscopic exposure of the upper tract. When the surgeon is familiar with the exposure, he can proceed to more difficult nephrectomies: pretransplant and partial nephrectomy.

Time can only be limited by training. Today, training is easily available in many centers of adult and pediatric surgery. Experienced peers are also available to accompany the surgeon in his initial experience, especially in the era of telerobotic surgery.[66] Mentored laparoscopic teaching is a safe way to introduce advanced urologic laparoscopic procedures in the pediatric urology department.[67] This might improve the results of the surgeon's initial experience with laparoscopy and encourage its development among a larger number of pediatric urologists.

# References

1. Warady BA, Hebert D, Sullivan EK, et al. Renal transplantation, chronic dialysis, and chronic renal insufficiency in children and adolescents. The 1995 Annual Report of the North American Pediatric Renal Transplant Cooperative Study. Pediatr Nephrol 1997; 11:49–64.

2. Woolf AS, Winyard PJD. Gene expression and cell turn over in human renal dysplasia. Histol Histopathol 2000; 15:159–66.

3. El-Ghoneimi A, Berrebi D, Levacher B, et al. Glial cell line derived neurotrophic factor is expressed by the epithelia of human renal dysplasia. J Urol 2002; 168:2424–8.

4. Glassberg K. Normal and abnormal development of the kidney: a clinician's interpretation of current knowledge. J Urol 2002; 167:2339–51.

5. Woolf AS, Winyard PJD. Advances in the cell biology and genetics of human kidney malformations. J Am Soc Nephrol 1998; 9:1114–25.

6. Winyard P, Chitty L. Dysplastic and polycystic kidneys: diagnosis, associations and management. Prenat Diagn 2001; 21:924–35.

7. Lifson BJ, Teichman JM, Hulbert JC. Role and long-term results of laparoscopic decortication in solitary cystic and autosomal dominant polycystic kidney disease. J Urol 1998; 159:702–5.

8. Dunn MD, Portis AJ, Naughton C, et al. Laparoscopic cyst marsupialization in patients with autosomal dominant polycystic kidney disease. J Urol 2001; 165:1888–92.

9. Belk RA, Thomas DF, Mueller RF, et al. A family study and the natural history of prenatally detected unilateral multicystic dysplastic kidney. J Urol 2002; 167:666–9.

10. Bolduc S, Upadhyay J, Restrepo R, et al. Renal ultrasonography and nuclear renal scintigraphy in the evaluation of duplex systems predict the extent of histological lesions. Br J Urol Int 2002; 89(s2):38.

11. Van Eijk L, Cohen-Overbeek TE, Den Hollander NS, et al. Unilateral multicystic dysplastic kidney: a combined pre- and postnatal assessment. Ultrasound Obstet Gynecol 2002; 19:180–3.

12. Hiraoka M, Tsukahara H, Ohshima Y, et al. Renal aplasia is the predominant cause of congenital solitary kidneys. Kidney Int 2002; 61:1840–4.

13. Lazebnik N, Bellinger MF, Ferguson JE 2nd. Insights into the pathogenesis and natural history of fetuses with multicystic dysplastic kidney disease. Prenat Diagn 1999; 19:418–23.

14. Deeb A, Robertson A, MacColl G, et al. Multicystic dysplastic kidney and Kallmann's syndrome: a new association? Nephrol Dial Transplant 2001; 16:1170–5.

15. Weiser AC, Amukele SA, Palmer LS. Metachronous presentation of ureterovesical junction obstruction contralateral to a multicystic dysplastic kidney. J Urol 2002; 167:2538–9.

16. Ranke A, Schmitt M, Didier F, Droulle P. Antenatal diagnosis of multicystic renal dysplasia. Eur J Pediatr Surg 2001; 11:246–54.

17. Feldenberg LR, Siegel NJ. Clinical course and outcome for children with multicystic dysplastic kidneys. Pediatr Nephrol 2000; 14:1098–101.

18. Mathiot A, Liard A, Eurin D, Dacher J. [Prenatally detected multicystic renal dysplasia and the associated anomalies of the genito-urinary tract]. J Radiol 2002; 83:731–5.

19. Peters CA, Carr MC, Lais A, et al. The response of the fetal kidney to obstruction. J Urol 1992; 148:503–9.

20. Attar R, Quinn F, Winyard PJ et al. Short-term urinary flow impairment deregulates PAX2 and PCNA expression and cell survival in fetal sheep kidneys. Am J Pathol 1998; 152:1225–35.

21. Oliveira EA, Diniz JS, Vilasboas AS, et al. Multicystic dysplastic kidney detected by fetal sonography: conservative management and follow-up. Pediatr Surg Int 2001; 17:54–7.

22. Rudnik-Schoneborn S, John U, Deget F, et al. Clinical features of unilateral multicystic renal dysplasia in children. Eur J Pediatr 1998; 157:666–72.

23. Ambrose SS, Gould RA, Trulock TS, Parrott TS. Unilateral multicystic renal disease in adults. J Urol 1982; 128:366–9.

24. Holloway WR, Weinstein SH. Percutaneous decompression: treatment for respiratory distress secondary to multicystic dysplastic kidney. J Urol 1990; 144:113–15.

25. Shah MS, Glassberg KI. Multicystic dysplastic kidney disease. In: Gearhart JP, Rink RC, Mouriquand PDE, eds. Pediatric urology. Philadelphia: WB Saunders, 2001:279–87.

26. Elder JS, Hladky D, Selzman AA. Outpatient nephrectomy for nonfunctioning kidneys. J Urol 1995; 154:712–14.

27. Seeman T, John U, Blahova K, et al. Ambulatory blood pressure monitoring in children with unilateral multicystic dysplastic kidney. Eur J Pediatr 2001; 160:78–83.

28. Homsy YL, Anderson JH, Oudjhane K, Russo P. Wilms tumor and multicystic dysplastic kidney disease. J Urol 1997; 158:2256–9.

29. Minevich E, Wacksman J, Phipps L, et al. The importance of accurate diagnosis and early close followup in patients with suspected multicystic dysplastic kidney. J Urol 1997; 158:1301–4.

30. Perez LM, Naidu SI, Joseph DB. Outcome and cost analysis of operative versus nonoperative management of neonatal multicystic dysplastic kidneys. J Urol 1998; 160:1207–11.

31. Zerin J. Computed tomography and magnetic resonance imaging of the kidneys in children. In: Gearhart JP, Rink R, Mouriquand PDE, eds. Pediatric urology. Philadelphia: WB Saunders 2001:124–39.

32. Joshi VV, Beckwith JB. Multilocular cyst of the kidney (cystic nephroma) and cystic, partially differentiated nephroblastoma. Terminology and criteria for diagnosis. Cancer 1989; 64:466–79.

33. Blazer S, Zimmer EZ, Blumenfeld Z, et al. Natural history of fetal simple renal cysts detected in early pregnancy. J Urol 1999; 162:812–14.

34. Hayden Ck Jr, Swischuk LE, Smith TH, Armstrong EA. Renal cystic disease in childhood. Radiographics 1986; 6:97–116.

35. Morgan C Jr, Rader D. Laparoscopic unroofing of a renal cyst. J Urol 1992; 148:1835–6.

36. El-Ghoneimi A, Valla JS, Steyaert H, Aigrain Y. Laparoscopic renal surgery via a retroperitoneal approach in children. J Urol 1998; 160:1138–41.

37. Micali S, Caione P, Virgili G, et al. Retroperitoneal laparoscopic access in children using a direct vision technique. J Urol 2001; 165:229–32.

38. Clayman RV, Kavoussi LR, Soper NJ, et al. Laparoscopic nephrectomy: initial case report. J Urol 1991; 146:278–82.

39. Ehrlich RM, Gershman A, Mee S, Fuchs G. Laparoscopic nephrectomy in a child: expanding horizons for laparoscopy in pediatric urology. J Endourol 1992; 6:463.

40. Das S, Keizur JJ, Tashima M. Laparoscopic nephroureterectomy for end-stage reflux nephropathy in a child. Surg Laparosc Endosc 1993; 3:462–5.

41. Ehrlich RM, Gershman A, Fuchs G. Laparoscopic renal surgery in children. J Urol 1994; 151:735–9.

42. Roberts J. Retroperitoneal endoscopy. J Med Primatol 1976; 5:124–7.

43. Gaur D. Laparoscopic operative retroperitoneoscopy: use of a new device. J Urol 1992; 148:1137–9.

44. Doublet JD, Barreto HS, Degremont AC, et al. Retroperitoneal nephrectomy: comparison of laparoscopy with open surgery. World J Surg 1996; 20:713–16.

45. Guilloneau B, Ballanger P, Lugagne PM, et al. Laparoscopic versus lumboscopic nephrectomy. Eur Urol 1996; 29:288–91.

46. Valla JS, Guilloneau B, Montupet P, et al. Retroperitoneal laparoscopic nephrectomy in children. Preliminary report of 18 cases. Eur Urol 1996; 30:490–3.

47. Abbou C, Cicco A, Gasman D, et al. Retroperitoneal laparoscopic versus open radical nephrectomy. J Urol 1999; 61:1776–80.

48. Hemal AK, Gupta NP, Wadhwa SN, et al. Retroperitoneoscopic nephrectomy and nephroureterectomy for benign nonfunctioning kidneys: a single-center experience. Urology 2001; 57(4):644–9.

49. Borer JG, Cisek LJ, Atala A, et al. Pediatric retroperitoneoscopic nephrectomy using 2 mm. instrumentation. J Urol 1999; 162:1725–9; discussion 1730.

50. Kobashi KC, Chamberlin DA, Rajpoot D, Shanberg AM. Retroperitoneal laparoscopic nephrectomy in children. J Urol 1998; 160:1142–4.

51. Shanberg AM, Sanderson K, Rajpoot D, Duel B. Laparoscopic retroperitoneal renal and adrenal surgery in children. BJU Int 2001; 87(6):521–4.

52. El-Ghoneimi A, Sauty L, Maintenant J, et al. Laparoscopic retroperitoneal nephrectomy in high risk children. J Urol 2000; 164:1076–9.

53. Diemunsch P, Becmeur F, Meyer P. Retroperitoneoscopy versus laparoscopy in piglets: ventilatory and thermic repercussions. J Pediatr Surg 1999; 34:1514–17.

54. Bales GT, Fellner SK, Chodak GW, Rukstalis DB. Laparoscopic bilateral nephrectomy for renin-mediated hypertension. Urology 1994; 43:874–7.

55. Peters C. Laparoendoscopic renal surgery in children. J Endourol 2000; 14:841–7.

56. Borzi P. A comparison of the lateral and posterior retroperitoneoscopic approach for complete and partial nephroureterectomy in children. BJU Int 2001; 87:517–20.

57. Adams JB, Micali S, Moore RG, et al. Complications of extraperitoneal balloon dilation. J Endourol 1996; 10:375–8.

58. Hamilton BD, Gatti JM, Cartwright PC, Snow BW. Comparison of laparoscopic versus open nephrectomy in the pediatric population. J Urol 2000; 163:937–9.

59. York GB, Robertson FM, Cofer BR, et al. Laparoscopic nephrectomy in children. Surg Endosc 2000; 14:469–72.

60. Yao D, Poppas DP. A clinical series of laparoscopic nephrectomy, nephroureterectomy and heminephroureterectomy in the pediatric population. J Urol 2000; 163:1531–5.

61. Fornara P, Doehn C, Friedrich HJ, Jocham D. Nonrandomized comparison of open flank versus laparoscopic nephrectomy in 249 patients with benign renal disease. Eur Urol 2001; 40:24–31.

62. Peters CA. Complications in pediatric urological laparoscopy: results of a survey. J Urol 1996; 155:1070–3.

63. Rassweiler J, Fornara P, Weber M, et al. Laparoscopic nephrectomy: the experience of the laparoscopy working group of the German Urologic Association. J Urol 1998; 160:18–21.

64. Soulie M, Seguin P, Richeux L, et al. Urological complications of laparoscopic surgery: experience with 350 procedures at a single center. J Urol 2001; 165:1960–63.

65. Kumar M, Kumar R, Hemal AK, Gupta NP. Complications of retroperitoneoscopic surgery at one centre. BJU Int 2001; 87:607–12.

66. Docimo SG, Moore RG, Adams J, et al. Early experience with telerobotic surgery in children. J Telemed Telecare 1996; 2:48–50.

67. El-Ghoneimi A, Farhat W, Bagli D, et al. Mentored retroperitoneal laparoscopic renal surgery in children: a safe approach to learning. BJU Int 2002; 89(s2):78.

# 11

# Pediatric lower urinary tract minimally invasive surgery

Patrick C Cartwright, Brent W Snow, and Todd Renschler

## Endoscopic management of reflux

The least invasive procedures for the treatment of vesico-ureteral reflux require no incision at all. In the early 1970s, Teflon (polytetrafluoroethylene paste) was first cystoscopically injected into the bladder neck to treat urinary incontinence. Matouschek introduced the idea of Teflon injection to treat reflux in 1981.[1] The subureteric injection was popularized by O'Donnell and Puri in the early 1980s and termed the STING procedure.[2] Since that time, multiple injectable substances have been developed and studied in order to provide the ideal treatment for reflux. This ideal substance should be nonimmunogenic, nonmigratory, noninflammatory, stable over time, and deliverable via a cystoscope. Although the injectable substances vary, the technique is essentially the same for all subureteric injection procedures.

The procedure usually lasts about 15 min and is performed under general anesthesia via the cystoscope. A needle perforates the mucosa 3–4 mm distal to the ureteral orifice at the 6 o'clock position. The needle is then advanced 5–8 mm prior to injection, with the targeted space being the lamina propria. The needle is left in place for about 30 s after injection to prevent extrusion after needle removal. Visually, the final goal of injection is an inverted crescent shape to the ureteral orifice. Ureteral catheterization may be used to facilitate the injection, and either the lower pole ureteral orifice or both may be injected for duplicated systems. Results have varied using this same technique with different substances, and most debate regarding endoscopic treatment of reflux deals with the specific safety profile and efficacy of those substances.

## Teflon

Subureteric Teflon injection or STING is the oldest of these procedures and hence has the longest follow-up to date.

Teflon consists of polytetrafluoroethylene (PTFE) particles in a 50% suspension with glycerine. After injection, the glycerine is absorbed, leaving the PTFE particles in place permanently. A fibrous capsule then forms around the Teflon plug. The STING procedure has been mainly performed in Europe. With 11–17 years of follow-up reported in one series by Chertin et al, 393 ureters in 258 patients were injected with Teflon, with a mean follow-up of 13.5 years.[3] Preoperatively, reflux was graded as follows: grade II 4.1%, grade III 64%, grade IV 25%, and grade V 7%. Reflux resolved after one injection in 76.8% and converted to grade I or II in 4.8%, requiring no further treatment. A cumulative success rate of 90.3% was achieved after a second injection, 92.9% after a third, and 93.4% after a fourth. Open ureteroneocystotomy was required in 1.8% of ureters that were refractory to STING treatment. No adverse effects related to the Teflon were noted, and there was no particular difficulty with the post-STING reimplants. A 5% long-term recurrence was described, and these patients were observed for low-grade reflux and subjected to a repeat procedure.

A large, multicenter European survey yielded similar results to the Dublin data:[4] 53 pediatric surgeons in 41 centers responded to the survey and were able to amass a STING database of 12,251 ureters in 8332 children with a median follow-up of 6 years; 75.3% and 87.4% ureteral resolution rates were seen after one and two injections, respectively. Open ureteral reimplantation was required in 4.5% because of failed STING and in 0.33% because of post-STING obstruction. The STING procedure has also been shown to have slightly poorer results for STING after failed reimplant and in duplex systems.[5–7]

The main concern that has arisen since the introduction of STING has been the safety profile of injecting a non-biologic substance into children. Aaronson et al showed the ability of Teflon to migrate to the lungs and brains in dogs who had their bladders injected.[8] Three cases of Teflon migration to pelvic lymph nodes in post-STING children have also been reported.[9] Most concerning is a case of ischemic brain injury that occurred in a 6-year-old girl 1 year after STING, although her stroke could not be definitively linked to Teflon migration. Because of the concerns of Teflon migration, the STING procedure has gained limited acceptance in the United States. However, proponents of the procedure note that no adverse effect of Teflon migration has been noted in their large series of patients with extended follow-up.

## Collagen

Bovine collagen has also been investigated as a biologic alternative to Teflon. Bovine collagen is treated with pepsin to decrease antigenicity and cross-linked with glutaraldehyde (a combination termed GAX) to prevent breakdown. After injection, histology reveals a foreign body reaction with fibroblast invasion and human collagen.[10] Although collagen is a biologic substance which inherently seems safe, there are immunologic concerns with injection of bovine collagen. All candidates should be skin tested 4 weeks prior to the procedure. Three percent will demonstrate a delayed hypersensitivity reaction and are not eligible for the procedure termed SCIN (subureteric collagen injection). After injection, 22–30% will develop antibovine collagen antibodies, predominantly immunoglobulin G (IgG) type.[11,12] There have been no documented cases of autoimmune disorders with SCIN, although this remains a concern and theoretical possibility. The only known immunologic complication in pediatric patients is a local inflammatory reaction after repeat injection in a seropositive girl.[12]

Even with these immunologic possibilities, the greatest obstacle to widespread SCIN is its lower resolution rates and lack of long-term durability. Frey et al performed SCIN in 132 patients and 204 ureters.[13] At a median follow-up of 33 months, reflux resolved in 62.7% of ureters after a single injection and 66 ureters underwent a second injection with a 54.5% resolution rate; furthermore, 10% developed a late recurrence of reflux. The tendency of reflux to recur late in collagen injection patients was marked in another study of 58 refluxing ureters in 36 patients.[14] Initial reflux resolution was 95%, but declined to 35% at 1 year and only 9% after 37 months. The explanation for the long-term failure of collagen injections is bovine collagen breakdown and volume loss of the subureteral plug. The collagen preparation used routinely has a final collagen concentration of 35 mg/ml (GAX 35), and has been shown in a pig model to decrease its size by 27% at 6 months after injection. A 65 mg/ml paste (GAX 65) has been developed to prevent breakdown and, in the same porcine model, implant volume decreased by only 0.1%.[15] GAX 65 injections were performed in 28 ureters

with a 3-month resolution rate of 87.5%.[16] However, long-term studies have not been published and cannot address the biggest concern of SCIN, which is the question of long-term durability.

## Polydimethylsiloxane (Macroplastique)

Polydimethylsiloxane is a solid, silicone elastomer that has also been investigated as an injectable substance. Macroplastique consists of these particles suspended in a hydrogel with a mean particle size of 209 μm.[17] The larger particle size provides a theoretical advantage to limiting migration of the material, since macrophages are unable to phagocytose particles greater than 80 μm. Histologically, a fibrous capsule develops around the implant, surrounding a foreign body reaction. Clinical results reveal 81% overall reflux resolution rate after a single injection and 18 months median follow-up.[18] This rate increased to 90% after two injections. Interestingly, resolution rates declined as reflux grade increased, with a major decrease in efficacy for grade IV reflux (45% resolution). In children with bilateral reflux, patient resolution rates decreased to 74% after one injection and 87% after two. Long-term recurrent and de-novo reflux developed in 3% and 3% of patients, respectively. Other clinical series have similar resolution rates in a similar short follow-up period.[19]

In much the same way Teflon is viewed, polydimethylsiloxane has considerable clinical success but also raises concerns of patient safety. Smith et al demonstrated particle migration locally and distantly to the spleen in dogs after subureteral injection.[20] Periurethral injections in another dog study revealed migration to a lung venule. Lymph node migration after subureteral injection in a 10-month-old girl has also been reported.[21] These findings, coupled with a troubled past of silicone implants in the United States, no doubt will be a formidable obstacle to the widespread use of Macroplastique in the United States despite its relative clinical efficacy.

## Deflux

Because it consists of a biologic material with a theoretically better safety profile, Deflux has received greater recent attention and enthusiasm in the United States. The injectable paste consists of 80–120 μm microspheres of dextranomer (a polysaccharide of dextran) suspended in hyaluronic acid. Because of its relatively larger size, Deflux is theoretically less likely to migrate beyond the subureteral space. In a rabbit model, the dextranomer spheres did not demonstrate migration to other organs.[22] Even if Deflux were to migrate, it would probably be hydrolyzed to glucose and water. After implantation, histologic findings of the distal ureter reveal granulomatous inflammation with multinucleated giant cells and other inflammatory cells. The implant site is surrounded by a fibrotic pseudocapsule containing dextranomer at different stages of resorption and calcification as well as eosinophils in some patients but not others.[23]

The demonstration of dextranomer resorption in vivo raises the question of long-term durability. However, relatively long-term follow-up is available after Deflux injection. A retrospective review of 221 patients with 334 refluxing ureters was performed with a mean follow-up of 5 years.[24] Overall, 68% of patients and 75% of ureters had a positive response (grade I or less) at time of last follow-up. Only 54% of patients demonstrated grade I or less reflux after a single injection. A 4% long-term recurrence rate was also demonstrated. No obstruction or hydronephrosis developed as well. As with other materials, resolution rates tended to be higher for lower grades of reflux. Other studies with shorter follow-up times reveal only slightly better results.[25,26]

Based on the above clinical results, a computer model was developed to compare cost of traditional reflux management to different clinical scenarios that included endoscopic injection with Deflux. Although methodology of the study may be questioned, it does point out the potential savings in the overall cost of correcting reflux when using subureteric injection approaches, with savings ranging from $889 to $2218 per patient, depending upon the clinical scenario.[27]

## Other materials and issues

In addition to the injectable substances used most commonly, other materials are being investigated currently. Urocol paste consists of triple calcium phosphate ceramic suspended in a gel. At 6 months follow-up, 71% success has been reported in 346 ureters.[28] Coaptite is a similar calcium hydroxylapatite suspension that has been used in 40 patients. Initial 3-month cure rates for grade II, III, and IV were 95%, 55%, and 42%, respectively.[29] Autologous chondrocytes have also been injected. They have the advantage of avoiding concerns about foreign materials but do require a second anesthetic to harvest the chondrocytes. Results at 3 months show a 57% success rate for a single injection. At 1 year after multiple injections, 70% of ureters and 65% of patients are cured.[30] All of these newer materials lack long-term follow-up, but may prove to be comparably better substances.

Another issue that has been raised by Capozza et al has been the use of endoscopic injection in children with voiding dysfunction. They hypothesize that high voiding pressures cause displacement of the implant material and are responsible for many treatment failures. Based on voiding dysfunction questionnaires, they have shown that success rates decline as the degree of voiding dysfunction increases. The authors have concluded that endoscopic injection should not be performed in untreated dysfunctional voiders.[31]

## Summary

The combination of antibiotic prophylaxis and open surgical ureteral reimplantation has had great success in the management of vesicoureteral reflux. Many children, especially with low-grade reflux, can be spared any manipulation with prophylaxis as their reflux resolves naturally with time. Open reimplantation has a remarkable success rate, with relatively rare complications and minimal morbidity. Most children are discharged from the hospital in 1 to 2 days with low pain medication requirements. Certainly, the bar is high for other management techniques. Even with these successes, we should still continue to find ways to improve and limit the discomfort that our treatment strategies have on our young patients. Current goals include decreasing hospital stay, limiting cystography, minimizing pain, and lowering costs of treatment. Endoscopic management holds great promise because it may accomplish many of these goals. However, questions as to the long-term stability and safety of the procedure remain. Injections of Teflon and silicone particles have the highest resolution rates and seem to be more durable, but particles have been shown to migrate in children. Many physicians have a great sense of unease about implanting a foreign material that will remain with the child for a lifetime. Alternatively, biologic materials have been employed, but are hampered with durability issues as the body breaks down the implant over time. Studies on collagen injections have clearly shown that long-term recurrence is an obstacle to its widespread use. Deflux appears to maintain its implant volume for longer periods of time, but histologic studies show that the material is resorbed from the implant site, although at a lesser rate than bovine collagen. At the current time, Deflux has a growing number of proponents. Surgeons are willing to accept the lower success rates for a greater safety profile. The reflux resolution rates can also be maximized by applying the procedure to select patients: namely, those with lesser grades who lack voiding dysfunction.

In its current state, endoscopic management is seen as a substitute or alternative to open reimplantation. However, because of its minimally morbid nature, subureteral injection may alter the way we approach reflux completely. This technique could easily be applied in early treatment as an alternative to antibiotic prophylaxis. One study has already demonstrated higher resolution rates with Deflux when prospectively compared to antibiotic prophylaxis in short follow-up. More research on the application of current materials as well as the development of new materials is warranted.

# Origins of percutaneous bladder procedures

The smaller bony structure of the pelvis in children causes the bladder to assume an intra-abdominal position. This creates relatively easy access to this area for minimally invasive procedures. For decades, suprapubic access to the bladder for urine aspiration and culture has been a standard practice in young children. As instrumentation has improved, a variety of problems have been approached in this manner, including things such as antegrade ablation of posterior urethral valves via a trocar placed into the bladder.[32] More recently, it has been suggested that placing a scope through such an access port may be of value in observing the bladder neck while periurethral injection of bulking agents is performed. Additionally, suprapubic access is valuable as an adjunct to ureteroscopy or ureteral catheterization in patients with an altered ureteral positioning, such as those having undergone cross-trigonal reimplants[33] or renal transplantation where transurethral approaches may fail. Experience with occasional transvesical procedures such as these inevitably led pediatric urologists to apply these techniques to the correction of the common problem of vesicoureteral reflux.

# Extravesical ureteral reimplantation

Initial attempts at laparoscopic correction of reflux were made transperitoneally using a modified Lich reimplant technique.[34] The techniques were initially reported in 1993–94 in a porcine model.[35,36] Since vesicoureteral reflux does not naturally occur in most animals, the reflux had to be first created by making an endoscopic incision of the ureteral tunnel. One camera port and two or three other transperitoneal working ports were utilized and the posterior bladder wall was exposed. Detrusor incisions were made superolateral to the ureteral hiatus, detrusor muscle was separated from the epithelium, the ureter was positioned within the trough, and the detrusor was closed over the ureter with absorbable sutures or staples. In these studies, 13–15 laparoscopic reimplanted ureters were free of reflux at 3–6 months after surgery, while one ureter became obstructed. The average operating times were 132 and 141 min in the two respective studies.[35,36]

In 1994, Ehrlich et al reported on two patients with successful outcomes from laparoscopic extravesical reimplantation.[37] Shortly after, Janetschek and coworkers reported outcomes in 6 children,[38] one of whom required postoperative ureteral stenting for 6 weeks. The authors felt that the procedure was complex and unwieldy and offered no significant advantage to the patients. Despite this, others have pursued extravesical laparoscopic reimplantation in children. Fung and colleagues have more recently reported 36 ureters repaired in 26 children (ages 4–13 years old).[39] Their technique involved utilizing four ports; only one patient had persistent reflux at 3 months and the operative time was about 1.5 hours per ureter. Even with improved techniques, the overall recovery from a laparoscopic extravesical reimplant seems to be not significantly easier or quicker than that following open extravesical reimplant procedures, except possibly in the amount of pain medicine required. Because of the difficulty in fully visualizing the deep retrovesical space and the steep procedural learning curve involved, this technique has not gained widespread acceptance.

# Transvesical ureteral reimplantation

Following the initial reports of laparoscopic extravesical reimplantation, two groups reported on experience with combined laparoscopic (transvesical) and cystoscopic (transurethral) reimplantation in adults and children.[40,41] These procedures were initially based upon the Gil-Vernet trigonoplasty technique[42] and have been termed endoscopic trigonoplasty or percutaneous endoscopic trigonoplasty (PET procedure).

The technique of the combined transvesical/ transurethral approach to reimplantation begins with cystoscopy to assess the bladder. Two small transvesical trocars are placed under cystoscopic guidance at the 10 and 2 o'clock positions near the dome of the bladder (Figure 11.1). An Endoclose needle (Ethicon) is used to pass a 2-0 polyglactin suture just beside the trocar through the rectus fascia and muscle and into the bladder. A cystoscopic grasper retrieves the free end of the suture within the bladder and the empty needle is withdrawn and passed again on the opposite side of the trocar. The grasper then passes the suture to the empty Endoclose needle and the suture is drawn up through the fascia to the skin (Figure 11.2). The suture is tied loosely around the trocar and prevents the bladder wall from slipping off of the trocar during the procedure. The same is done for each trocar placed into the bladder. This placement technique will allow for single suture closure of the bladder wall and rectus fascia and muscle.

The bladder is then drained and 'pneumobladder' is created with $CO_2$ insufflation. The cystoscope may be used

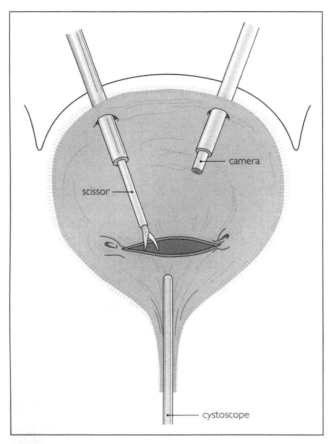

scissor

camera

cystoscope

**Figure 11.1**

Two transvesical trocars are placed under direct cystoscopic guidance at the 10 and 2 o'clock position near the dome of the bladder (12 o'clock position).

for suction of the operative site or, with the grasper inserted, for retraction during the procedure. During endoscopic trigonoplasty, the bladder epithelium between the two ureteral orifices, along the interureteric ridge, is cauterized and then using the miniature laparoscopic scissors the bladder epithelium is elevated both on the superior and inferior edges to create a 1 cm wide trough (Figure 11.3). Then, 3-0 polyglactin sutures (2) are placed on the medial edge of each ureteral orifice in such a fashion as to bury the knot when the suture is tied (Figure 11.4). This draws the ureteral orifices to the midline over exposed bladder muscle (Figure 11.5). Interrupted 4-0 polyglactin sutures are then used to reappose the bladder epithelium in the midline and complete the reimplant. Catheter drainage is used postoperatively, leaving either a small tube via a trocar site as a suprapubic tube or placing a urethral catheter. The trocars are removed and the sutures tied, which creates a watertight bladder wall closure and closes the fascia at the same time.

## Combined endoscopic/transvesical reimplant results

In 1995, Okamura and associates reported outcomes in 12 adult patients with low- and moderate-grade vesicoureteral reflux utilizing the endoscopic trigonoplasty technique.[40] Their technique differed slightly from the one described with the two suprapubic trocars placed in the vertical midline of the bladder and suturing being done with a 'ski' needle via the cystoscopic grasper rather than with a needle holder placed through a port. A single horizontal mattress suture was used and early cystogram showed resolution in all patients. In 1996, Cartwright et al reported their experience of 22 children having the percutaneous endoscopic trigonoplasty procedure.[41] Reflux was of a moderate grade in most and a high grade in a few. There was no ureteral obstruction encountered and no reflux immediately after the procedure. As follow-up was extended to 6 months, reflux resolved in 20 of the 32 ureters, for a resolution rate of 62.5%. Success could not be correlated to patient age, laterality, initial grade of reflux, or preoperative bladder instability. Complications were encountered, including significant hyponatremia and a perivesical urine collection requiring drainage. It was the authors' opinion that this was technically feasible but the learning curve was significant and technical modifications were necessary to improve the modest success rate to an acceptable level.

Pursuing the transvesical laparoscopic reimplant one step further, Gatti et al modified the procedure by completely mobilizing the ureters.[43] Trocar placements were similar and a stent was placed within the ureteral orifice and sewn to mucosa. Using the cystoscopic graspers, the orifice could be retracted, aiding greatly in the dissection. Using the miniature laparoscopic scissors, 2.5 cm of ureteral mobility was obtained; there was a technical concern that further dissection extravesically would allow $CO_2$ to escape in large amounts into the retroperitoneum, causing collapse of the working space within the lumen of the bladder. Tunnels for reimplanting the ureters were created by incising and dissecting the mucosa to create an appropriate crosstrigonal orientation. The dissected muscular hiatus was closed and the ureters were drawn across the bladder and secured with polyglactin sutures and epithelium closed over them. Subepithelial tunnel lengths of 2–2.5 cm were obtained. At 1 year follow-up, 10 of the 12 ureters showed no vesicoureteral reflux (5 of 7 patients). Yeung and Borzi have also performed cross-trigonal reimplants in 4 patients with good results.[44]

In 1997, Okumura and associates published a study with follow-up on 28 patients, many of whom were children who had undergone their endoscopic trigonoplasty.[45] Their resolution rates at 1–3 months were 95%, which had

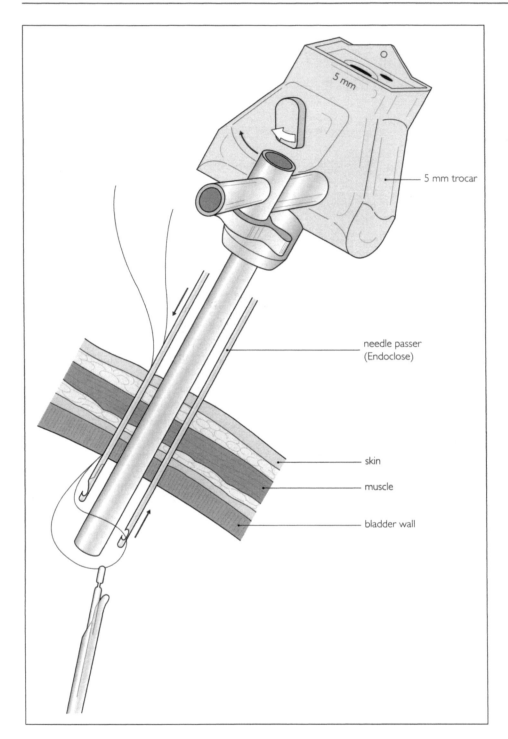

**Figure 11.2**
Prevent the bladder wall from slipping off of the canulla by passing a 2-0 polyglactin suture alongside the trocar through the rectus fascia and muscle and into the bladder. The suture is grasped and withdrawn on the opposite side of the trocar. The suture is tied loosely around the trocar insufflations side arm. This is repeated with the other transvesical trocar. This same suture is utilized to close the bladder wall and rectus fascia at the conclusion of the procedure.

decreased to 79% at 12 months. As Okumura et al did cystoscopy to evaluate their surgical repair, they found that the trigone had split in 5 of their patients, resulting in recurrent reflux in 3 patients. This same group continues to work on technique alterations to improve the outcome, being convinced that the recovery is better than that in open reimplant surgery (especially in adults).[46–48]

## Bladder autoaugmentation

Another minimally invasive operation that has been performed on the bladder is bladder autoaugmentation or detrusor myectomy. This has generally been carried out transperitoneally, exposing the dome of the bladder and taking great care to dissect away detrusor fibers while

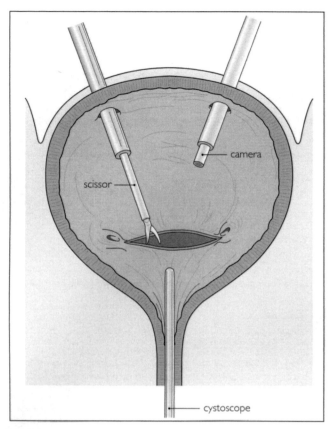

**Figure 11.3**
During endoscopic trigonoplasty, the bladder epithelium between the two ureteral orifices is incised with electrocautery, along the interureteric ridge. The trough is developed by elevating the superior and inferior edges with mini-laparoscopic scissors to create a 1 cm wide trough.

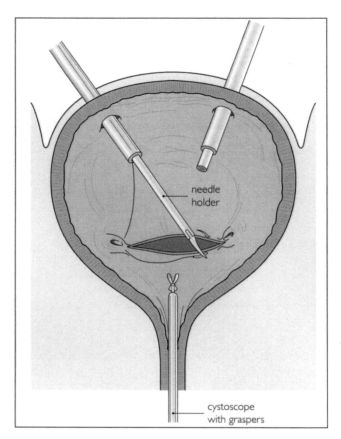

**Figure 11.4**
Utilizing mini-laparoscopic needle drivers, a 3-0 polyglactin suture (2) is placed on the medial edge of each ureteral orifice in such a fashion as to bury the knot.

keeping the epithelium intact and using either cautery or laser to divide the fibers. This allows the bladder epithelium to bulge into the peritoneal cavity, creating a bladder diverticulum at the dome in hopes of lessening filling pressures, minimizing detrusor instability, and (at times) to increase bladder capacity.[49,50] In general, results of laparoscopic autoaugmentation mirror those of open surgery.

## Miscellaneous procedures

There are unusual circumstances in which minimally invasive techniques may be creatively applied. One of the authors laparoscopically repaired an injury to the bladder neck and urethra discovered during laparoscopic partial colectomy and pull through (with mucosal proctectomy) in a 1-month-old baby. Placement of a transvesical trocar, in addition to the peritoneal trocars, allowed for guiding the difficult placement of a catheter across the injured area. In addition, laparoscopy has been used by the authors to close isolated bladder dome rupture from trauma.

## Perspective

Laparoscopic surgery in children carries the significant benefit of improved cosmesis, creating only small trocar site scars. However, the benefit of rapid recovery and return to full activity, which is well documented in the adult literature, is less well defined or demonstrable in this group. Younger children often bounce back so promptly from modest open procedures that the room for improvement in this regard is smaller than in adults. Indeed, in our practice, we will often perform unilateral, extravesical open reimplant as an outpatient procedure in younger children.

This said, as more precise and pediatric-specific laparoscopic equipment is designed, there is reason to think that our current techniques will be improved. In addition, the development of staples and clips that do not become the nidus for stone formation in the urinary tract would be of great utility. The current and mounting experience with robotic laparoscopic systems seems to hold great promise for the precise reconstructive ability required for good

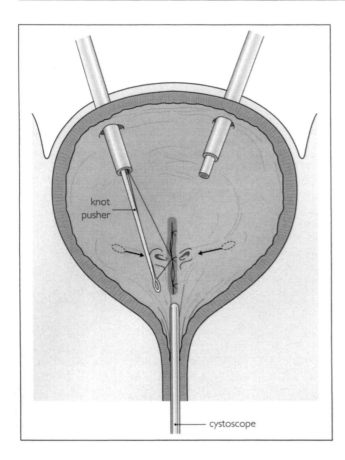

knot pusher

cystoscope

**Figure 11.5**
After placing and tying the suture, both ureteral orifices will be drawn closer to the midline.

outcomes in children. It appears clear that minimally invasive approaches to bladder surgery in children will continue to be pursued and will probably become, with time and experience, common surgical approaches.

# References

1. Matouschek E. Die Behandlund des Vesilorenalen Refluxes durch Transurethrale Einstritzung von Teflonpaste. Urolege 1981; 20:263.

2. O'Donnell B, Puri, P. Treatment of vesicoureteric reflux by endoscopic injection of Teflon. Br Med J 1984; 289:7.

3. Chertin B, Colhoun E, Velayudham M, Puri P. Endoscopic treatment of vesicoureteral reflux: 11 to 17 years of followup. J Urol 2002; 167:1443.

4. Puri P, Granata C. Multicenter survey of endoscopic treatment of vesicoureteral reflux using polytetrafluoroethylene. J Urol 1998; 160:1007.

5. Kumar R, Puri P. Endoscopic correction of vesicoureteric reflux in failed reimplanted ureters. Eur Urol 1998; 33:98.

6. Miyakita H, Ninan GK, Puri P. Endoscopic correction of vesico-ureteric reflux in duplex systems. Eur Urol 1993; 24:111.

7. Steinbrecher HA, Edwards B, Malon PSJ. The STING in the refluxing duplex system. Br J Urol 1995; 76:165.

8. Aaronson IA, Rames RA, Green WB, et al. Endoscopic treatment of reflux: migration of Teflon to the lungs and brain. Eur Urol 1993; 23:394.

9. Aragona F, D'Urso L, Scremin E, et al. Polytetrafluoroethylene giant granuloma and adenopathy: long-term complications following suburetal polytetrafluoroethylene injection for the treatment of vesicoureteral reflux in children. J Urol 1997; 158:1539.

10. Frey P, Lutz N, Berger D, Herzog B. Histological behavior of glutaraldehyde cross-linked bovine collagen injected into the human bladder for the treatment of vesicoureteral reflux. J Urol 1994; 152:632.

11. Inoue K, Nakamoto T, Usui A, Usui T. Evaluation of antibody class in response to endoscopic suburetal collagen injection in patients with vesicoureteral reflux. J Urol 2001; 165:555.

12. Leonard MP, Decter A, Hills K, Mix LW. Endoscopic suburetal collagen injection: are immunological concerns justified? J Urol 1998; 160:1012.

13. Frey P, Lutx N, Jenny P, Herzog B. Endoscopic suburetal collagen injection for the treatment of vesicoureteral reflux in infants and children. J Urol 1995; 154:804.

14. Haferkamp A, Contractor H, Mohring K, et al. Failure of suburetal bovine collagen injection for the endoscopic treatment of primary vesicoureteral reflux in long-term follow-up. Urology 2000; 55:759.

15. Frey P, Mangold S. Physical and histological behavior of a new injectable collagen (GAX 65) implanted into the submucosal space of the mini-pig bladder. J Urol 1995; 154:812.

16. Frey P, Gudinchet F, Jenny P. GAX 65: a new injectable cross-linked collagen for the endoscopic treatment of vesicoureteral reflux – a double-blind study evaluating its efficiency in children. J Urol 1997; 158:1210.

17. Solomon LX, Birch BR, Cooper, AJ, et al. Nonhomologous bioinjectable material in urology: size matters? BJU Int 2000; 85:641.

18. Herz D, Hafez A, Bagli D, et al. Efficacy of endoscopic suburetal polydimethylsiloxane injection for treatment of vesicoureteral reflux in children: a North American clinical report. J Urol 2001; 166:1880.

19. Al-Hunayean AA, Kehinde EO, Elsalam MA, Al-Mukhtar RS. Outcome of endoscopic treatment for vesicoureteral reflux in children using polydimethylsiloxane. J Urol 2002; 168:2181.

20. Smith DP, Kaplan WE, Oyasu R. Evaluation of polydimethylsiloxane as an alternative in the endoscopic treatment of vesicoureteral reflux. J Urol 1994; 152:1221.

21. Dewan PA, Hoebeke P, Hall HE, Chow CW, Edwards GA, Terlet J. Migration of particulate silicone after ureteric injection with silicone. BJU Int 2000; 85:557.

22. Stenberg A, Sundin A, Larsson BS, et al. Lack of distant migration after injection of a 125 iodine labeled dextranomer based implant into the rabbit bladder. J Urol 1997; 158:1937.

23. Stenberg A, Larsson E, Lackgren G. Endoscopic treatment with dextranomer-hyaluronic acid for vesicoureteral reflux: histological findings. J Urol 2003; 169:1109.

24. Lackgren G, Wahlin N, Skoldenber E, Stenberg A. Long-term followup of children treated with dextranomer/hyaluronic acid copolymer for vesicoureteral reflux. J Urol 2001; 166:1887.

25. Capoxxa N, Caione P. Dextranomer/hyaluronic acid copolymer implantation for vesico-ureteral reflux; a randomized comparison with antibiotic prophylaxis. J Pediatr 2002; 140:230.

26. Oswald J, Riccabona M, Lusuardi L, Bartsch G, Radmayr C. Prospective comparison and 1-year follow-up of a single endoscopic subureteral polydimethylsiloxane versus dextranomer/hyaluronic acid copolymer injection for treatment of vesicoureteral reflux in children. Urology 2002; 60:894.

27. Kobelt G, Canning DA, Hensle TW, Lackgren G. The cost-effectiveness of endoscopic injection of dextranomer/hyaluronic acid copolymer for vesicoureteral reflux. J Urol 2003; 169:1480.

28. Kajbafzadeh A, Habibi Z. Endoscopic subureteric urocol injection in treatment of vesicoureteral reflux in children. J Urol Suppl 2003; 169:170.

29. Mevorach R, Rabinowitz R, Beck C, Hulbert W. Endoscopic treatment of vesicoureteral reflux with coaptite. J Urol Suppl 2002; 167:107.

30. Caldamone AA, Diamond DA. Long-term results of the endoscopic correction of vesicoureteral reflux in children using autologous chondrocytes. J Urol 2001; 165:2224.

31. Capozza N, Patricolo M, Matarazzo AL, Paione P. Endoscopic treatment of vesico-ureteral reflux: twelve years' experience. Urol Int 2001; 67:228.

32. Zaontz MR, Firlit CF. Percutaneous antegrade oblation of posterior urethral valves in infants with small caliber urethras: an alternative to urinary diversion. J Urol 1986; 136:247.

33. Cohen SJ. Ureterozystoneostomie, eine neue Antireflux-technik. Aktvel Urol 1975; 6:1.

34. Lich R, Howerton LW, Davis LA. Recurrent urosepsis in children. J Urol 1961; 86:851.

35. Atala A, Kavoussi L, Goldstein D et al. Laparoscopic correction of vesicoureteral reflux. J Urol 1993; 150(2Pt 2):748.

36. Schimberg W, Wacksman J, Rudd R, et al. Laparoscopic correction of vesicoureteral reflux in the pig. J Urol 1994; 151(6):1664.

37. Ehrlich RM, Gershman A, Fuchs S. Laparoscopic vesico-ureteroplasty in children: initial case reports. Urology 1994; 43(2):255.

38. Janetschek G, Radmayr C, Bartsch G., Laparoscopic ureteral anti-reflux plasty reimplantation: first clinical experience. Annales d'Urologie 1995; 29(2):101.

39. Lakshmanan Y, Fung LC. Laparoscopic extravesicular ureteral reimplantation for vesicoureteral reflux: recent technical advances. J Endourol 2000; 14(7):589.

40. Okamura K. Ono Y, Yamada Y, Kato T, et al. Endoscopic trigonoplasty for primary vesicoureteric reflux. Br J Urol 1995; 75(3):390.

41. Cartwright P, Snow B, Mansfield J, et al. Percutaneous endoscopic trigonoplasty: a minimally invasive approach to correct vesicoureteral reflux. J Urol 1996; 156(2 Pt2):661.

42. Gil-Vernet, JM. New technique for surgical correction of vesicoureteral reflux. J Urol 1984; 131:456.

43. Gatti J, Cartwright P, Hamilton B, Snow B. Percutaneous endoscopic trigonoplasty in children: long term outcomes and modifications in technique. J Endourol 1999; 13(b):581.

44. Yeung CK, Borzi PA. Endoscopic transtrigonal ureteric reimplantation for refluxing and obstructive megaureters under carbon dioxide pneumovesicum: a novel technique. Abstract 24, AAP, Urology, San Francisco, California, 2001.

45. Okamura K, Kato N, Takamura S, et al. Trigonal splitting as a major complication of endoscopic trigonoplasty at one year follow-up. J Urol 1997; 157:1423.

46. Okamura K. Endoscopic trigonoplasty in pediatric patient with primary vesicoureteral reflux: preliminary report. J Urol 1996; 156:198.

47. Okamura K, Kato N, Tsuji, Y, et al. A comparitive study of endoscopic trigonoplasty for vesicoureteral reflux in children and in adults. Int J Urol 1999; 6(11):562.

48. Okamura K, Yamada Y, Kato T, et al. Trigonoplasty for vesicoureteral reflux – from open surgery to endoscopic surgery. Nippon Hinyokika Gakkai Zasshi 1994; 85(9):1368.

49. McDougall E, Clayman R, Figensham R, et al. Laparoscopic retropubic autoaugmentation of the bladder. J Urol 1995; 153:123.

50. Britanisky RG, Poppas DP, Schichman SN, et al. Laparoscopic laser-assisted bladder autoaugmentation. Urology 1995; 46:31.

# 12

# Pediatric voiding dysfunction, neurogenic bladder, and posterior urethral valves

Victor Braren

## Introduction

The lower urinary tract in children has long been approached using minimally invasive treatment techniques. The challenges of posterior urethral valves (PUV) and abnormalities of the bladder neck were well suited to these methods of management. Endoscopic approaches to lower urinary tract anatomy have required pediatric urologists to adapt miniaturized equipment and fine tune techniques for treatment of anomalies of this area. This has even allowed treatment of newborns.

As is so often the case, terminology becomes a problem in dealing with the lower urinary tract. Unacceptable, oxymoronic neologisms and misnomers such as 'non-neurogenic neurogenic bladder' have unfortunately made their way into the literature. Even the term 'voiding dysfunction' has been criticized as covering only a part of the impairment spectrum, disregarding the storage and other lower tract functions that may become deranged. However, if one assumes that storage must occur in order for voiding to take place, the term 'voiding dysfunction' becomes inclusive and will be used by this author throughout this discussion.

## Voiding function and dysfunction: Anatomy, histology, physiology, and pharmacology

Both the normal and pathologic anatomy and the histology of the lower urinary tract have been well delineated.

The function of the lower urinary tract is to allow efficient collection, storage, and voluntary, complete voiding of urine. During normal bladder filling there is a minimal rise in intravesical pressure despite the ongoing increase in volume; at the same time, a gradual increase in urethral resistance occurs. In the normal circumstance, there is no involuntary contractile detrusor activity and increases in intra-abdominal pressure do not cause urinary leakage. Prior to reaching bladder capacity, the sensation of bladder filling is perceived by the child and urination is voluntarily initiated; micturition proceeds to completion, with a decrease in bladder outlet resistance and contraction of the bladder smooth musculature.

Wein has observed[1] that the pathophysiology produced by an abnormal clinical state can often be explained according to a part of one theory of voiding but one should not take this to mean that the entirety of the theory is correct. After reviewing the literature, which contains many conflicting models of urinary tract function, the reader will have to adopt those precepts that are clinically and/or scientifically most useful to the situation at hand.

## Anatomy of the bladder

Both Galen and daVinci were interested in how human beings 'collected' urine and how the bladder emptied itself. Early on, the observation was made that the bladder contained three layers: an outer connective tissue layer, a set of smooth muscle layers, and mucosa lining the interior of the bladder. Classically, the smooth muscle of the bladder is considered to have two components: the detrusor and the trigone. The trigone is that region of the posterior bladder wall generally considered to be between the ureteral orifices and the bladder neck; it is further divided into the superficial area and deep trigone. Most observers believe that the detrusor is organized at the bladder base as an outer longitudinal, a middle circumferential, and an inner longitudinal layer. The superficial layer of the trigone is usually considered to be ureteral in origin, whereas the remainder of the outer musculature is endodermal. The anatomy of the ureteral orifice is considered elsewhere in this book.

## Anatomy of the urethra

The male and female urethras differ from each other considerably and will be described separately. The pediatric female urethra varies in length from about 8 mm in a term female to upwards of 4 cm in length and 6 mm in diameter in a postpubertal adolescent girl. It is embedded in the anterior aspect of the vagina, and consists of an outer muscular layer and an epithelium. The urethral epithelium at rest consists of longitudinal folds that are apposed to each other during the storage phase of the bladder. There is an inner longitudinal smooth muscle portion which extends throughout the length of the female child's urethra and there may or may not be an outer circular or semicircular layer; this is debated among anatomists. The smooth muscle of the pediatric female urethra is embedded in a matrix of collagen that is considered by most to be the major structural component.

The male urethra in a child is classically divided into anatomic segments. The preprostatitic urethra is only a few millimeters in length in the newborn male child but grows to 1.5 cm in length in adolescence. It contains smooth muscle bundles generally oriented in a circular arrangement that becomes continuous distally with the prostatic capsule; these muscle bundles are separated by connective tissue. The prostatic urethra is between 6 and 8 mm in length in a newborn male, growing to 2 cm in length in an adolescent. The membranous urethra is only 1 mm or so in length in the newborn male and may extend distally into the bulb of the penis. Some anatomists perceive longitudinal and/or circular fibers in the membranous urethra, while other observers are not in agreement. The anterior urethra is distal to the membranous portion and functions purely as a conduit; it is generally considered not to have a role in either maintaining continence or facilitating bladder emptying.

There is continuity between the bladder and urethra. The extension of the supravesical trigone layer into the urethral wall has been well described, and suggests that the opening of the bladder neck and proximal urethra during active bladder contraction is based in part on passive anatomic factors. The external sphincter has a voluntary striated muscle component that allows interruption of urinary flow in normal children.

In the male, the sphincter is described as completely annular, although decreased in its posterior component, as it blends with the fibers of the prostatic capsule, while in the female the area is described as tapering considerably and being deficient posteriorly. The intrinsic segment is often referred to as the rhabdosphincter and readers are referred to more in-depth discussions of the functional anatomy.[2] In both boys and girls, the caudal end of the striated component is adjacent to a bulky skeletal muscle structure oriented in the horizontal plane in the pelvic floor encircling the membranous urethra. This corresponds to what is described in standard anatomy textbooks as the external urethral sphincter. The presence of an intrinsic striated component is also agreed upon by most observers. The striated sphincter is generally considered to comprise both the intramural and intrinsic striated components of the female child's urethra and the posterior urethra in the male child.

Despite older observations in the literature, it is now generally regarded that the bladder neck does not contain an anatomic sphincter. Pseudosphincteric action at the bladder neck is thought to be due to the inherent tension exerted by elastic fibers in this area on the lumen of the bladder neck.

An understanding of the physiology and cellular biology of smooth and striated muscle relevant to the lower urinary tract is important in understanding the normal function of this region. Not only are structural innervation and neural control of muscle function important but also one must be aware of more basic concepts such as tonus, excitation–contraction coupling, and viscoelasticity. Knowledge of neurotransmission and receptors is also crucial. These issues are beyond the scope of this chapter.

## Anatomy of the gross peripheral innervation of the lower urinary tract

The bladder and urethra are supplied by efferent parasympathetic and sympathetic neurons through the pelvic and hypogastric nerves. Both of these bear afferent (sensory) neurons from the bladder and urethra back to the spinal cord. The pelvic nerve usually has three or four trunks that branch on either side of the rectum. Efferent sympathetic nerves traverse lumbar sympathetic ganglia and join the presacral nerve. This complex then divides into the left and right hypogastric nerves. The inferior hypogastric plexus is formed by a meeting of the hypogastric and pelvic nerves. Various branches of this plexus innervate the pelvic organs. Afferent neurons are borne by both the hypogastric and pelvic nerves to the lumbosacral spinal cord and by dorsal columns, reaching the spinal cord through either dorsal or ventral roots.

Efferent innervation of the striated sphincter is derived from the sacral spinal cord by means of the pudendal nerve. Whether the pudendal nucleus is the only motor center or not is debatable. The autonomic nervous system may also help innervate these muscles. Neural and humoral influences on lower urinary tract function, including receptor distribution, stimulation, and blockade, are being elucidated through the use of animal models, and are beyond the scope of this discussion.[3]

# Central nervous system control of the lower urinary tract

Voiding is a function of the peripheral autonomic nervous system. Final definitive control of lower urinary tract function however resides at higher neurologic levels. The spinal cord, brainstem, cerebellum, and basal ganglia may all exert functional control of the lower urinary tract. Likewise, very sophisticated laboratory experimentation has shown that there is a role for the thalamus, hypothalamus, limbic system, and cerebral cortex. Organization of the micturition reflex, including the possible role of the supraspinal micturition center and sacral areas, are key to the understanding of both normal and abnormal voiding. There are at least six component reflexes of micturition.[4]

## Clinical considerations

Wein et al have delineated several functional questions regarding urinary tract function.[5] The following questions and answers are based on these queries.

**What determines bladder response during filling?** The normal bladder responding to filling at a physiologic rate produces minimal change in intravesical pressure until capacity is approached. Normally, excellent compliance is brought about during the early stages of bladder filling by quiescent characteristics of the bladder wall. When the filling volume exceeds the rate of stress relaxation, the viscoelastic properties of the bladder wall allow for an increase in intravesical pressure. Therefore, there is little or no rise in bladder pressure until bladder capacity is approached. These phenomena can be explained by the classically demonstrated inherent responses of smooth muscle to stretch.

Partial bladder outlet obstruction can bring about a reduction in bladder capacity and compliance. This is thought to be due to intramural infiltration of connective tissue. We have previously documented that this can result in poor compliance that is unresponsive to pharmacologic manipulation, and this group may require bladder augmentation.[6]

The interplay of inhibitory neural mechanisms and prostaglandin release contributes significantly to both the filling and storage phase of micturition. Wein and Hanno have pointed out the existence in animals of a spinal sympathetic reflex, which is evoked by bladder filling.[7]

**What determines outlet response during filling?** Landmark experimentation, occurring through the 1960s into the 1980s, brought about agreement that there is a gradual rise in urethral/bladder neck pressure during bladder filling. Unfortunately, both in an experimental and clinical setting, the measurements of urethral pressure and concomitant definitions are difficult and nonstandardized. Separation of the smooth and striated muscular contributions to urethral pressure is unreliable. Various authors have tried to arrive at estimates of urethral pressure components by looking not only at striated and smooth muscle but also at vasculature and connective tissue; these derivations have not produced a consensus.

There is a demonstrable interaction of the passive properties of the urethral wall with a continuity of smooth muscle from the bladder base. Most observers believe that bladder filling increases bladder neck tension and that this is then conveyed to the urethra and mirrored by tonal changes in the urethral wall. Prostaglandins released from the bladder mucosa and bladder musculature during filling may also raise urethral resistance.

**Why does urinary leakage not occur with increases in intra-abdominal pressure?** It has been well demonstrated that during voluntary micturition, bladder pressure becomes higher than outlet pressure; thereby, accommodative changes occur in the configuration of the bladder outlet, and urine passes into and through the proximal urethra. It has been pointed out that coordinated bladder contraction does not occur in response to changes such as intra-abdominal pressure brought about by Valsalva maneuver. Urine flows into the proximal urethra by coordinated bladder neck relaxation along with an increase in intravesical pressure. This comes about through a neurally mediated reflex mechanism that is associated with resistance changes in the bladder neck and proximal urethra. It has been further demonstrated that any increase in intra-abdominal pressure is uniformly transmitted to the proximal urethra. It has also been shown that increases in urethral closure pressure noted with incremental extrinsic pressure applied to the abdomen are greater than the extrinsic pressure employed. This indicates that there is active muscular function in addition to simple passive pressure transmission involved. Both the smooth muscle and striated sphincter are thought to be involved.

If one considers the bladder neck and proximal urethra as a sphincter unit, the anatomic location of the structure helps explain positive transmission. At least in the female, the sphincter unit is thought to be abdominal as opposed to pelvic in location and thereby permits pressure transmission. There are, however, those who have questioned the validity of these explanations.

**Why does voiding ensue with a normal bladder contraction?** It has been confirmed that there is reflex correlation between a voluntarily induced bladder contraction of adequate magnitude and the active response of the proximal urethra. Electromyography (EMG) has clearly demonstrated a decrease in pelvic floor striated muscle tonus before voluntary bladder contraction initiation, which suggests that this decrease is brought about by a reflex mechanism involving the striated sphincter and mediated through the pudendal nerve. It is also most often thought that a similar coordination of smooth muscle sphincter activity comes about, presenting itself as a decrease in efferent hypogastric nerve activity. Whether this mechanism is brought about by excitation of adrenergic receptors or not is debatable.

## Diagnosis and classification of voiding dysfunction

One of the most difficult aspects of the treatment of voiding dysfunction in children is determining whether one is dealing with what will be a self-limiting problem or whether the voiding dysfunction is a symptom complex of a more severe underlying problem. A thorough history is required, stressing whether the problem occurs day and/or night; whether there is urgency, frequency, hesitancy, 'pressure', or dysuria; whether the child wets the bed at night or self-arouses and then voids (true nocturia); whether a family member has observed the child's urinary stream; and whether the child is ever noted to strain to void (stranguria). It is important to know whether the child has ever had a documented urinary tract infection (UTI) or not. Time of onset of the symptoms (primary or secondary) is important. Also, one must ask if the symptoms have changed over time and if so, how?

A complete physical examination is necessary, with a 'quick' genitourinary neurologic examination (Table 12.1). Special attention should be paid to the back and sacrum. Often in severe, recalcitrant cases, the author will suggest consultation with a pediatric neurologist. Both a dipstick and a microscopic urinalysis are performed. Urine culture and sensitivity is only undertaken in the case of an abnormal urinalysis or a history of UTI. A simple ultrasonic residual urine should be obtained on the initial visit.

In cases of nocturnal enuresis only, the evaluation may stop here and treatment ensue. In more complicated cases, modest imaging may be ordered, such as a renal and pelvic ultrasound; special attention should be paid to the thickness of the bladder wall on pelvic ultrasound. A voiding cystourethrogram (VCUG) is ordered if the child has had a UTI. Suspected back/spinal abnormalities are evaluated by bony films and magnetic resonance imaging (MRI) if needed. Endoscopic evaluation is limited to refractory cases or if an obstructive component is suspected. The author employs a fairly high index of suspicion for obstructive causes of micturitional abnormalities, having seen a plethora of these overlooked by previous treating urologists. There seems to be an unwarranted avoidance of simple cystoscopy in this group, bringing about delayed diagnosis and treatment.

Urodynamics are used only if initial empiric therapy fails or the case is severe. Attention is drawn to the algorithm of Wahl et al (Figure 12.1). Repeat urodynamics after several weeks/months of treatment are often helpful but the child's symptomatic response is a better gauge of therapy success.

Special urodynamic tests such as those relying on supersensitivity to parasympathomimetic agents, or anticholinergic stimulation may be helpful but this author has found them hard to interpret and cumbersome. Electromyography and evoked potentials may be helpful and this author leaves those studies to the neurologist; these investigations are less popular now than previously as they have been found to be of minimal therapeutic benefit. Simple flow rate determination, on the other hand, may be very useful and it is the recommendation of this author that all pediatric urologists have that capability readily available.

Historically, numerous attempts have been made to classify voiding dysfunction. All classification systems have their champions and detractors, but they all suffer from

**Table 12.1** *'Quick' genitourinary neurologic examination*

| Test | Normal response | Abnormal response |
|------|-----------------|-------------------|
| Back examination | Grossly normal spine | Dimple(s), hair tufts, hemangioma |
| Lower extremity deep tendon reflexes | Normal | Absent or clonic |
| Bulbocavernosus/clitoroanal reflex | Present | Absent or hyperactive |
| Genital pinprick | Normal | Absent |
| Perigenital light touch | Normal | Absent or paresthetic |
| Hot/cold water | Normal | Absent or paresthetic |
| Anal tone | Present | Lax or clonic |
| Observation of ambulation | Normal gait | Various forms of abnormal gait |

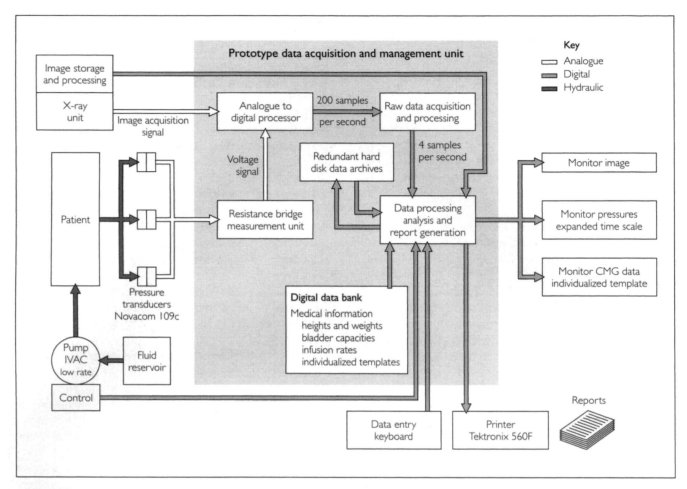

**Figure 12.1**
Wahl's urodynamic methodology. (Reproduced with permission of Wahl.)

some deficiency. This author prefers the functional system shown in Table 12.2. As one initially evaluates a child, then looks for landmarks of success or failure of the treatment regimens, reliance on this classification is most clinically relevant.

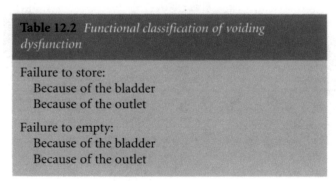

**Table 12.2** *Functional classification of voiding dysfunction*

Failure to store:
　Because of the bladder
　Because of the outlet

Failure to empty:
　Because of the bladder
　Because of the outlet

*Source*: Modified from Wein et al.[5]

## Treatment of voiding dysfunction

The old adage that 'children are not small adults' is applicable here: not only are the problems different but also one is dealing with the role of organ maturation and changing physiology as the child grows. Goals of management should always be clearly understood by the care team and the family (Table 12.3). The author will give a brief overview of current pharmacologic intervention options, review some behavior modification techniques, but will not, for instance, re-examine all the surgical options available, only the more recent minimally invasive ones.

Anticholinergics have long been our mainstay when using the pharmacologic option for control of voiding dysfunction. Oral oxybutynin has led the way since its introduction; its extended-release formulation is helpful in older children. Anticholinergic agents developed earlier serve as second-line therapy. More recently introduced, tolterodine can be very effective, but does not come as a

**Table 12.3** *Goals of treatment in voiding dysfunction*

Normal bladder control
No catheter or stoma
Preservation of renal function
Absence of urinary tract infection
Adequate urine storage at low pressure
Complete urine emptying at low pressure
Educational/vocational adaptability
Social/peer group satisfaction

liquid, so is limited as to age usage. When compared to oxybutynin, the author has found fewer side-effects with tolterodine in age/symptom-matched patients, especially dry mouth.

In children with neurologically or functionally increased outlet resistance, α-adrenergic blocking agents may play a role.

When incomplete bladder emptying is part of the clinical picture, oral bethanechol continues to be the pharmacologic mainstay, but again is limited in the pediatric population because of a lack of a liquid form. Intermittent catheterization continues to be useful in select patients.

Increased outlet resistance is needed in some children with poor bladder neck/urethral tone and this can often be accomplished with either physiotherapy (modified Kegel's exercises) or pharmacologically with agents such as pseudoephedrine. Success rates with both these approaches can be excellent, although one has to watch the patient's blood pressure closely when using pseudoephedrine.

Collagen-derivative injection therapy to the bladder neck and proximal urethra to 'bulk up' the outlet has met with, at best, only modest success. Open procedures such as vesicourethral suspension, 'slings', and use of the artificial sphincter have limited but definitive roles in managing these children and treating physicians should be well versed in these techniques.

## Innovations in minimally invasive management of voiding dysfunction

**Diagnostics**. No matter what new treatment modalities may arise, the applicability of such treatments only attains a level of success if based on the soundest, most-reliable information obtained from diagnostic tools. Urodynamics must be improved, especially in ways that are minimally invasive; per urethram urodynamics are self evidently nonphysiologic due to the presence of a foreign body in the bladder. Noninvasive, suprapubic ultrasonic sensing equipment is being developed and, if made reliable, will add considerably to the diagnostic armamentarium. The role of uroflowmetry will continue to be paramount; more

dependable, cost-effective flowmetric instrumentation is being developed.

**Newer pharmacologic agents.** For the foreseeable future, anticholinergics will continue to be the pharmaceutical of choice when detrusor relaxation is needed. The extended-release forms now available are of considerable help. Two new forms of oxybutynin are in development: a topical transdermal delivery patch and S-oxybutynin, which is formulated to improve tolerability when compared to the currently available form.

Further work is also being done with other pharmacologic agents for improved formulations and alternative delivery systems, production of selective receptor antagonists, neuronal desensitizing agents, CNS receptor remodelers, and channel-active agents. Several pharmaceutical houses are also trying to develop dual-acting or combination therapies. Time-release intravesical anticholinergics may soon be inserted once a month, the way urethral suppositories were in the past.

**Endoscopic/injection therapy advancements.** As has already been mentioned, manufacturers of cystoscopes and laparoscopic equipment are diligently striving to develop small-caliber instrumentation with finer optics, although 2 mm is the smallest attainable so far. Even those instruments are difficult to use because of their malleability and fragility.

Like most observers, this author has been displeased with injection therapy for incontinence using collagen derivatives. Other intrinsically natural agents such as autologous fat, myoblasts, and chondrocystes have been used with minimal success. Polytetrafluoroethylene (Teflon) has been used with moderate success, although it has received bad press because of particle migration. Our European colleagues have achieved very good results with endoscopic injection of polydimethyl siloxane (Macroplastique) and authorization for use of this agent in the United States is being sought.

The approval of newer bulking agents such as pyrolytic carbon-coated zirconium beads (Durasphere) and dextranomer/hyaluronic acid microspheres (Deflux) seems to offer promise, although usage and long-term evaluation in children is still on the horizon. Other compounds tried with limited success have been ethylene vinyl alcohol, bioglass, and silicone microballoons.

**Laparoscopic bladder procedures.** Two procedures have gained some favor. Our group has been very pleased with the long-term results of laparoscopic bladder autoaugmentation (LBAA) (Figure 12.2). We have performed 17 LBAAs with good-to-excellent results in all but 2 children. Patient selection and preventing postoperative urinary extravasation are the two predictors of successful outcome.[8]

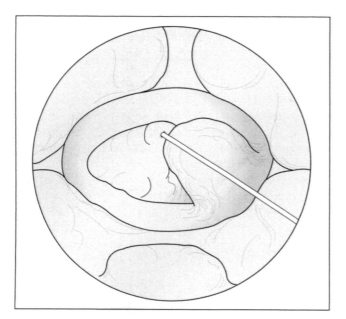

**Figure 12.2**
Laparoscopic bladder autoaugmentation. The bladder is seen through an umbilical camera port looking down into the pelvis. The top is anterior, the bottom (rectum in view) is posterior. The laparoscopic grasper is holding the detrusor elliptical flap, which has been partially dissected off the mucosa; the mucosa can be seen bulging to the left of the flap.

Laparoscopic bladder neck suspension (modified Burch) has been used in a few older girls with true stress incontinence and in a few spina bifida females. After some early enthusiasm, indications have been more limited, as, in most hands, the laparoscopic approach offers much less long-term success than open procedures.

**Biofeedback and neuromodulation.**    Behavioral modification has taken a step forward with the development of game-playing software for children. The group which advanced the software has reported excellent results with its use.

Neuromodulation embraces a wide variety of treatment modalities. Down-regulation of the sacral reflex arc which influences voiding is the goal of all these forms of therapy. Bower et al[9] recently reported their experience with adjunctive neuromodulation in children. Further developments in this area are to be expected.

**Robotic surgery/computer assisted surgery.**    The future of robotic surgery and computer-assisted surgery holds unlimited opportunities. It is not too far removed from robotic biopsy – which has already been done – to robotic resection.

Microelectrical mechanical systems (MEMS) also offer advances in pediatric urologic surgery. Most of these devices are less than the size of a human hair. The future of these modalities as both sensors and actuators is limitless. Stereotactic radiosurgery combined with telemedicine may allow totally off-site surgery in the future.

# Posterior urethral valves

If one defines posterior urethral valves (PUV) as any congenital narrowing of the distal prostatic urethra, a considerable spectrum of abnormalities presents itself. Historically, Young et al[10] classified three types of PUV, only one of which is now universally recognized to exist. The diagnosis and treatment of PUV has always been a significant challenge. Accepted endpoints of management are not agreed upon other than generally endorsing the view that normal micturitional control and preservation of renal function are conclusive goals.

Treatment of PUV with minimally invasive techniques was an accepted challenge from the onset of diagnosis of the entity. Early treatment often involved performing a cytotomy and fulgurating the valves from above.

The incidence of valves seems to correlate closely with one's predilection for diagnosing them: the more open one is to the possibility that any narrowing in the posterior urethra may be valves, the higher one accepts the incidence thereof. The best postulation the author can arrive at from various sources is that valves have an incidence range of 1 in 5000–8000 boys.

## Embryology

PUV have no known genetic basis and are rarely familial; however, there are a few reports of twins with valves and the author has seen 3 male siblings with PUV. Even in identical twins, only one may be affected. Uncommonly, other organ system anomalies may be reported.

To understand the embryology of PUV, one must be grounded in the formation of the normal genitourinary tract. Many theories as to how PUV evolve have been proposed. One of the earliest, and still a theory with many adherents, is that PUV are a persistence of normal urethral folds. This serves as at least a partial explanation of Young's type I valves but does not explain, among other presentations, diaphragmatic valves.

It is also believed by some that valves are remnants of the urogenital membrane or that valves are a result of an abnormal melding of the ejaculatory duct, which is wolffian in origin, and the prostatic utricle (müllerian in origin). Causation by an abnormal insertion and persistence of the distal aspect of the wolffian system has also been postulated.

## Diagnosis and classification

Diagnosis of PUV is now often made in utero and, on occasion, also treated before birth.

There are overabundant presenting signs and symptoms in any group of boys found to have valves. Urinary symptoms can be as meager as 'urinary dribbling' and as striking as urinary extravasation and ascites. UTIs are a common presentation. Uncommonly, neonatal hematuria and azotemia may be seen in babies later found to have valves. Nonurinary manifestations such as vomiting (and other gastrointestinal symptoms), respiratory distress, edema, failure to thrive, and seizure disorders may be seen.

Older boys tend to present with a wider array of symptoms and often the symptoms may be less definitively urologic, such as malaise and growth retardation. Enuresis and vague voiding dysfunction are also often seen at presentation in older boys.

Abnormal physical findings may vary from palpable kidneys and an ascitic abdomen to a palpable bladder. A distended abdomen may be seen, and perhaps noted not uncommonly are signs suggesting renal insufficiency. On occasion, no abnormal physical findings are described.

Laboratory studies are usually not helpful at time of diagnosis but are needed as baselines to follow the child with valves. A serum creatinine, a set of electrolytes, and a complete blood count (CBC; especially looking for anemia) are all initially necessary. The urine should be serially evaluated for protein, blood, and the presence of infection.

The VCUG is the study of choice for diagnosing PUV. Several other abnormalities need to be considered in the differential diagnosis of PUV. Various discoordinate types of voiding dysfunction, especially external sphincter dyssynergia, may produce cystographic patterns similar to PUV. Conditions such as variants of mixed incomplete abdominal musculature (prune-belly syndrome) may also radiographically appear similar to PUV. Polyps of the verumontanum are uncommon, but not rare. Also, on occasion, VCUG patterns seen in boys with neurogenic bladder and meatal stenosis may mimic PUV. Boys with severe non-neurogenic voiding dysfunction (the Hinman syndrome) may in certain circumstances have VCUGs easily confused with PUV.

To further perplex the issue, there are boys with mild PUV who may have a misrepresentative appearance of the urethra on VCUG. These are often older children with enuresis. At cystoscopy, the valves may be visually quite pronounced and not correlative with the VCUG. There are many anecdotal reports of this phenomenon.

Cystoscopy plays a paramount role in the diagnosis and treatment of PUV. One should have a high index of suspicion for the existence of valves in boys who have not responded to empirical treatment for such entities as voiding dysfunction. One should also be prepared to endo-scopically treat valves at the time of cystoscopy to avoid a second anesthesia/sedation. The variant endoscopic appearances of PUV are well documented in the literature and will not be further discussed here.

Urodynamics may play a role in deciding how urgently to treat a child with PUV and also may be critical in the long-term management of the sundry aberrances of 'valve bladder'. A set of baseline urodynamics has been advocated by some in all boys with PUV so as to have a predetermined reference data set for comparison with future treatment. One is referred to the earlier discussion of urodynamics in this chapter.

## Management of posterior urethral valves

Complete obliteration of obstructive valve tissue is the goal of all types of treatment. Prior to the invention of the infant resectoscope, open techniques for excision with surgical exposure of the posterior urethra were carried out. This often involved symphysiotomy. Due to bleeding, poor visualization in the surgical field was often encountered, the valves inadequately visualized, and frequently open resection was insufficient, leaving behind obstructive valve remnants. Postoperatively, it was not infrequently noted that the sphincter had been damaged.

Now, endoscopic resection or incision of the valves is usually a straightforward procedure in the hands of adequately trained pediatric urologists. Often it is the only treatment necessary to abolish the valves and problems concomitant to them.

Refinement of the techniques and miniaturization of instrumentation for endoscopic management of PUV have allowed the treating surgeon to successfully carry out valve ablation in most boys, save the very smallest premature male infants. This has been one of the most rewarding developments in minimally invasive surgery in pediatric urology. These advancements will be dealt with below.

While such preparations are being undertaken, or as a part of the initial treatment, bladder drainage may be necessary. Historically, this has been accomplished by temporary per urethram placement of an appropriate-size polyethylene feeding tube. Lately, as manufacturing techniques have been perfected, Foley catheters as small as 6F have been universally available (in some locales, 4F Foley catheters are being used). Foley catheterization may be preferred for a closed system in all but the most premature infant. Cutaneous vesicostomy may be necessary in some children, although the indications for such have greatly narrowed over the last few years.

Children with PUV who have concomitant hydro-ureteronephrosis have always presented formidable and controversial management problems. Mild-to-moderate hydroureteronephrosis often resolves after valve ablation. But in children with severely dilated, possibly aperistaltic ureters, management is much more challenging. After valve ablation, some of these children will resolve their ureteral dilation, but unremitting severe hydroureteronephrosis may in the long run contribute to renal insufficiency in some PUV children and require interventional drainage. Dialysis and renal transplantation continue to be required in a subset of boys with PUV no matter how well they are managed early on.

It is the author's advice that when a decision has been made for upper tract diversion, percutaneous approaches are preferred over open techniques such as loop ureterostomies or pyelostomies.[11] Often percutaneous techniques can be employed without requiring a full general anesthesia, using only local procaine-derivative injection with anesthesia standby with sedation. All forms of upper urinary tract diversion, however, must be looked upon with a jaundiced eye, as many institutions have reported that such diversion did not improve the child's long-term outlook.

## Minimally invasive valve ablation techniques

Historically, ablation of PUV was quite cumbersome and resulted not infrequently in damage to the urethra with an iatrogenically induced lifelong problem with urethral stricture disease, among the likelihood of other problems. One malady – PUV – was traded for another – a urethral stricture. Often, instruments used were the smallest adult resectoscopes, originally designed for resection of adult benign prostatic hyperplasia or bladder tumors.

As the instruments were too large in caliber to be inserted per urethram, a perineal urethrostomy was advocated by some. Open resection from a retropubic approach was promoted by others. Use of an otoscope and 'blind' valve destruction with sounds, metal stylets, or hook electrodes – some employing diathermy – also had their adherents. Rupture with balloon catheters was advocated. On occasion, crude (by today's standards) radiographic techniques were used to assist, converting these techniques to 'semi-blind'. Even wishful thinking was employed in hopes that an indwelling Foley catheter 'for some weeks' would lead to destruction of the valvular folds by ulceration.[12]

This author's technique involves taking the child to the cystoscopic suite and having the pediatric anesthesiologist administer a light general anesthetic, usually by face mask or LMA (laryngeal mask airway) unless the child has renal insufficiency/electrolyte problems – then an endotracheal tube may be used. If the child is not in hospital, the procedure is done as an outpatient/same-day surgery. In babies, the 9F infant resectoscope is introduced into the bladder; a

larger scope is used for older boys. A meatotomy may be necessary. The obturator is left in the sheath, which is heavily lubricated prior to passage. The obturator is removed, the bladder drained, and the working element with 30° Hopkins optics inserted. Either a video camera or direct telescopic examination may be carried out; the author recommends one use whichever method gives the resectionist the best vision. The bladder is closely inspected for trabeculations, ureteral orifice configuration, or other abnormalities and the scope is then pulled gently down the urethra until the valves are visualized. The bladder neck and prostatic urethra are evaluated en passant, paying close attention to any contracture or hypertrophy of the former and the degree of dilation in the latter. Optics are then changed to the 0° lens to allow the resectionist at least two different views of the valvular structure.

One valve at a time is then engaged with the right-angle electrode at either the 5 o'clock position (left valve), or the 7 o'clock position (right valve) (Figure 12.3). While the author prefers the right-angle electrode, a loop, bugbee, or other type electrode may produce equal results in the hands of others. Endoscopic solution should be flowing antegrade through the open scope port to balloon-out the valve. Close attention is paid to the location of the external urinary sphincter and assurance attained that it is not violated during the procedure.

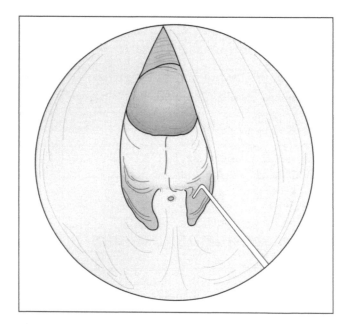

**Figure 12.3**
View of the posterior urethra with valve leaflets on either side. The tip of the pediatric resectoscope is just inside the sphincter. The elevated, hypertrophic bladder neck may be seen distally, the verumontanum proximally, and the moderately dilated prostatic urethra between. The right-angle electrode is preparing to engage the left valve leaflet (to the viewer's right).

The valve is then 'pop-buzz' incised. Pop-buzz involves using fairly high cutting current and very rapidly tapping of the power source foot pedal while the valve is engaged under minimal pressure. This usually destroys the valve, much as cutting a billow of a parachute. The floor of the urethra where the incision occurred is then closely inspected to be sure the entire valve leaflet has been destroyed. Additional pop-buzz swipes may be necessary. Care is taken to be sure the swipes are not too deep. When each of the valves is destroyed in this fashion, the 12 o'clock position of the urethra is closely scrutinized and if any obstructive tissue is noted, it is dealt with in the same manner. Any bleeding is strictly controlled by turning off the solution flow and inspecting the base of the incision area, gently coagulating it with low current as necessary. A Foley catheter is rarely left in, only if the resection has been difficult, or bleeding control challenging. The child is discharged home as soon as he voids.

The author has used this technique for resection of PUV in 105 boys, 11 of which were secondary resections following continued obstruction after primary resection by other urologists. A catheter has been left only six times (94.3% catheter-free resections). On one occasion, a child bled 20 hours post-resection, was catheterized, and did well with the catheter removed 2 days later. Long-term outcome has been excellent, as per voiding and renal function criteria. Only 3 boys have required repeat ablation (2.9%).

In follow-up, close attention is paid to voiding habits, flow rate, and residual urine (measured by ultrasound). A post-resection cystogram is not necessary if the ablation was straightforward, the child is asymptomatic with normal micturitional control, the upper tracts and serum chemical parameters were normal, and there were no/nil bladder trabeculations noted at cystoscopy prior to ablation. If these criteria are not met, follow-up cystography may be indicated. 'Routine' post-ablation cystograms only serve to reassure the physician and are most often unnecessary.

## Future unique innovations

Better treatment of PUV in the future with less operative complications is contingent upon the ability to further miniaturize the instrumentation employed. It may be that up to two-thirds of PUV are now diagnosed prenatally. In future, that may rise to > 90%. Better maternal/fetal diagnostic ultrasonography is to be expected. The challenge however is to determine whether earlier management will ameliorate long-term outcome.

Other prognostic modalities will need to improve to aid in better management of PUV. Advances in noninvasive sonographic diagnosis will continue to be made.[13]

Likewise, progress in applications of MRI to urethral abnormalities will proceed.[14] The evolution of miniaturization of pediatric urologic instruments has been one of our greatest technological advances. This progress continues. There is now a 4.5F blunt needle cystoscope commercially available. Companies in the endoscopic market continue to work to develop resectoscopes smaller than 9F and prototypes are obtainable. Instrumentation as small as 2 mm has been successfully used in laparoscopy and one would hope such could be eventually applied to transurethral devices. A cut-down version of a 6.9F semi-rigid ureteroscope has been adapted for use in treating PUV (pers comm).

Several commercial experimental analyses of newer power sources for application to valve ablation are being considered. The Harmonic Scalpel (Ethicon Endo-Surgery, Inc., Cincinnati, Ohio), already with many accepted applications in laparoscopy, is undergoing testing for transurethral adaptation. Pulsed radiofrequency waves may also offer PUV treatment prospects. Various laser sources are always under consideration with the major difficulty encountered in transurethral use in children being the limiting of depth penetration of the laser and resultant periurethral damage.

## References

1. Wein AJ. Overactive bladder: defining the disease. Am J Manag Care 2000; 6(Suppl): S559–64.

2. DiSanto ME, Wein AJ, Chacko S. Lower urinary tract physiology and pharmacology. Curr Urol Rep 2000; 1:227–34.

3. Ghafar MA, Shabsigh, Chichestr P, et al. Effects of chronic partial outlet obstruction on blood flow and oxygenation of the rat bladder. J Urol 2002; 167:1508–12.

4. Blok BF. Central pathways controlling micturition and urinary continence. Urology 2002; 59(Suppl 1):13–17.

5. Wein AJ, Levin, RM, Barrett DM. Voiding function and dysfunction: relevant anatomy, physiology, and pharmacology. In: Gillenwater JY, Grayhack JT, Howards SS, Duckett JW, eds. Adult and pediatric urology, 2nd edn. St. Louis: Mosby Year Book, 1991:981–8.

6. Braren V, Bishop MR. Laparoscopic bladder auto-augmentation in children. Urol Clin North Am 1998; 25:533–40.

7. Wein AJ, Hanno, PM. Targets for therapy of the painful bladder. Urology 2002; 59(Suppl 1):68–73.

8. Braren V. Laparoscopic bladder auto-augmentation in children: an update. Dialog Ped Urol 2001; 24:7–8.

9. Bower WF, Moore KH, Adams RD. A pilot study of the home application of transcutaneous neuromodulation in children with urgency or urge incontinence. J Urol 2001; 166:2420–2.

10. Young HH, Frontz WA, Baldwin JC. Congenital obstruction of the posterior urethra. J Urol 1919; 3:289–365.

11. Winfield AC, Kirchner SG, Brun M, et al. Percutaneous nephrostomy in neonates, infants, and children. Radiology 1984; 151:617–22.

12. Innes Williams D. The male bladder neck and urethra. In: Innes Williams D, ed. Paediatric urology. Butterworths: London, 1968:262.

13. Kaefer M, Barnewolt C, Retik AB, Peters CA. The sonographic diagnosis of infravesical obstruction in children: evaluation of bladder wall thickness indexed to bladder filling. J Urol 1997; 157:989–91.

14. Miller OF, Lashley DB, McAleer IM, Kaplan, GW. Diagnosis of urethral obstruction with prenatal magnetic imaging. J Urol 2002; 168:1158–9.

# 13

# Intersex

Thomas F Kolon

## Diagnosis

An individual's chromosomal sex is established at fertilization; chromosomal sex then directs the undifferentiated gonads to develop into either testes or ovaries. A patient's phenotypic sex results from the differentiation of internal ducts and external genitalia under the influence of hormones and transcription factors. If there is any discordance among these processes (i.e. chromosomal, gonadal, or phenotypic sex determination), then ambiguous genitalia or intersexuality develop. Currently, there are four main categories of intersex that are described: female pseudohermaphroditism (FPH); male pseudohermaphroditism (MPH); gonadal dysgenesis, either pure (PGD) or mixed (MGD); and true hermaphroditism (TH).[1–3]

## Female pseudohermaphroditism

Female pseudohermaphroditism is the most common intersex disorder. The patient's ovaries and müllerian derivatives are normal and the sexual ambiguity that is seen is limited to masculinization of the external genitalia. A female fetus is masculinized only if she is exposed to androgens and that degree of masculinization is determined by the stage of sexual differentiation at the time of exposure (Figure 13.1). Masculinization may also uncommonly be secondary to exogenous maternal steroids.

Congenital adrenal hyperplasia (CAH) accounts for the majority of FPH patients. Inactivating or loss of function mutations in five genes involved in steroid biosynthesis can cause CAH: CYP21, CYP11B1, CYP17, HSD3B2, and StAR (Figure 13.2). While all six of these biochemical defects are characterized by impaired cortisol secretion, only CYP21 and CYP11B1 are predominantly masculinizing disorders, with HSD3B2 to a lesser extent. Although the female fetus is masculinized due to overproduction of adrenal androgens and precursors, the affected males have no genital abnormalities. In contrast, HSD3B2, CYP17, and StAR deficiencies block cortisol synthesis and gonadal steroid production. Thus, affected males have varying degrees of MPH while females generally have normal external genitalia. Each of

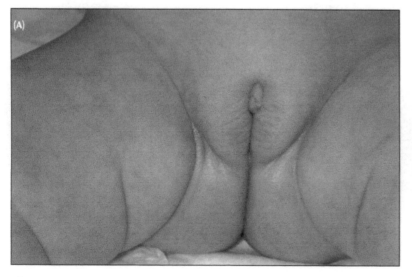
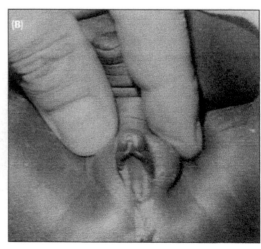

**Figure 13.1**
46XX patients with mild (A) and moderate (B) masculinization due to congenital adrenal hyperplasia.

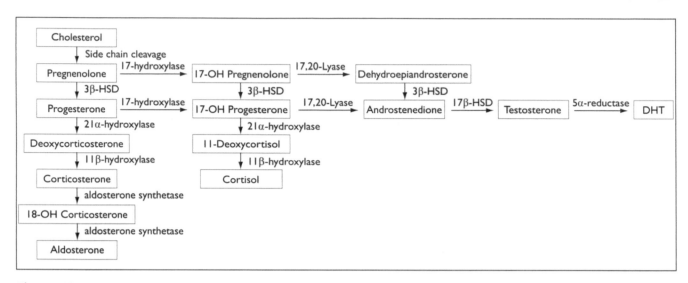

**Figure 13.2**
The intersex steroid biosynthetic pathways with responsible enzymes. 3β-HSD = 3β-hydroxysteroid dehydrogenase; 17β-HSD = 17β-hydroxysteroid dehydrogenase; DHT = dihydrotestosterone.

these genetic defects are inherited in an autosomal recessive pattern.[4–6]

Deficiency of CYP21 is the most common cause of genital ambiguity. Two CYP21 genes are located on chromosome 6 between HLA-B and HLA-DR: a functional CYP21B gene and a CYP21A pseudogene that is nonfunctional due to its encoding of multiple stop codons. Recombination between CYP21B and the homologous but inactive CYP21A accounts for approximately 95% of 21α-hydroxylase deficiency mutations.[7] A transfer of CYP21A sequences to CYP21B is present in 80% of patients resulting in a variable decrease in 21α-hydroxylase activity. These conversions usually involve the transfer of inherent CYP21A mutations. Patients with simple masculinizing 21α-hydroxylase deficiency have been identified with a conversion mutation causing severely decreased enzyme activity but sufficient aldosterone production to prevent salt wasting.[8–10]

CYP11B1 encodes 11β-hydroxylase, which converts 11-deoxycorticosterone to corticosterone and 11-deoxycortisol to cortisol.[9] Alternatively, CYP11B2 encodes for aldosterone synthetase, which converts deoxycorticosterone (DOC) to corticosterone and 18-hydroxycorticosterone to aldosterone. It is expressed in the zona glomerulosa and is under the influence of angiotensin II and potassium. Cortisol deficiency results in increased secretion of 11-deoxycortisol, DOC, corticosterone, and androgen by the adrenal gland. Hypertension, which occurs in about two-thirds of patients, is presumptively a consequence of excess DOC, with resultant salt and water retention. Excess androgen secretion in utero masculinizes the external genitalia of the female fetus. After birth, untreated males and females progressively virilize and experience rapid somatic growth and skeletal maturation.

3β-hydroxysteroid dehydrogenase (3β-HSD) catalyzes pregnenolone to progesterone and dehydroepiandrosterone (DHEA) into androstenedione.[6] Complete deficiency of 3β-HSD impairs synthesis of adrenal aldosterone and cortisol and gonadal testosterone and estradiol. These newborns have severe CAH and exhibit signs of mineralocorticoid and glucocorticoid deficiency in the first week of life. Affected females have mild-to-moderate clitorimegaly and males exhibit ambiguous genitalia with variable degrees of MPH (hypospadias, cryptorchidism, penoscrotal transposition, blind vaginal pouch). Masculinization occurs as a result of DHEA conversion to testosterone in fetal placenta and peripheral tissues. This results in too much masculinization in the female and insufficient masculinization in the male fetus. As with 21α-hydroxylase deficiency, a spectrum of phenotypes exist, including classic salt-wasting, non-salt-wasting, and non-classic, late-onset forms.

Enzyme CYP17 (P450) catalyzes two reactions:

1.  17α-hydroxylation of pregnenolone
2.  17,20-lyase (side-chain cleavage) of 17-hydroxypregnenolone and 17-hydroxyprogesterone.[6]

This rare autosomal recessive disorder occurs in two forms: combined 17α-hydroxylase and 17,20-lyase deficiency (most common) and isolated 17,20-lyase deficiency. Phenotypically, affected females have normal internal and external genitalia, but demonstrate sexual infantilism due to an inability of the ovaries to secrete estrogens at puberty. In both forms of the disorder, males display a developmental spectrum from a normal female phenotype to an ambiguous hypospadiac male. The magnitude of the decreased masculinization in the male infant correlates with the severity of the block in 17α-hydroxylation. In mild defects, aldosterone secretion may be normal and hypertension absent.[11]

Also called lipoid adrenal hyperplasia, StAR deficiency is a rare form of CAH and is the most severe genetic defect in steroidogenesis. It is associated with severe glucocorticoid and mineralocorticoid deficiency due to failure to convert cholesterol to pregnenolone.[5,6] Affected males have female external genitalia with a blind vaginal pouch, while females demonstrate normal internal and external genitalia. Many patients die in infancy, while about 33% survive with replacement therapy. While 46XY patients have severe testosterone deficiencies, 46XX females can enter puberty and menstruate, although they later develop polycystic ovaries and progressive ovarian failure. No surviving 46XY patient has demonstrated testis function at puberty.

## Gonadal dysgenesis

Mixed gonadal dysgenesis is the next most common intersex disorder. In general, gonadal dysgenesis disorders comprise a spectrum of anomalies ranging from complete absence of gonadal development to delayed gonadal failure. Complete or partial gonadal dysgenesis includes failed gonadal development in genetic males and females due to abnormalities of sex or autosomal chromosomes. This involves a gonad that has not properly developed into a testis or an ovary such as a dysgenetic testis or a streak gonad.

Complete gonadal dysgenesis describes a 46XX child with streak gonads or, more commonly, a child with Turner's syndrome (45X or 45X/46XX). 45X/46XX mosaicism may be seen in up to 75% of patients with Turner's syndrome.[12] Another uncommon form of pure gonadal dysgenesis is called Swyer syndrome. The child looks female externally and has a uterus and fallopian tubes; however, the karyotype is 46XY with a Y chromosome that usually does not work and two dysgenetic gonads in the abdomen.[13]

Partial gonadal dysgenesis refers to disorders with partial testicular development, including mixed gonadal dysgenesis, dysgenetic male pseudohermaphroditism, and some forms of testicular or ovarian regression. Mixed or partial gonadal dysgenesis (45X/46XY or 46XY) involves a streak gonad on one side and a testis, often dysgenetic, on the other side. A patient with a Y chromosome in the karyotype is at a higher risk than the general population to develop a tumor in the streak or dysgenetic gonad. Gonadoblastoma is the most common tumor.[14] Although it is a benign growth, it can give rise to a malig-

nant tumor called a dysgerminoma.[15] The risk of tumor is about 20–25% and is age-related. Surgical removal of the gonad is therefore recommended. The patient with a 45X/46XY karyotype and normal testis biopsy could retain his testis if it is scrotal or can be placed in the scrotum. This child would then need a very close follow-up of the testis, usually by monthly self-examination for tumor formation.

## True hermaphroditism

True hermaphroditism describes expression of both ovarian and testicular tissue in the individual. True hermaphroditism can result from sex chromosome mosaicism, chimerism, or a Y chromosome translocation. The most common karyotype in the United States is 46XX, although 46XY or mosaicism or chimerism (46XX/46XY) can occur. While a mosaicism may occur from a chromosomal nondisjunction, chimerism may result from a double fertilization (an X and a Y sperm) or from fusion of two fertilized eggs. Some patients with 46XX true hermaphroditism have the SRY gene translocated from the Y to the X chromosome. However, for most patients, the genes responsible are not yet identified.[16,17] This fairly uncommon condition can be further classified into three groups:

- lateral TH has a testis on one side and an ovary on the contralateral (usually left) side
- bilateral TH has an ovotestis on each side
- unilateral TH, which is the most common form, has an ovotestis on one side and either a testis or an ovary on the contralateral side.

The genital development in TH patients is ambiguous, with the phenotypic expression of hypospadias, cryptorchidism, and incomplete fusion of the labioscrotal folds. The genital duct differentiation in these patients generally follows that of the ipsilateral gonad on that side, such as a female fallopian tube with an ovary and a male vas deferens with a testis.[18]

## Male pseudohermaphroditism

Male pseudohermaphroditism is a heterogeneous disorder in which testes are present but the internal ducts system and/or the external genitalia are incompletely masculinized (Figure 13.3). The phenotype is variable and ranges from completely female external genitalia to mild male ambiguity such as hypospadias or cryptorchidism. Male pseudohermaphroditism can be classified into eight basic etiologic categories:

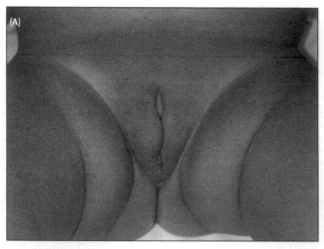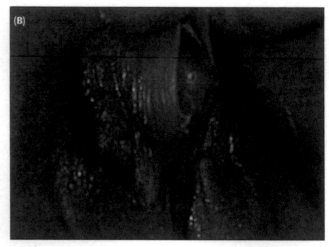

**Figure 13.3**
(A and B) 46XY patient with severe hypospadias and unilateral cryptorchidism due to dysgenetic male pseudohermaphroditism.

1. Leydig cell failure
2. testosterone biosynthesis defects
3. androgen insensitivity syndrome
4. 5α-reductase deficiency
5. persistent müllerian duct syndrome
6. testicular dysgenesis
7. primary testicular failure or vanishing testes syndrome
8. exogenous insults.

## Leydig cell failure

Male pseudohermaphroditism can result from Leydig cell unresponsiveness to human chorionic gonadotropin (hCG) and luteinizing hormone (LH), since the production of testosterone by the Leydig cells is critical to male differentiation of the wolffian ducts and the external genitalia. The phenotypes of these patients vary from normal female to hypoplastic external male genitalia.

## Testosterone biosynthesis enzyme defects

Defects in four of the steps of the steroid biosynthetic pathway from cholesterol to testosterone may produce genital ambiguity in the male[5,6] (Figure 13.2). These include the less common forms of CAH: 3β-HSD, CYP17 17α-hydroxylase/17,20-lyase), steroidogenic acute regulatory (StAR) protein deficiency, and 17β-HSD deficiencies. Complete deficiency of 3β-HSD impairs the synthesis of adrenal and cortisol and also gonadal testosterone and estradiol.[19–21] These newborns demonstrate severe CAH and exhibit signs of mineralocorticoid and glucocorticoid deficiency in the first week of life. Affected female infants have mild-to-moderate clitorimegaly. Male infants exhibit ambiguous genitalia with variable degrees of hypospadias, cryptorchidism, penoscrotal transposition, and a blind vaginal pouch. Masculinization occurs in these infants as a result of DHEA conversion to testosterone in the fetal placenta and peripheral tissues. This results in too much masculinization in a female and insufficient masculinization in the male fetus. Females with 17α-hydroxylase or 17,20-lyase deficiency have normal internal and external genitalia but demonstrate sexual infantilism due to an inability of the ovaries to secrete estrogen at puberty. In both forms of the disorder, males display a developmental spectrum from the normal female phenotype to the ambiguous hypospadiac male.[11,22] Affected males with StAR deficiency have female external genitalia with a blind vaginal pouch, whereas females demonstrate normal internal and external genitalia.[23,24] The affected 46XY males with 17β-HSD deficiency have external female genitalia, inguinal testes, internal male ducts, and a blind vaginal pouch. At puberty, these patients demonstrate an increase in their levels of gonadatropins, androstenedione, estrone, and testosterone. Delayed virilization may ensue if some testosterone levels approach the normal range.[25,26]

## Androgen insensitivity syndrome

The broad phenotypic spectrum of androgen sensitivity syndrome (AIS) includes 46XY patients that vary from normal female external genitalia that is seen in AIS7 or testicular feminization to normal males with infertility such as an AIS1. This disorder affects 1 in 20,000 live male births and the patients demonstrate a maternal inheritance pattern since the androgen receptor gene is located on the long arm of the X chromosome.[27] The amino terminal domain of the gene is encoded by exon 1 and is critical to target gene transcription regulation. Exons 2 and 3 encode the DNA-binding domain and the 5′ region of exon 4 encodes the hinge region containing the nuclear targeting signal. The 3′ region of exon 4 and exons 5–8 encodes the steroid-binding domain that confers ligand specificity. Binding of dihydrotestosterone or testosterone to this receptor ligand-binding domain results in activation of the receptor.[28] The majority of androgen receptor gene mutations affect the steroid-binding domain and result in receptors unable to bind androgens or receptors that bind androgens but exhibit qualitative abnormalities and do not function well. Exons 5 and 7 are the sites of many of the point mutations and the distribution of these alterations is similar for patients with either complete or partial androgen resistance.[29–31]

A child with complete androgen insensitivity externally resembles a girl, although the karyotype is XY and testes are located internally. Traditionally, these children have been raised as girls. Most children are not diagnosed until a work-up is performed when primary amenorrhea occurs at puberty. Occasionally, this condition is also discovered at the time of inguinal hernia repair or, more recently, when a prenatal karyotype does not match the external phenotype of the newborn child (Figure 13.4). An interesting finding is the phenotypic variability of families with affected males with partial AIS. This suggests that other factors in the sex differentiation cascade influence the phenotypic manifestation of gene mutations.

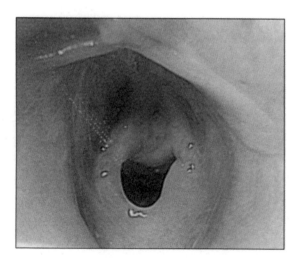

**Figure 13.4**
Abdominal testis identified at time of inguinal hernia repair in 46XY patient with complete androgen insensitivity syndrome.

## 5α-Reductase deficiency

5α-Reductase deficiency was first described by Nowakowski and Lenz in 1961 as pseudovaginal perineal scrotal hypospadias.[32] This is an autosomal recessive condition and these patients have a defect in the conversion of testosterone to its 5α-reduced metabolite, dihydrotestosterone (DHT). These patients have a 46XY karyotype and ambiguous external genitalia but normally differentiated testes with male internal ducts. However, at puberty, significant virilization occurs as testosterone levels increase into the adult male range while DHT remains disproportionately low. The SRD5A2 gene on chromosome 2 accounts for most fetal 5α-reductase activity. There are three genetic isolates of this disorder that have been described: they are found in the Dominican Republic, the New Guinea Samba Tribe, and in Turkey. Many of these patients undergo a change of their gender identity from female to male after puberty.[33,34] The patients with SRD5A2 gene deletions have measurable DHT levels at puberty, probably due to the peripheral conversion of testosterone to DHT. Virilization can be secondary to slightly increased plasma DHT levels and to the chronic effect of adult testosterone (T) levels on the androgen receptor.

## Persistent müllerian duct syndrome

Antimüllerian hormone (AMH), which is also termed müllerian inhibitory substance (MIS), is secreted by the Sertoli cells from the time of fetal seminiferous tubule differentiation until puberty. MIS binds to a receptor in the mesenchyme surrounding the müllerian ducts before 8 weeks gestation, causing apoptosis and regression of the müllerian duct.[35] The diagnosis of persistent müllerian duct syndrome is often made at the time of inguinal hernia repair or orchiopexy: hence the term hernia uteri inguinale (Figure 13.5). Persistent müllerian duct syndrome (PMDS) can occur from a failure of the testes to synthesize or secrete MIS due to an AMH gene mutation or from a defect in the response of the duct to MIS (AMH2 receptor mutation). PMDS is inherited in a sex-linked autosomal recessive manner and AMH mutations are most common in Mediterranean or Arab countries with high rates of consanguinity.[36] Most of these familial mutations are homozygous and the patients have low or undetectable levels of serum MIS. In contrast, AMH2 receptor mutations are often heterozygous and are more common in France and Northern Europe. These patients usually have high-normal or elevated MIS concentrations.[12]

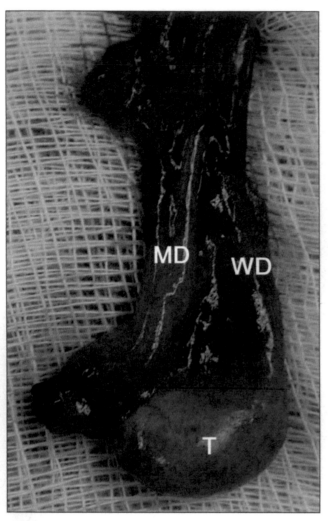

**Figure 13.5**
Retained müllerian structures in 46XY patient with unilateral cryptorchidism and persistent müllerian duct syndrome (MD = Müllerian duct, WD=wolffian duct. T = testis).

## Testicular dysgenesis

Dysgenetic male pseudohermaphroditism or dysgenetic testes can result from mutations or deletions of any of the genes involved in the testis determination cascade. These patients with dysgenetic gonads exhibit ambiguous development of the internal genital ducts, the urogenital sinus, and the external genitalia. The SRY gene is a single exon gene located on the short arm of the Y chromosome near the pseudoautosomal region.[37] SRY gene mutations usually result in complete gonadal dysgenesis and sex reversal as seen in XY sex reversal, or Swyer syndrome. Histologic analysis of dysgenetic gonads of XY males revealed that those with normal SRY had some element of rete testis and tubular function, whereas those with SRY mutations had completely undifferentiated gonads similar to those of 45X or Turner's syndrome individuals. Thus, it

is seen that SRY may have a direct role in testicular formation in addition to its indirect role in initiating the male differentiation cascade. The DSS locus (*dosage sensitive sex-reversal*) has been mapped to the Xp21 region, which contains the DAX1 gene. Duplication of the DSS locus has been associated with dysgenetic MPH and other anomalies. The DSS locus has been theorized to contain a wolffian inhibitory factor, which acts as an inhibitory gene of the testis determination pathway.[38] Swain et al have shown that DAX1 antagonizes SRY action in mammalian sex determination.[39] Male patients with Denys–Drash syndrome have ambiguous genitalia with streak or dysgenetic gonads, progressive neuropathy, and Wilms' tumor. Analysis of these patients revealed heterozygous mutations of the Wilms' tumor suppressor gene (WT1) at 11p13.[40] The WAGR syndrome (Wilms' tumor, aniridia, genitourinary abnormalities, mental retardation) is also associated with WT1 alterations.[41] The genitourinary anomalies seen in the WAGR syndrome are usually less severe than in Denys–Drash syndrome. The SOX9 gene has been associated with campomelic dysplasia, an often lethal skeletal malformation with dysgenetic MPH.[42] Affected 46XY males have phenotypic variability from normal males to normal females, depending on the function of the gonads.

## Congenital anorchia

Congenital anorchia or vanishing testes syndrome encompasses a spectrum of anomalies resulting from cessation of testicular function.[43] A loss of testes prior to 8 weeks gestation results in 46XY patients with female external and internal genitalia and either no gonads or streak gonads. A loss of testes at 8–10 weeks in development leads to ambiguous genitalia and variable ductal development. A loss of testis function after the critical male differentiation period, which is at 12–14 weeks gestation, results in a normal male phenotype externally, along with anorchia internally (Figure 13.6). Both sporadic and familial forms of anorchia exist. The familial cases, including some reports of monozygotic twins, support the presence of an as-yet unidentified mutant gene in some patients with the syndrome.

## Exogenous source

Exogenous insults to normal male development include maternal ingestion of progesterone or estrogen or various environmental hazards. As early as 1942, Courrier and Jost[44] demonstrated an antiandrogen effect on the male fetus induced by a synthetic progestagen and, more recently, Silver et al[45] showed an increased incidence of hypospadias in male offspring conceived by in-vitro fertilization. They hypothesized that the increased risk may be secondary to maternal progesterone ingestion. Sharpe and Skakkebaek have further postulated that the increase in

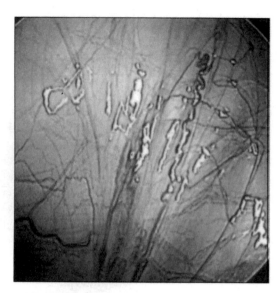

**Figure 13.6**
Atretic gonadal vessels seen by laparoscopy in 46XY patient with congenital anorchia.

reproductive abnormalities in men is related to an increase in the in-utero exposure to environmental estrogens.[46]

## Sex chromosome anomalies

Sex chromosome anomalies comprise another category of patients with intersexuality. Klinefelter's syndrome (47XXY) usually becomes evident during adolescence as the patient develops gynecomastia, variable androgen deficiency, and small atrophic testes with hyalinization of the seminiferous tubules. These patients demonstrate aspermatogenesis and increasing gonadotropin levels. 47XXY males may develop through nondisjunction of the sex chromosomes during the first or second meiotic division in either parent or, less commonly, through mitotic nondisjunction in the zygote at or after fertilization. These abnormalities almost always occur in parents with normal sex chromosomes. 46XY/47XXY mosaicism is the most common form of the Klinefelter variants. The mosaics, in general, manifest a much milder phenotype than classic Klinefelter patients. A differentiation of testes and a lack of ovarian development in these patients indicates that a single Y chromosome with SRY expression is enough for testis organogenesis and male sex differentiation in the presence of as many as four X chromosomes in some Klinefelter patients. These testes are not truly normal, however, since they are usually small and azoospermic. Although there are sporadic reports of paternity, most fertile Klinefelter individuals have had sex chromosome mosaicism.[47–49]

## Sex reversal

Categories of 46XX sex reversal include classic XX male individuals with apparently normal phenotypes, nonclassic XX males with some degree of sexual ambiguity, and XX true hermaphrodites.[50] Eighty to ninety percent of 46XX males result from an anomalous Y to X translocation involving the SRY gene during meiosis. In general, the greater amount of Y DNA present, the more masculinized the phenotype. Eight to twenty percent of XX males have no detectable Y sequences, including SRY. About 1 in 20,000 phenotypic males have a 46XX karyotype. Most of these patients have ambiguous genitalia, but reports of classic XX males without the SRY gene do exist.[38,50,51] This phenomenon again raises the possibility of mutation of a downstream wolffian inhibitory factor when cases of normal masculinization are seen without the presence of the SRY gene.

## History and physical examination

Patient history should include the level of prematurity; ingestion of exogenous maternal hormones, such as those used in assisted reproductive techniques, and maternal use of oral contraceptives during pregnancy. A family history is also useful for any urologic abnormalities, neonatal deaths, precocious puberty, infertility, or consanguinity. Any abnormal masculinization or cushingoid appearance of the child's mother should also be noted. Abnormalities of the prenatal maternal ultrasound are also helpful, such as discordance of the fetal karyotype with the genitalia by sonogram (Figure 13.7).

On physical examination, one should note any dysmorphic features, including a short broad neck or widely spaced nipples. The patient should be examined in a warm

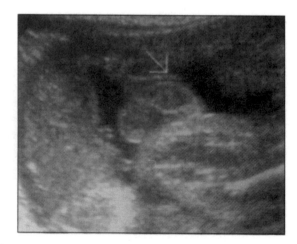

**Figure 13.7**
Prenatal ultrasound in 45X fetus showing discordant (male) genitalia (arrow).

room supine in the frog leg position with both legs free. An abnormal phallic size should be documented by width and stretched length measurements. One should describe the position of the urethral meatus and the amount of chordee (ventral curvature) and note the number of orifices: 3 in normal girls (urethra, vagina, and anus) or 2 in boys (urethra, anus). A rectal examination should also be performed for palpation of a uterus. With warmed hands, one should begin the inguinal examination at the anterior superior iliac crest and sweep the groin from lateral to medial with a nondominant hand. Once a gonad is palpated, grasp it with the dominant hand and continue to sweep toward the scrotum with the other hand to attempt to bring the gonad to the scrotum. Occasionally, some soap or lubricant on the fingertips may aid in this examination. It is important to check size, location, and texture of both gonads if palpable. The undescended testis may be found in the inguinal canal, the superficial inguinal pouch, at the upper scrotum, or rarely in the femoral, perineal, or contralateral scrotal regions. One should also note the development and pigmentation of the labioscrotal folds along with any other congenital anomalies of other body systems.

For differential diagnosis and treatment purposes, the distinction needs to be made whether or not the gonad is palpable. Unless associated with a patent processus vaginalis, ovaries and streak gonads do not descend while testes and rarely an ovotestis may be palpable. If no gonads are palpable, all four categories are possible (FPH, MPH, GD, and TH). Of these, FPH is most commonly seen, followed by MGD. If one gonad is palpable, FPH and PGD are ruled out, while MGD, TH, and MPH remain possibilities. If two gonads are palpable, MPH and rarely TH are the most likely diagnoses. In 46XY boys, hypospadias and cryptorchidism without an underlying intersex etiology would be a diagnosis of exclusion after a full evaluation.

## Patient evaluation

All patients require laboratory evaluation by serum electrolytes, 17-hydroxyprogesterone, testosterone, LH, and follicle-stimulating hormone (FSH) levels. A karyotype is also immediately performed. If the 17-hydroxyprogesterone level is elevated, 11-deoxycortisol and deoxycorticosterone levels will help differentiate 21α-hydroxylase deficiency from 11β-hydroxylase deficiency. If the 17-hydroxyprogesterone level is normal, a testosterone to DHT ratio, along with androgen precursors before and after hCG stimulation, will help elucidate the MPH etiology. During the first 60–90 days of life, there is a normal gonadotropic surge, with a resultant increase in the testosterone level of the infant. During this specific time period, one can forego the hCG stimulation for the androgen evaluation. A failure to respond to hCG, in combination with elevated LH and FSH levels, is consistent with anorchia.

An ultrasound can detect gonads in the inguinal region, where they are also most easily palpable, but it is only 50% accurate in showing intra-abdominal testes (Figure 13.8). A computed tomography (CT) scan and a magnetic resonance imaging (MRI) scan may also help to delineate the anatomy, although they are more expensive. These tests are also helpful in identifying a uterus. A genitogram should be performed to evaluate a urogenital sinus, including the entry of the urethra in the vagina. A cervical impression can be identified on the vaginogram[52] (Figure 13.9). Infants in whom TH, MGD, or MPH is considered will require an open or laparoscopic exploration with bilateral deep longitudinal gonadal biopsies for histologic evaluation.

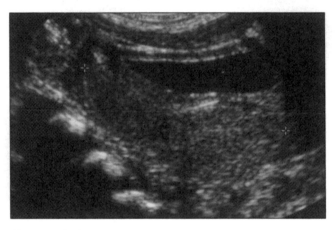

**Figure 13.8**
Postnatal ultrasound showing large uterus filled with debris (between cursors) behind the bladder.

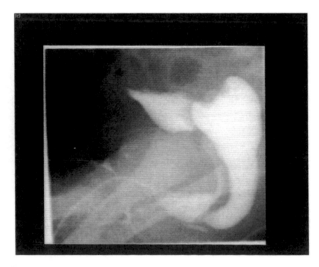

**Figure 13.9**
Genitogram showing superior cervical impression in vagina emptying into a urogenital sinus.

# Treatment options and indications

Much current research is aimed at understanding the influence of androgens on the fetal and newborn brain and its relationship to gender identity. Diagnosis and management of these children is very individualized and should always involve a team approach, which includes the pediatric urologist, endocrinologist, geneticist, and the child's parents immediately after birth.

## *Female pseudohermaphroditism*

Treatment of the newborn with CAH involves the correction of dehydration and salt loss by electrolyte and fluid therapy with mineralocorticoid replacement.[4] Glucocorticoid replacement is then generally added upon confirmation of the diagnosis. Infants that are going to be raised as girls usually undergo clitoral reduction and vulvovaginoplasty in early infancy, but controversy exists on the timing of surgery and all aspects must be weighed prior to decision making. Surgery can be performed for an infant, toddler, or adolescent. Many surgeons advocate early surgery for both technical and psychologic reasons, realizing that vaginal revision may be needed after puberty. Surgery has three main aims:

- reducing the size of the enlarged masculinized clitoris
- reconstructing the female labia
- increasing the opening and possibly length of the vagina.

These procedures have gone through many changes during the history of surgery. Surgical technique continues to be revised to optimize the girl's external appearance and functional size, while maintaining adequate sensation. Clitorectomy, which involves removing the entire clitoris, is long out of practice, as is clitoral recession without reduction, since it is associated with painful erections upon stimulation. Reduction clitoroplasty is the operation of choice for most infants with clitorimegaly. The central portions of the corporal bodies are excised and the surgeon preserves the dorsal neurovascular bundles by incising Buck's fascia laterally at the 3 o'clock and 9 o'clock positions. The corporal bodies need to be dissected beyond the bifurcation to the inferior pubic rami, where they are transected. The remaining proximal and distal portions of the bodies are then reapproximated and placed in the investing fascia: this optimizes future erectile function. Occasionally, a glansplasty is required for an extremely large glans and this is accomplished by excising a triangle of tissue on the dorsum of the glans. A vulvoplasty is carried out by extending the incision for the clitoroplasty on either side of the midline strip of tissue down to the level of the vaginal orifice. Redundant labial scrotal skin is brought down as preputial flaps to form the labia minora.[53-58]

The position of the vagina should be accurately determined preoperatively by the genitogram as part of the work-up for intersex. There are four main types of vaginal repair:

- a simple cutback of the perineum
- a flap vaginoplasty
- a pull-through vaginoplasty
- a more extensive rotation of skin flaps or segmental bowel interposition.

Usually, a low vaginoplasty can be performed at the same time as the clitoroplasty. When the vagina opens very low, a simple cutback with a vertical midline incision may be all that is needed to open the introitus. Usually, however, a posterior based U-shaped flap is necessary for a tension-free anastomosis, reducing the risks of postoperative vaginal stenosis.[53] Exposure of the high vagina requires either a perineal approach (Hendren operation, Passerini-Glazel operation), a posterior vaginoplasty as recommended by Pena, or an anterior sagittal transanorectal vaginoplasty as described by Domini. When the vagina is extremely high and small, replacement with a bowel segment will be necessary, usually with the sigmoid colon.[57-60]

## *Gonadal dysgenesis*

A streak gonad does not descend but it may be palpable as a small remnant of tissue in an inguinal hernia sac. If the testis is in the inguinal position, it can be removed using an incision in the groin, as for a traditional orchiopexy or hernia repair. If the gonad is in the abdomen, as is usually the case with the gonadal dysgenesis, then the treatment options include open abdominal exploration and removal of the gonads or laparoscopic gonadectomy, which is the usual preference. When a purely female anatomy exists, such as in Turner's syndrome or Swyer syndrome, no treatment may be necessary. These girls have sexual infantilism at puberty marked by no onset of secondary sexual development. Some degree of female development, however, may be seen in up to 20–25%. Since gonadoblastoma does not occur in the absence of Y chromosome material, removal of the streak gonads is not required.[14] Growth hormone is usually recommended early in childhood and estrogen therapy is begun after puberty to optimize the patient's height. Rare cases of spontaneous pregnancy have been reported, although infertility is the norm. Pregnancy may thus be possible using donor eggs and assisted reproductive techniques.

## True hermaphroditism

Generally, a female sex has been assigned to most patients due to the presence of a vagina, uterus, and ovarian tissue. Less commonly, the patient has a 46XY karyotype with adequate penile development and without a uterus present, so a male sex assignment would be more appropriate. The decision of sex of rearing should always be deferred until the child has had an adequate evaluation of his genitourinary system. Usually, the internal organs need to be visualized and the gonads biopsied. This can be done through an open abdominal exploration or accomplished with the use of the laparoscope. If raised as a female, the child should have dysgenetic testicular tissue removed due to the risk of malignancy. The possible need for vaginoplasty can be performed early or deferred until puberty. If the child is raised as a boy, he should have any hypospadias or cryptorchidism repaired as an infant. Testosterone supplementation may be needed if the amount of testicular tissue present is inadequate to begin or continue puberty. A persistent müllerian duct, such as a uterus and fallopian tubes, has usually not fully regressed and connects to the urethra near the bladder at the verumontanum. If there is a decision to rear the child as a boy, the structures are generally removed, taking care not to injure the vas deferens, which usually runs alongside the uterus. Extensive dissection behind the bladder neck and up to the area where the müllerian structures insert into the urethra is usually contraindicated in order to avoid damage to the sphincter mechanism, risking incontinence. Both open and laparoscopic excisions have been reported.[61-63] Arguments for removal of the müllerian structures include the possibility of cyclic hematuria post puberty, or the formation of stones or chronic urinary tract infections if the continuity with the urethra is maintained and stasis occurs in a dilated müllerian remnant.[61-64] Arguments against removal maintain that complications from the structures are uncommon and their removal risks injury to the vas deferens, the bladder neck, and the urethral sphincter.[65]

## Male pseudohermaphroditism

Decreased masculinization (hypospadias with cryptorchidism or more ambiguous development) is seen in most patients with MPH. In untreated patients with 5α-reductase deficiency, significant virilization occurs at puberty, as testosterone levels increase into the adult male range while DHT remains disproportionately low. Treatment is currently unclear for this enzyme deficiency when diagnosed in infancy. Male gender assignment has been recommended because the natural history of this deficiency is virilization at puberty with subsequent change to male gender. However, this decision requires

surgical hypospadias repair and orchiopexy with male hormonal replacement.

Rarely do patients with dysgenetic testes have fully masculinized external genitalia. The surgical issues are very dependent on the degree of masculinization in each individual case, which also influences the decision process of sex assignment. If a 46XY infant with testicular dysgenesis is going to be raised as a male, he will need a hypospadias repair, orchiopexy, or possibly orchiectomy. Müllerian ducts have usually not fully regressed and may be fully or partially removed at the time of other repairs in order to facilitate orchiopexies. As previously discussed, retained female structures have the potential for urinary tract infections, stones, or even cyclic hematuria at puberty. Dysgenetic testes may appear normal grossly but microscopically are disorganized and poorly formed; thus, a biopsy of the gonad is recommended in most children undergoing intersex evaluation. Currently, the recommendation is to remove an undescended dysgenetic testis because of the risk of malignancy.[66,67] In 45X/46XY patients, if the biopsy is normal and the testis is scrotal or can be placed in the scrotum, it should not be removed, but a risk of malignancy correlates with the extent of testicular descent. Tumors have also been reported in scrotal dysgenetic testes. A scrotal testis needs to be followed very closely for this reason. The possibility does exist of a male gender in these patients who would require a hypospadias repair yet would have removal of severely dysgenetic testis requiring replacement hormones. It would seem obvious that treatment in these cases needs to be individualized. The child's parents should discuss with the pediatric urologist, endocrinologist, geneticist, and psychiatrist the issues of testosterone imprinting in utero, the need for hormones pre- and postpuberty, the degree of masculinization, the function of the testis, and the extent of surgery that is required.

Affected boys with errors in testosterone production are undermasculinized, with varied degrees of hypospadias, cryptorchidism, bifid scrotum, or a blind vaginal pouch. For the patient reared as a boy, testosterone therapy may be indicated to augment penile size and to aid in the hypospadias repair. The natural history in some of these patients when untreated is virilization at puberty with a gender role change from female to male.[25,26,68,69] Therefore, many recommend a male gender assignment diagnosis. Some enzyme deficiencies require glucocorticoid and mineralocorticoid replacement and all of these patients need testosterone replacement at puberty for masculinization. Gonadectomy is required in 46XY patients raised as girls in order to address the risk of tumor formation in the future.

Traditionally, a child with a complete androgen insensitivity syndrome would be raised as a girl. Most of these children are not diagnosed until a work-up is performed when amenorrhea occurs at puberty. Occasionally, it is discovered at the time of inguinal hernia repair and more recently when a prenatal karyotype does not match the external phenotype of the newborn child. If the child is to be raised female, an orchiectomy is required. The testes are at risk for cancer development and the incidence of malignant tumors is estimated to be 5–10%.[70,71] Seminoma is the most common tumor seen, but nonseminomatous germ cell tumors and other malignancies have also been reported. Tumor risk appears to be greater in older patients and in those with complete rather than partial AIS, and tumor formation appears to occur postpuberty. Intratubular germ cell neoplasia has been identified in prepubertal boys with partial AIS but not complete AIS.[71] If an AIS patient presents with an inguinal hernia, the gonads are usually removed during the hernia repair for diagnosis and cancer risks. Vaginal dilation or vaginal augmentation may or may not be needed: usually this is reserved until after puberty and a number of techniques are available. In patients with partial AIS, orchiectomy is recommended as soon as the diagnosis is made to avoid further virilization in patients who will be raised in the female gender. Male gender assignment is usually successful in patients with a predominantly male phenotype; however, predicting the adequacy of masculinization in adulthood may not be possible based on the maternal family history or characterization of the androgen receptor genetic defect. Some children respond well to high-dose androgen therapy, but its durability is not yet clear.

Controversy exists concerning the best time to perform the orchiectomy. Traditionally, in an infant with complete AIS, the testes are left in place until after puberty to take advantage of the hormonal function and, in this way, natural female pubertal changes can occur by testosterone conversion to estrogen. After puberty is completed, the testes would be removed and replacement estrogen begun. Risks with this approach are as follows: no cancers have been reported in prepubertal children, but carcinoma-in-situ has been uncommonly seen. If the testes happen to be in the inguinal region, they can be easily injured. One also needs to explain to a mature postpubertal patient of the need to remove the testes. Of course, delaying the surgery also further increases the risks of testis cancer if the patient is lost to follow-up care. If orchiectomy is performed early, replacement hormones are then required for pubertal changes.

## Patient and preoperative preparation

Gonadectomy or orchiectomy is performed due to the malignant potential for patients assigned to female gender. If the patient is to be assigned a male gender and the gonads consist of testicular elements, they can be preserved and orchiopexies performed early. As previously discussed, an early prophylactic orchiectomy can be performed if patients are to be raised as female rather than undergoing a therapeutic orchiectomy after puberty. Inappropriate müllerian structures in males should be removed if needed to aid in orchiopexy or if needed for cyclic hematuria or urinary stones. Laparoscopy has been very useful both as a diagnostic and therapeutic procedure in boys with nonpalpable gonads. In the cases of intersex, laparoscopy is also helpful in defining the internal duct structures, removing structures contrary to the current gender assignment, helping in gonadal biopsies, or removing gonads with an increased malignant potential. However, open laparotomy through a Pfannenstiel incision is better suited for deep longitudinal gonadal biopsies, which are generally preferred over a superficial forceps biopsy that would be used laparoscopically. Open laparotomy also facilitates a partial gonadectomy, which may be performed in cases of true hermaphroditism.

In general, diagnostic laparoscopy or a laparoscopic orchiopexy and laparoscopic gonadectomy are performed on an outpatient basis under general anesthesia. The child is placed supine with the arms tucked on the sides. The child is secured to the table in order to allow the table to be adjusted into the Trendelenburg position as needed. The position and draping of the child are suitable for an open abdominal procedure if this becomes necessary. A urethral catheter is inserted and left in for the entire case. An orogastric tube is used to decompress the stomach and we generally advise our anesthesiologist to avoid nitrous oxide in order to limit the potential for dilation of the bowel.

## Recommended equipment or instruments

I generally use a 5 mm lens system for most laparoscopic procedures. However, a 3 mm lens system provides adequate visualization for simple diagnostic laparoscopy. There is a greater assortment of 5 mm instruments available at this time, but as the mini-laparoscopic systems improve, most centers will probably convert to 3 mm working ports. The instrument that is most used is a 5 mm atraumatic grasper. Cautery is used sparingly during a laparoscopic orchiopexy since coagulation within 2 mm of a vessel can injure the vessel wall, possibly leading to thrombosis. A 5 mm vascular clip applier is used through the 5 mm cannulas. At this point 3 mm clipping devices are not commonly available. Laparoscopic scissors that may be used with or without cautery are also necessary. If one prefers to bring a testicle down into the scrotum through a 10 mm cannula, then this should be available as well as the previously mentioned 5 mm ports. Some centers also use Amplatz dilators to enlarge the scrotal canal for an orchiopexy.

# Approach and helpful tips

Cystoscopy will help elucidate a müllerian remnant entering the urethra. Catheterization of the verumontanum and injection of contrast can highlight the retained structures (Figure 13.10). If there is a history of chronic urinary infection, cystoscopy and basket stone extraction 13.11).

Initial laparoscopic access is usually achieved at the infraumbilical position. However, some surgeons prefer the supraumbilical incision to avoid the umbilical vessels during open trocar placement. After incising the skin, the subcuticular tissues are spread, exposing the fascia, which is tagged with sutures and then incised. The peritoneum is identified and opened and a 5 mm insufflation port is then placed into the abdomen; 3 mm instruments are placed with cannulas, which resemble large Veress needles – thus, one does not use open access for placement of the 3 mm cannula. Open trocar placement is seen as the safest method of entering the abdomen in small children and minimizes complications of placement of a Veress needle into the bowel or major blood vessels.

The peritoneal cavity can be inspected with the lens attached to the camera prior to insufflation to ensure that the cannula placement is correct. Once an adequate pneumoperitoneum is achieved through insufflation, the surgeon takes note of all vessels, vas deferens, intra-abdominal gonads, and presence of any müllerian structures. If a patent processus vaginalis is noted, pressure on the inguinal canal can push peeping testes back into the abdomen for visualization. If the internal inguinal ring is closed, the surgeon examines for a blind-ending vas deferens close to blind-ending spermatic vessels. The finding of a blind-ending vas deferens alone does not prove a testis has vanished and further laparoscopic exploration is needed up to the origin of the gonadal vessels near the kidneys. A high abdominal testis can be either removed or brought down to the scrotum in a primary or staged fashion. Correct placement of the laparoscopic ports is important. The camera port is generally in the infraumbilical incision. This may be all that is needed for a diagnostic laparoscopy. However, further procedures generally require placement of two other working ports. These working ports are placed at the midclavicular line just below or even with the umbilicus. To work on the right inguinal region, the left lower quadrant port is generally placed slightly lower and vice versa for the left side. However, in cases of intersex, work may be done on both sides and both ports can be placed slightly below the umbilicus in the midclavicular line on the right and left sides. In very small children, it is helpful to place the working ports above the level of the umbilicus in order to avoid crossing the instruments and to facilitate their use.

The surgeon stands on the side opposite to the undescended testis or gonad in question. The child is placed in a mild Trendelenburg position with the lateral tilt away from the side that is being examined. A laparoscopic incision with scissors is made on the anterior lip of the patent processus vaginalis and continued laterally.[72] This incision is then carried medially to the adjacent gonadal vessels. The incision from the anterior lip is continued medially and extended further along the path of the vas deferens with care to leave a wide strip in order to preserve the paravasal vasculature. Elevating the gonadal vessels by grasping the local tissue or gonad with atraumatic grasping forceps allows for further dissection distally

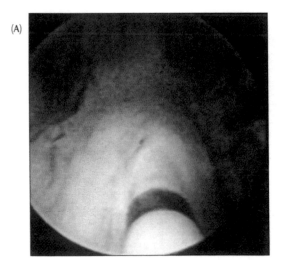

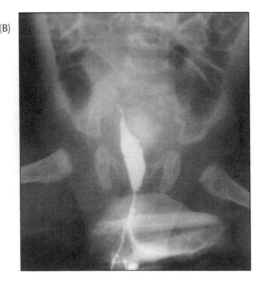

**Figure 13.10**
(A and B) Cystoscopic catheterization of utricular opening in urethra (A) and contrast study demonstrating uterus and right fallopian tube (B).

along the sac of a patent processus vaginalis if present. This is especially helpful in a peeping or high inguinal testis. The gonadal vessels are on the medial posterior aspect of the hernia sac. With an undescended testis, care must be taken to define a caudal extent of the vas deferens if there is a long looping vas. Since gubernacular attachments are very vascular, they are divided with cautery. Incision in the peritoneum is extended laterally along the gonadal vessels toward the kidney. Further dissection along the medial aspect of the vas deferens creates a triangular flap of peritoneum containing the juncture of the vas gonadal vessels and testis. When the testis has been sufficiently mobilized, it can then be prepared for orchiopexy into the scrotum or removal in cases of AIS. For gonadectomy, 5 mm vascular clips are placed on the gonadal vessels proximal to the gonad. A similar clip is placed on the vas deferens. If a staged orchiopexy is needed, a clip can be placed on the gonadal vessels as far rostral as possible, allowing for a communication between the arteries of the vas deferens and the most distal spermatic vessels to increase over the next 6 months. Koff and Sephic, however, suggest that the communication between the caudal spermatic vessels and the arteries to the vas occur within the testes or close to the testicular hilum.[73] They therefore recommend placing the clip close to the testes in order to improve the mechanics of transfer provided by division of the spermatic vessels.

For relocation of the testis to the hemiscrotum, a small transverse incision is created on the hemiscrotum and a subdartos pouch is dissected. We use a 5 mm port advanced through the hemiscrotum and pass it into the peritoneal cavity medial to the medial umbilical ligament but lateral to the bladder. Some centers employ graspers through the 5 mm port, others change over to a 10 mm cannula, and yet others simply advance a hemostat into the peritoneal cavity in order to grasp the testis and bring it down to the scrotum where it is anchored in place. In the small child, all cannula sites are closed, including 3 mm or 5 mm sites, since a cannula site omental herniation has been described in a 3.5 mm cannula site in an infant. The umbilical cannula site is closed after all carbon dioxide has been removed from the abdomen.

Various laparoscopic techniques have been described for intersex procedures. Laparoscopic gonadectomy, as previously described, has become our standard approach for 46XY AIS patients who have complete testicular feminization and also in cases of 46XY Swyer syndrome or gonadal dysgenesis with the Y component in a mosaic karyotype in order to prevent gonadal tumor formation (Figure 13.12). These techniques have been reported by many institutions.[74–76] Cystoscopy for complete AIS reveals a blind-ending vaginal pouch without a cervix, and laparoscopy

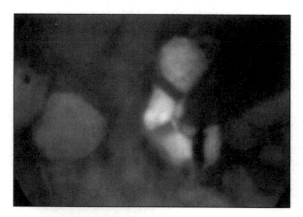

**Figure 13.11**
Cystoscopy of large utricle with basket stone extraction.

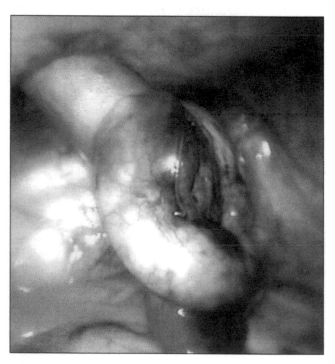

**Figure 13.12**
Laparoscopic orchiectomy of abdominal testis in 46XY patient with complete androgen insensitivity syndrome.

for gonadectomy shows absence of the cervix behind the bladder (Figure 13.13).

For true hermaphroditism, we prefer to convert a diagnostic laparoscopy to open gonadal biopsy in order to obtain a deep longitudinal gonadal biopsy. In most ovotestes, a polar distribution is seen with a clear demarcation between the two components. Rarely, however, the

(A)

(B)

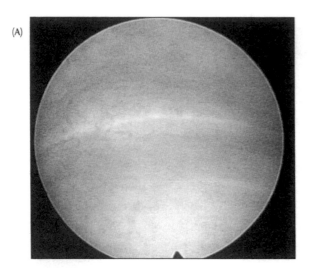

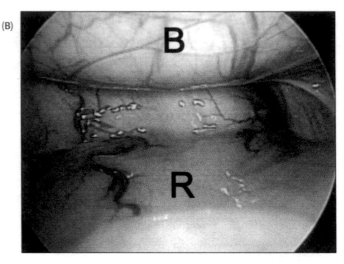

**Figure 13.13**
46XY patient complete androgen insensitivity syndrome: vaginoscopy (A) showing absence of cervix and laparoscopy (B) showing absence of uterus between the bladder (B) and rectum (R).

gonad may contain an outer ovarian cortex with an inner medullary zone of testicular tissue, which might be missed with a simple laparoscopic forceps biopsy, although this technique has been described[61,65,77] (Figure 13.14). In cases of retained müllerian structures, such as in PMDS, a hysterectomy can be performed by dissection of the hypoplastic uterus in the medial confluence of the streak gonads behind the bladder without sectioning of the wolffian ductal structures. Lateral to the uterine body, there are blood vessels that need to be cauterized. After incision of the peritoneal cul-de-sac, distal dissection of the uterus can be performed in the retrovesical space. The bladder facilitates this process. To remove all of the components, traction on the uterus enables the entire gonad duct and uterus complex to be removed en bloc.[61] Completion of this dissection usually requires removal through a 10 mm trochar. In cases of PMDS, however, the undescended testes need to be relocated to the scrotum. Extreme care must be taken when dissecting along the lateral edges of the uterine body, since this is where the vas deferens runs and injury may occur. It must be noted, however, that there are also some areas of vasal atresia in cases of PMDS. We may simply remove as much of the uterine body as needed in order to facilitate the orchiopexy. In contrast, others have simply bivalved the uterine body in the middle in order to allow both testes to reach the scrotum without tension (Figure 13.15). Various laparoscopic treatment options for orchiopexy with retained müllerian structures employing laparoscopic, laparoscopic assisted, or open methods through a Pfannenstiel incision have also been described. Ng and Koh describe three laparoscopic treatment options – division of the vas and oviduct and ipsilat-

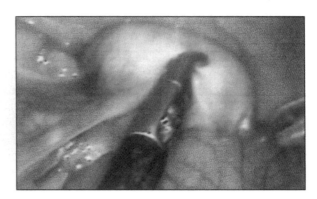

**Figure 13.14**
Laparoscopic biopsy of abdominal gonad.

eral orchiopexy; division of spermatic vessels, followed later by Ombrédanne operation; and a one-stage division of spermatic vessels and Ombrédanne operation.[78]

Vaginal agenesis is found as part of the Mayer–Rokitansky–Küster–Hauser syndrome and laparoscopic techniques for creation of a neovagina have been reported by a number of authors.[79,80] A neovagina might also be required in severe cases of 46XX CAH and other cases of severe genital ambiguity without formation of any female structures. The Vecchietti procedure for creation of a neovagina was described for treatment of Rokitansky–Kuster–Hauser syndrome in 1970 and has since been referred by many through both laparoscopic and open techniques.[79] Chabre et al described a bilateral laparoscopic adrenalectomy for CAH in an adult with severe hypertension. This patient had two novel mutations in the splice donor sites of the CYP11B1 gene. The surgery

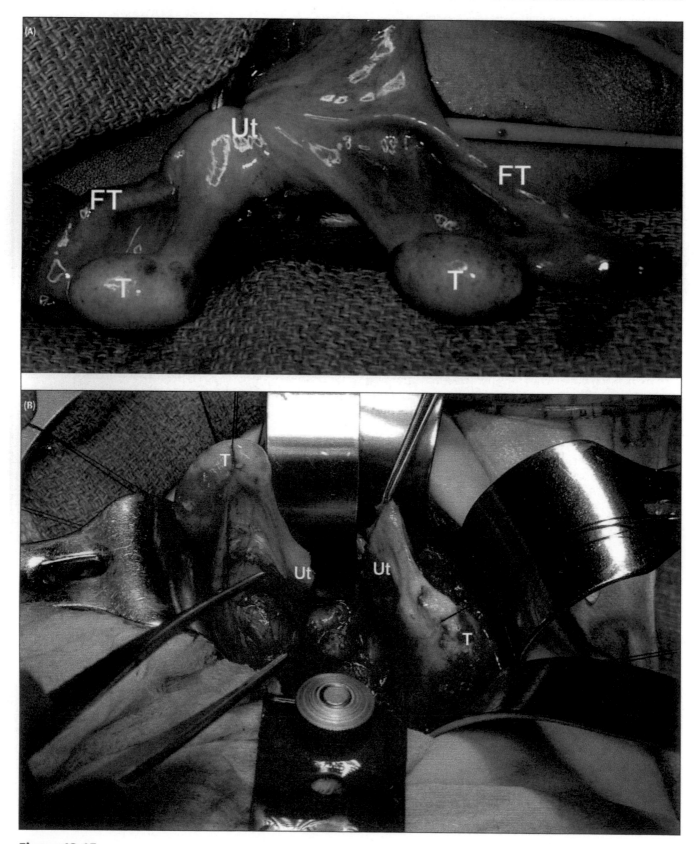

**Figure 13.15**

(A and B) 46XY patient with persistent müllerian duct syndrome (A) and open bivalve of uterus to enable orchiopexies of bilateral abdominal testes (Ut = uterus, FT = fallopian tube, T = testis).

was followed by normalization of blood pressure and good compliance with a glucocorticoid and androgen substitution therapies.[81]

# Common and unusual intraoperative and acute postoperative problems

The most common initial difficulty encountered with Veress needle is improper placement, resulting in injuries to the stomach, bowel, bladder, and major vessels.[82] Very thin patients, infants, and adolescents are at particular risk of vascular injuries, since there is less distance between the anterior abdominal wall and the great vessels. In adults, the site of injury should be re-examined during and at the end of the laparoscopic procedure. Usually in children, and if there is any question regarding the injury, an immediate open laparotomy is performed and the perforation examined directly and repaired.

Carbon dioxide is the preferred agent for insufflation because it is readily available and inexpensive, suppresses combustion with cautery and lasers, and is rapidly absorbed. However, this absorption across the peritoneum may result in hypercarbia and acidosis. One disadvantage of carbon dioxide is that it may make the patient more prone to cardiac arrhythmias compared with other agents such as nitrous oxide. Nitrous oxide, however, is highly combustible and is insoluble in the blood. If it is directly injected into the bloodstream, serious embolism will occur. Pneumoperitoneum also exerts compression upon the vena cava, which may hinder cardiac return. Gas emboli, as previously described from $CO_2$ entering venous channels that are exposed during an operative dissection, can be fatal unless detected rapidly.

On placement of the Veress needle, if the angle of the needle is too oblique, it may slide down along the peritoneum without actually penetrating the peritoneum. Insufflation will then occur between the fascia and the peritoneum, with expansion of the preperitoneal space. Reinsertion of the Veress needle is required or one can convert to the open Hasson technique. One clue would be an elevated reading through the insufflation port (above 15 mmHg), since the carbon dioxide is being pumped into a closed space. Insufflated gas may also dissect along the extraperitoneal fascial planes and into the thoracic or pelvic regions, resulting in subcutaneous or scrotal emphysema or pneumomediastinum. This is not a serious problem and is easily diagnosed by palpating crepitus. Symptomatic pneumomediastinum or pneumothorax requires immediate termination of the procedure, evacuation of the peritoneal gas, and possibly further treatment with a tube thoracostomy. When performing procedures with a patent processus vaginalis, it is a good routine to manually compress the scrotum at the end of the procedure in order to release the pneumoscrotum.

Unlike injuries with the Veress needle, placement of a trocar into the intestinal tract, bladder, or a major blood vessel requires immediate open laparotomy and repair. The trocar and its sheath should be left in place while opening the abdomen in order to minimize bleeding or intestinal contamination and also to help identify the site of injury. An exploration for an abdominal gonad or extended dissection of gonadal vessels may place the ureter at risk especially near the beginning of the external iliac vein where the ureter crosses the bifurcation of the iliac artery. Development of gross hematuria or pneumaturia during a laparoscopic procedure usually suggests a bladder injury. Intravenous administration of methylene blue or indigo carmine can help identify a ureteral injury or placement of the dye into the bladder through a Foley catheter can help identify a bladder injury when the area is examined laparoscopically. Cystoscopy and retrograde ureterograms may be required. The ureter may be stented or directly repaired if needed. Minor bladder injuries usually require only Foley catheter drainage.[82,83]

In reconstructive surgery for CAH, a decrease in sensation to the clitoris may result despite microsurgical handling of the neurovascular supply. Urethral stricture or diverticulum formation have also been described, as in a male hypospadias repair.[84,85] Although uncommon, narrowing of the vaginal opening may develop from scar, and injury to the rectum or colon has also been described. As surgical techniques improve, so do outcomes. In each case, the repair is individualized and agreed upon only after extensive counseling by all physicians involved. The discussion with the family should include a full description of the current anatomy, the timing and types of surgery, the need for further treatment, and expectations after the repair.

All infants raised as boys will require a hypospadias repair and chordee correction. Most repairs are one-stage procedures, however, some severe cases may be performed by a two-stage urethroplasty. Orchiopexies are usually carried out at the same time as the hypospadias repair.

# Results

Although many of the procedures from 20 years ago are outdated and techniques have changed, long-term results of intersex surgery are scarce. No long-term results of infant reduction clitoroplasty are available. Gearhart et al studied patients who underwent reduction clitoroplasty with preservation of a dorsal neurovascular bundle and found that elicitation of evoked potentials was well preserved.[86] This confirms that the neurologic pathways are intact; however, it does not prove normal erotic sensation. Since sexual fulfillment is a complex subject that involves not only clitoral and vaginal sensation but also psychological factors, these mechanisms are still not fully understood.[86,87] Some women who have had a clitorectomy as infants have still been capable of orgasm, and approximately 20% of adult women who have never had any genital surgery are anorgasmic.

The most common complication after vaginoplasty is vaginal stenosis. An examination under anesthesia should be performed prior to puberty to ensure that normal menstruation can occur without obstruction. Adequate caliber for intercourse can usually be obtained by self serial dilation during late adolescence. Current available data suggest that many of the patients who undergo early vaginoplasty will need some sort of revision for stenosis of the introitus later in life.

Success rates for inguinal orchiopexy are 87–92%, with the higher rates for children less than 6 years old. Success rates for abdominal orchiopexies are slightly less, 74–82%.[88] Inadequate testis position occurs in up to 10% of cases and testicular atrophy is seen in about 5%. Damage to the vas deferens occurs in 1–2% and epididymoorchitis is uncommon. Baker et al described a multi-institutional analysis of laparoscopic orchiopexy.[89] Using information from 10 institutions, they noted a 15% loss to follow-up rate. Success rates included 97.2% for primary laparoscopic orchiopexy without vessel division, 74.1% for single-stage laparoscopic orchiopexy with division of the spermatic vessels, and 87.9% for a two-stage laparoscopic orchiopexy with a first-stage division of the vessels. There was an overall 92.8% success rate for laparoscopic surgery. This is higher than that historically ascribed to open orchiopexy. Single-stage laparoscopic orchiopexy with division of the vessels had a markedly higher atrophy rate than two-stage laparoscopic orchiopexy.

A successful hypospadias repair gives the patient a straight penis with a urethra at the end that allows the boy to stand to urinate and direct his urinary stream. After puberty, it also provides for an erect penis which will be sensitive and straight enough for adequate intercourse while allowing a forward deposit of semen with ejaculation. The two main complications of hypospadias surgery are a urethrocutaneous fistula and urethral meatal stenosis. They occur in about 10–15% of cases and are more prevalent in extensive or repeat hypospadias repair. Although less common, one may also see urethral stricture, urethral diverticulum, persistent chordee, or redundant shaft skin.[84,85]

Esposito et al reported on complications of pediatric urologic laparoscopy.[82] Over a 3-year period, 4350 laparoscopic procedures were performed at 8 Italian pediatric surgery centers: 414 cases were for cryptorchidism and 37 cases involved ambiguous genitalia. The majority of these cases were gonadectomy. Only a 2.7% complication rate, of which 6 cases required conversion to open surgery, was noted. There was no mortality in their series, with a maximum follow-up of 4 years, and only one of their complications requiring open conversion occurred during an orchiopexy.

Treatment of the child with intersex should not end with the first postoperative visit. A boy should be evaluated 1 year after orchiopexy for testes size, location, and viability. Starting at puberty, the boy should also be shown how to perform monthly testicular self-examinations. The parents should be made aware of the issues regarding cancer and infertility. Cryptorchidism places the patient at increased risks for malignant testicular tumor development (22 times the general population). Orchiopexy is not protective against testis cancer development, but it does allow easier palpation for subsequent physical examinations. Although intra-abdominal testes comprise only 10–15% of all undescended testes, they account for almost 50% of those testes which develop into cancer. The most common tumor in an undescended testes is a seminoma, which is also more common in abdominal vs inguinal testes. Up to 30% of dysgenetic testes may develop cancer, most commonly a benign tumor called gonadoblastoma. Although this tumor does not spread, it can develop into a malignant form called a dysgerminoma. Patients with a 45X/45XY mosaic karyotype also have an increased risk of carcinoma-in-situ (CIS). Some surgeons have recommended ultrasound and biopsy of a testis at puberty. Ultrasound is then performed yearly until age 20, when a repeat biopsy is performed. Absence of CIS at age 20 suggests that the risk of CIS is minimal.[14,15,70]

The patient with hypospadias repaired as a child should remain in follow-up with his physician in order to identify and correct any long-term complications of the surgery. It is also important to document adequate control of voiding and the force of urinary stream. There appear to be no decreases in fertility from a urethral point of view other than that previously described for cryptorchidism.

## Conclusion

Cosmetic and functional results improve yearly with advances in optical magnification, instrumentation and sutures, and tissue handling. Continuous research in this area allows the surgeon to refine his technique and provide the patient with the best repair possible. Girls who have undergone a feminizing genitoplasty again require long-term follow-up for issues of menstruation, intercourse, and sensation as previously described. With a proper assignment of sex of rearing and a continued management with continuity of care, intersex individuals should be able to lead well-adjusted lives and ultimately obtain sexual satisfaction. Simple, yet comprehensive discussions with all physicians involved and the parents must take into account parental anxieties, and social, cultural, and religious views in order to obtain appropriate gender assignment.

# References

1. Wiener JS, Marcelli M, Lamb DJ. Molecular determinants of sexual differentiation. World J Urol 1996; 14:278–94.

2. Kolon TF, Lamb DL. The molecular basis of intersex conditions. AUA Update Series 2001: XX(14):106–12.

3. Kolon TF, Lamb DJ. Gene transcription and translation. Cont Urol 1998; 10(11):42–67.

4. New MI. Congenital adrenal hyperplasia. In: De Groot L, ed. Endocrinology, 3rd edn. Philadelphia: WB Saunders, 1995:1813–35.

5. Donohue PA, Parker K, Migeon CJ. Congenital adrenal hyperplasia. In: Scriver CR, Beaudet AL, Sly WS, Valle D, eds. The metabolic and molecular basis of inherited disease. 7th edn. New York: McGraw-Hill, 1995:2929–66.

6. Miller WL, Tyrell JB. The adrenal cortex. In: Felig P, Baxter JD, Frohmer LA, eds. Endocrinology and metabolism, 3rd edn. New York: McGraw-Hill, 1995:555–711.

7. White PC, Grossberger D, Onufer BJ, et al. Two genes encoding steroid 21-hydroxylase are located near the genes encoding the fourth component of complement in man. Proc Natl Acad Sci USA 1985; 82:1089–93.

8. Miller WL. Genetics, diagnosis and management of 21-hydroxylase deficiency. J Clin Endocrinol Metab 1994; 78:241–6.

9. New MI, White PC. Genetic disorders of steroid hormone synthesis and metabolism. Baillières Clin Endocrinol Metab 1995; 9:525–54.

10. Speiser PW, Dupont J, Zhu D, et al. Disease expression and molecular genotype in congenital adrenal hyperplasia due to 21-hydroxylase deficiency. J Clin Invest 1992; 90:584–95.

11. Miura K, Yasuda K, Yanase K, et al. Mutation of cytochrome P-45017α gene (CYP17) in a Japanese patient previously reported as having glucocorticoid-responsive hyperaldosteronism: with a review of Japanese patients with mutations of CYP17. J Clin Endocrinol Metab 1996; 81:3797–801.

12. Hook EB, Warburton D. The distribution of chromosome genotypes associated with Turner's syndrome: livebirth prevalence rates and evidence for diminished fetal mortality and severity in genotypes associated with structural X abnormalities or mosaicism. Hum Genet 1983; 64:24–7.

13. Hsu LYF. Phenotype/karyotype correlations of Y chromosome aneuploidy with emphasis on structural aberrations in postnatally diagnosed cases. Am J Med Genet 1994; 53:108–40.

14. Jorgenson N, Muller J, Jaubert F, et al. Heterogeneity of gonadoblastoma germ cells: similarities with immature germ cells, spermatagonia, and testicular carcinoma in situ cells. Histopathology 1997; 30:177–86.

15. Casey AC, Bhodauria S, Shapter A, et al. Dysgerminoma: the role of conservative surgery. Gynecol Oncol 1996; 63:352–7.

16. Fechner PY, Rosenberg C, Stetten G, et al. Nonrandom inactivation of the Y-bearing X chromosome in a 46XX individual: evidence for the etiology of 46XX true hermaphroditism. Cytogenet Cell Genet 1994; 66:22–6.

17. Braun A, Kammerer S, Cleve A, et al. True hermaphroditism in a 46, XY individual, caused by a postzygotic somatic point mutation in the male gonadal sex-determining locus (SRY): molecular genetics and histological findings in a sporadic case. Am J Hum Genet 1993; 52:578–85.

18. Hadjiathanasion CG, Brauner R, Lortat-Jacob S, et al. True hermaphroditism: genetic variants and clinical management. J Pediatr 1994; 125:738–43.

19. La Chance Y, Luu The V, Verrault H, et al. Characterization of the human 3β-hydroxysteroid dehydrogenase/$\Delta^5$ – $\Delta^4$ isomerase gene and its expression in mammalian cells. J Biol Chem 1990; 265:469–75.

20. Simard J, Rheaume E, Mebarki F, et al. Molecular basis of human 3β-hydroxysteroid dehydrogenase deficiency. J Steroid Biochem Mol Biol 1995; 53:127–38.

21. Rheaume E, Simard J, Morel Y, et al. Congenital adrenal hyperplasia due to point mutations in the type II 3β-hydroxysteroid dehydrogenase gene. Nat Genet 1992; 1:239–45.

22. Geller DH, Auchus RJ, Mendonca BB, et al. The genetic and functional basis of isolated 17,20-lyase deficiency. Nat Genet 1997; 17:201–5.

23. Bose HS, Sugawara T, Strauss JF 3rd, Miller WL. The pathophysiology and genetics of congenital lipoid adrenal hyperplasia. International Congenital Lipoid Adrenal Hyperplasia Consortium. N Engl J Med 1996; 335:1870–8.

24. Matsuo N, Tsuzaki S, Anzo M, et al. The phenotypic definition of congenital lipoid adrenal hyperplasia: analysis of the 67 Japanese patients. Abstract 200. 33rd Annual European Society of Pediatric Endocrinology Meeting. Horm Res 1994; 41:106.

25. Geissler WM, Davis DL, Wu I, et al. Male pseudohermaphroditism caused by mutations of testicular 17β-hydroxysteroid dehydrogenase 3. Nat Genet 1994; 7:34–9.

26. Saez JM, de Peretti E, Morera AM, et al. Familial male pseudohermaphroditism with gynecomastia due to a testicular 17-ketosteroid reductase defect. I. In vivo studies. J Clin Endocrinol Metab 1971; 32:604–10.

27. Bangsboll S, Qvist I, Lebech PE, Lewinsky M. Testicular feminization syndrome and associated gonadal tumors in Denmark. Acta Obstet Gynecol Scand 1992; 71:63–6.

28. Lubahn DR, Joseph DR, Sar M, et al. The human androgen receptor: complementary deoxyribonucleic acid cloning, sequence analysis, and gene expression in prostate. Mol Endocrinol 1988; 2:1265–75.

29. La Spada AR, Wilson EM, Lubahn DB, et al. Androgen receptor gene mutations in X-linked spinal and bulbar muscular atrophy. Nature 1991; 352:77–9.

30. Patterson MN, McPhaul MJ, Hughes IA. Androgen insensitivity syndrome. Baillières Clin Endocrinol Metab 1994; 8:379–404.

31. MacLean HE, Warne GL, Zajac JD. Defects of androgen receptor function: from sex reversal to motor neurone disease. Mol Cell Endocrinol 1995; 112:133–41.

32. Nowakowski H, Lenz W. Genetic aspects in male hypogonadism. Recent Prog Horm Res 1961; 17:53–95.

33. Imperato-McGinley JL, Guerrero L, Gautier T, et al. Steroid 5α-reductase deficiency in man: an inherited form of male pseudohermaphroditism. Science 1974; 186:1213–15.

34. Boudon C, Lobaccaro JM, Lumbroso S, et al. A new deletion of 5α-reductase type 2 gene in a Turkish family with 5α-reductase deficiency. Clin Endocrinol 1995; 43:183–8.

35. Baarends WM, van Helmond MJ, Post M, et al. A novel member of the transmembrane serine/threonine kinase receptor family is specifically expressed in the gonads and in mesenchymal cells adjacent to the mullerian duct. Development 1994; 120:189–97.

36. Imbeaud S, Carre-Eusebe D, Rey R, et al. Molecular genetics of the persistent mullerian duct syndrome: a study of 19 families. Hum Mol Genet 1994; 3:125–31.

37. Goodfellow PA, Lovell-Badge R. SRY and sex determination in mammals. Ann Rev Genet 1993; 27:71–92.

38. Kolon TF, Ferrer FA, McKenna PH. Clinical and molecular analysis of XX sex reversed patients. J Urol 1998; 160:1169–72.

39. Swain A, Narvaez V, Burgoyne P, et al. DAX1 antagonizes SRY action in mammalian sex determination. Nature 1998; 391:761–7.

40. Pelletier J, Bruening W, Kashtan CE, et al. Germline mutations in the Wilms tumor suppressor gene are associated with abnormal urogenital development in Denys–Drash syndrome. Cell 1991; 67:437–47.

41. Von Heyninger V, Boyd PA, Seawright A, et al. Molecular analysis of chromosome 11 deletions in aniridia: Wilms Tumor Syndrome. Proc Natl Acad Sci USA 1996; 82:8592–6.

42. Foster JW, Dominguez-Steglich MA, Guioli S, et al. Campomelic dysplasia and autosomal sex reversal caused by mutations in an SRY-related gene. Nature 1994; 372:525–30.

43. Grumbach MM, Barr ML. Cytological tests of chromosomal sex in relation to sexual anomalies in man. Recent Prog Horm Res 1958; 14:255–334.

44. Courrier R, Jost A. Intersexualite totale provoque par la pregnenilone au cours de la grossesse. CR Soc Biol 1942; 136:395–6.

45. Silver RI, Rodriguez R, Chang TS, Gearhart JP. In vitro fertilization is associated with an increased risk of hypospadias. J Urol 1999; 161:1954–7.

46. Sharpe RM, Skakkebaek NE. Are oestrogens involved in falling sperm counts and disorders of the male reproductive tract? Lancet 1993; 341:1392–5.

47. Cozzi J, Chevret S, Rousseaux S, et al. Achievement of meiosis in XXY-germ cells: study of 543 sperm karyotypes from an XY/XXY mosaic patient. Hum Genet 1994; 93:32–4.

48. Jacobs PA, Hassold TJ, Whittington E, et al. Klinefelter's syndrome: an analysis of the origin of the additional sex chromosome using molecular probes. Ann Hum Genet 1988; 52:147–51.

49. Ferguson-Smith MA, Mack WS, Ellis PM, et al. Parental age and the source of the X chromosomes in XXY Klinefelter's syndrome. Lancet 1964; 1:46.

50. Boiseckkine C, Toublanc JE, Abbas N, et al. Clinical and anatomical spectrum in XX sex-reversed patients: relationship to the presence of Y-specific DNA sequences. Clin Endocrinol 1994; 40:733–42.

51. Palmer MS, Sinclair AH, Berta P, et al. Genetic evidence that ZFY is not the testis-determining factor. Nature 1989; 342:937–9.

52. Kolon TF. Intersex. In: Schwartz MW, ed. The 5-minute pediatric consult. New York: Lippincott, Williams & Wilkins, 2003:480–1.

53. Fortunoff S, Lattimer JK, Edson M. Vaginoplasty technique for female pseudohermaphrodites. Surg Gynecol Obstet 1964; 118:545–8.

54. Costa EMF, Mendonca BB, Inacio M, et al. Management of ambiguous genitalia in pseudohermaphrodites: new perspectives on vaginal dilation. Fertil Steril 1997; 67:229–32.

55. Newman K, Randolph J, Parson S. Functional results in young women having clitoral reconstruction as infants. J Pediatr Surg 1992; 27:180–3, discussion 183–4.

56. Donahoe PK, Gustafson ML. Early one-stage surgical reconstruction of the extremely high vagina in patients with congenital adrenal hyperplasia. J Pediatr Surg 1994; 29:352–6.

57. Hendren WH, Atala A. Repair of the high vagina in girls with severely masculinized anatomy from the adrenogenital syndrome. J Pediatr Surg 1995; 30:91–4.

58. Passerini-Glazel G. A new 1-stage procedure for clitorovaginoplasty in severely masculinized female pseudohermaphrodites. J Urol 1989; 142:565–8.

59. Domini R, Rossi F, Caccarelli PL, et al. Anterior sagittal transrectal approach to the urogenital sinus in adrenogenital syndrome: preliminary report. J Pediatr Surg 1997: 32: 714–16.

60. Pena A, Filmer B, Bonilla E, et al. Transanorectal approach for the treatment of urogenital sinus: preliminary report. J Pediatr Surg 1992; 27:681–5.

61. Denes FT, Medonca BB, and Arap S. Laparoscopic management of intersex states. Urol Clin North Am 2001; 28:31–42.

62. Colacurci N, Cardone A, DeFranciscis P, et al. Laparoscopic hysterectomy in a case of male pseudohermaphroditism with persistent Mullerian duct derivatives. Hum Reprod 1999; 12:272–4.

63. Wiener JS, Jordan GH, Gonzales ET Jr. Laparoscopic management of persistent Mullerian duct remnants associated with an abdominal testis. J Endocrinol 1997; 11:357–9.

64. Martin TV, Anderson KR, Weiss RM. Laparoscopic evaluation and management of a child with ambiguous genitalia, ectopic spleen, and Meckel's diverticulum. Tech Urol 1997; 3:49–50.

65. Yu TJ, Shu K, Kung FT, et al. Use of laparoscopy in intersex patients. J Urol 1995; 154:1193–6.

66. Williams JC, Merguerian PA, Schned HR, Amdur RJ. Bilateral testicular carcinoma-in-situ in persistent mullerian duct syndrome: a case report and review of the literature. Urology 1994; 44:595–8.

67. Rajfer J, Walsh PC. Mixed gonadal dysgenesis – dysgenetic male pseudohermaphroditism. Pediatr Adolesc Endocrinol 1981; 8:105–10.

68. Rosler A. Steroid 17β-hydroxysteroid dehydrogenase deficiency in man: an inherited form of male pseudohermaphroditism. J Steroid Biochem Mol Biol 1992; 43:989–1002.

69. Imperato-McGinley J, Peterson RE, Stoller R, et al. Male pseudohermaphroditism secondary to 17-hydroxysteroid dehydrogenase deficiency: gender role change with puberty. J Clin Endocrinol Metab 1979; 49:391–5.

70. Rutgers JL, Scully RE. Pathology of the testes in intersex syndromes. Semin Diagn Pathol 1987; 4:273–81.

71. Cassio A, Caccari EM, D'Errico A, et al. Incidence of intratubular germ cell neoplasia in androgen insensitivity syndrome. Acta Endocrinologia 1990; 123:416–20.

72. Jordan GH, Winslow BA. Laparoscopic single stage and staged orchiopexy. J Urol 1994; 152:1249–52.

73. Koff SH, Sephic PS. Treatment of high undescended testes by low spermatic vein ligation. J Urol 1996; 156:799–803.

74. McDougall EM, Clayman RV, Anderson K, et al. Laparoscopic gonadectomy in a case of testicular feminization. Urology 1993; 42:201–4.

75. Corsan GH, Jow W, Karacan M, Qasim S. Laparoscopic gonadectomy in complete androgen insensitivity syndrome. J Am Ass Gynecol Laparosc 1994; 2:87–9.

76. Wilson EE, Vuitch F and Carr BR. Laparoscopic removal of dysgenetic gonads containing a gonadoblastoma in a patient with Swyer syndrome. Obstet Gynecol 1992; 79:842–4.

77. Portuondo J, Negro J, Barral A, et al. Management of phenotypic female patients with an XY karyotype. J Reprod Med 1986; 31:611–15.

78. Ng JWJ, Koh GH. Laparoscopic orchiopexy for persistent mullerian duct syndrome. Pediatr Surg Int 1997; 12:522–5.

79. Vecchietti G, Ardillo L. La sindrome di Rokitansky-Kuster-Hauser: fisiopastologia e clinica. Aplasia vaginale-Lorni uterini rudimentali. Roma: Societi Editrice Universo 1970:83–8.

80. Borruto F, Chasen ST, Chervenak FA, Fedele L. The Vecchietti procedure for surgical treatment of vaginal agenesis: comparison of laparoscopy and laparotomy. Int J Gynecol Obstet 199; 64:153–8.

81. Chabre O, Porthat-Doyen S, Chaffanjon P, et al. Bilateral laparoscopic adrenalectomy for congenital adrenal hyperplasia with severe hypertension resulting from two novel mutations in splice donor sites of CYP11B1. J Clin Endocrinol Metab 2000; 85:4060–8.

82. Esposito C, Lima M, Girolamo M, et al. Complications of pediatric urological laparoscopy: mistakes and risks. J Urol 2003; 169:1490–2.

83. Peters CA. Complications in pediatric laparoscopy: results of a survey. J Urol 1996; 155:1070–4.

84. Asopa HS. New concepts in the management of hypospadias and its complications. Ann R Coll Surg Engl 1998; 80:161–4.

85. Retik AB, Keating M, Mandell J. Complications of hypospadias repair. Urol Clin North Am 1988; 15:223–40.

86. Gearhart JP, Burnett A, Owen JH. Measurement of pudendal evoked potentials during feminizing genitoplasty: technique and applications. J Urol 153:481–7.

87. Gooren L, Cohen-Kettenis PT. Development of male gender identity/role and a sexual orientation towards women in a 46,XY subject with an incomplete form of the androgen insensitivity syndrome. Arch Sex Behav 1991; 20: 459–70.

88. Docimo SG. The results of surgical therapy for cryptorchidism: a literature review and analysis. J Urol 1995; 154:1148–52.

89. Baker LA, Docimo SG, Surer I, et al. A multi-institutional analysis of laparoscopic orchidopexy. BJU Int 2001; 87: 484–9.

# 14

# Laparoscopy and cryptorchidism

Linda A Baker, Armando Lorenzo, Gerald H Jordan, and Steven G Docimo

## Introduction

The term cryptorchidism refers to the absence of a testicle in the scrotum. During embryonic life, the testis differentiates adjacent to the mesonephric kidneys and normally descends via the inguinal canal to its scrotal position. However, in 0.8–1.8% of 1-year-old boys,[1,2] this process is faulty, resulting in cryptorchidism. In the majority of cryptorchid boys, a testicle is palpable in the groin, but in about 20% a testicle is nonpalpable.[3] In these cases, the gonad might be absent, intra-abdominal (along the normal path of descent or ectopic) or within the inguinal canal (canalicular).[4,5] Prior to 1976, surgical management of the nonpalpable testicle consisted of inguinal exploration with extension of the exploration into the peritoneum if the testis, nubbin, or blind-ending vessels were not identified. The testicle was either absent, removed, positioned scrotally, or a rare worst case scenario, not located by the surgeon.

In 1976, Cortesi described diagnostic laparoscopy as a method to localize the nonpalpable testicle.[6] Soon thereafter, therapeutic laparoscopy was performed by Bloom,[7] Jordan et al,[8] and Bogaert et al.[9] With the introduction of these techniques, the management of the nonpalpable testicle has become a heated debate among pediatric urologists,[10–12] with camps divided for and against laparoscopic management. Nevertheless, as the years have passed, laparoscopic approaches to the nonpalpable testicle have become accepted and incorporated into daily practice by most pediatric urologists, both in the United States and abroad. In this chapter, we will review the preoperative issues, goals, timing, management decisions, procedures, and outcomes of laparoscopic management of the nonpalpable testis.

## Preoperative assessment

At initial evaluation of the patient, a history of palpable gonads, hypospadias, genital surgery or inguinal herniorrhaphy should be obtained. A careful, nonthreatening physical examination in a warm environment with warm lubricant on the groin is often crucial to identify a difficult-to-feel testicle. Note is made of the size of the contralateral testicle, if descended. If the contralateral descended testicle manifests compensatory hypertrophy (as judged by growth comparison to standard nomograms), this may indicate the lack of functioning testicular tissue on the nonpalpable side.[13,14] However, this finding is not absolutely accurate, and therefore the nonpalpable side must be further evaluated. Bilateral nonpalpable testicles represent a distinct subgroup that is discussed later.

Several diagnostic modalities have been used preoperatively in the evaluation of the patient with a nonpalpable testicle, including hormonal challenge and/or radiologic tests. Any diagnostic test that is utilized for the diagnosis of the nonpalpable testicle must uniformly and unequivocally determine the presence or absence of gonadal tissue, and localize it. Only laparoscopy uniformly accomplishes these goals.[5,15,16]

## Hormonal challenge

Hormonal therapy has promoted testicular descent in some nonpalpable cases, rendering some testicles palpable and even rarely fully descended.[17] Although rarely therapeutic, this therapy is best applied to the patient with bilateral nonpalpable testes (discussed below). The use of hormonal therapy in an attempt to promote descent, to our knowledge, in no way complicates either open orchiopexy or laparoscopic orchiopexy. The cost-effectiveness of this approach has been called into question, however.[18]

## Radiological evaluation

Many radiologic techniques, such as ultrasound, venography, computed tomography (CT), and magnetic resonance imaging (MRI), have been employed to locate the non-palpable testis, but unfortunately all of these modalities lack sufficient sensitivity to be solely relied upon.[2,19–22] Herniography, venography, and arteriography may give indirect evidence, but none equivocally define the gonad. Radiographic localizing studies suffer from the inability to rule out the presence of an intra-abdominal testis;[19] therefore, they cannot preclude surgery in the child with a nonpalpable testicle. Granted, ultrasound does image the nonpalpable undescended testicle in some cases; however, many an inguinal orchiopexy has been undertaken when an ultrasound has shown an 'inguinal gonad' which turns out to be a lymph node. While MRI or gadolinium-enhanced magnetic resonance angiography (MRA) has better sensitivity,[23] it is still not nearly as accurate as laparoscopy has been shown to be. Any utility of MRI and MRA is completely negated due to cost issues and the requirement of an anesthetic. Surgical exploration is still required.

Radiographic imaging studies may be useful in certain clinical circumstances. Inguinal ultrasound may help identify nonpalpable inguinal and abdominal testicles in select patients who are likely to derive maximal benefit from laparoscopy,[21] although examination under anesthesia at the time of orchiopexy is probably equally helpful.[5] Imaging is also used for unusual cases, such as the overweight boy with a nonpalpable inguinal testis and the follow-up of adolescents who, because of comorbid conditions, are not surgical candidates.

## Timing of surgery

At birth and into the first year of life, undescended testicles have been shown to have normal histology, including a normal population of germ cells. However, beyond 18 months of age, both light and electron microscopy demonstrate histologic changes, suggesting deterioration of the germ cell population of the testis.[24,25] Some reports have even noted testicular damage as early as 6 months in the human cryptorchid testis. Histology correlates with testicular position, with worse features seen in higher testicles. On the other hand, spontaneous testicular descent has been noted postnatally as late as 4–6 months of age. Therefore, the current recommendation concerning timing of orchiopexy would be between ages 6 and 12 months, since the risks of anesthesia in a healthy 6-month-old child are similar to that of a healthy adult. In addition, there may be anatomic and technical advantages to orchiopexy within the first 6 months, especially in patients with high undescended testicles with prune-belly syndrome. This approach maximizes the opportunity for those few testicles that will descend during the first year of life, while preventing the histologic changes that occur in those testicles that remain maldescended beyond the first

year of life. Data supporting this 'early orchiopexy' recommendation are being reported; testicular growth is more common in children operated prior to 18 months than when older,[26] and early orchiopexy seems to benefit adulthood Leydig cell function, thereby potentially enhancing fertility.[27]

Decisions regarding orchiopexy after age 2 years old are based on the risks/benefits of the testicle to the individual. Although an undescended testis may function poorly for fertility, the usefulness in terms of androgen production must be considered, especially in cases of a solitary testicle.

Occasionally, a postpubertal male is found to have an undescended testis, palpable or nonpalpable. Rarely are sperm noted in these testes[28] and these testes are at significant risk for malignant change. An updated analysis of the anesthetic risks of orchiectomy vs the lifetime risk of germ cell cancer was performed by Kibel and colleagues.[29] They advocate orchiectomy in all healthy, cryptorchid males until age 50 years. For some patients with comorbid conditions, the risks of surgery may be significant even before this age is reached. If not palpable, diagnostic laparoscopy with laparoscopic orchiectomy (especially if combined with another surgical procedure) is an optimal means of management that minimizes pain and time away from work, and scarring.

## Laparoscopic management of the nonpalpable testis

### Definitions, goals, and indications

Laparoscopy has been found to be useful for both the diagnosis of the unilateral or bilateral nonpalpable testicle (diagnostic laparoscopy) as well as for the management of the nonpalpable testicle (therapeutic laparoscopy). Laparoscopy is an excellent diagnostic approach to verify the existence and to locate the nonpalpable testicle.[30–33] The principal goal of diagnostic laparoscopy is to determine if there is nonpalpable testicular tissue. If there is nonpalpable testicular tissue, then the decision must be made as to whether the testicle is suitable for orchiopexy or better removed. In addition, mobility of the testis, its vas deferens, and its vascular supply is assessed, a crucial feature in planning the therapeutic surgical approach. The goal of therapeutic laparoscopy for the undescended testicle is either removal of the poor testicle or permanent fixation of the testicle in the scrotum. Therapeutic laparoscopy thus encompasses the options of laparoscopic orchiectomy, primary laparoscopic orchiopexy, laparoscopic one-stage Fowler–Stephens orchiopexy, or laparoscopic two-stage Fowler–Stephens orchiopexy. The indications/goals of laparoscopic orchiopexy are identical to the goals of open orchiopexy: namely, to improve fertility (and possibly diminish malignant transformation potential), relocate the testicle to the scrotum for easier examination, correct the associated inguinal hernia, prevent testicular torsion, and alleviate possible psychological trauma resulting from an empty hemiscrotum.[34]

## Alternative therapy

Management of the nonpalpable testis can be medical (hormonal therapy as previously described) or surgical. Surgical options include open techniques (inguinal exploration with the extension of the inguinal incision proximally to explore the abdomen or primary open abdominal approach), or laparoscopic techniques. Both techniques offer significant advantages and disadvantages.

## Disadvantages to open inguinal exploration

Serious concerns exist in the reliability of an open inguinal exploration to rule out an intra-abdominal testis. Pooling data from five series,[32,35–39] laparoscopy has identified 42 testicles in 86 'negative' open explorations for a nonpalpable testicle. Although a large sampling bias is expected in such reports, the fact that testicles are missed by open inguinal exploration but found by laparoscopy cannot be ignored, considering intra-abdominal testes are at highest risk for malignant degeneration.

Moreover, a critical assessment of the surgical outcomes of open orchiopexy for the intra-abdominal testicle reveals the need for improvement.[40,41] At present, therapeutic laparoscopy offers the highest success rate for orchiopexy for the intra-abdominal testicle.[38]

## Disadvantages to diagnostic and therapeutic laparoscopy

Opponents of therapeutic laparoscopic orchiopexy have voiced concerns about the long incision in the peritoneum, lengthy operation, higher operating room costs, potential injury to intra-abdominal or retroperitoneal organs, and the long-term risk of adhesions.[42] Operating room costs can be diminished by the use of reusable equipment[43] and countered by shorter and simpler hospitalization.[44] The incidence of adhesion formation from pediatric urologic laparoscopic procedures is lower than that expected with open exploration.[45,46] Clearly, as with any surgical approach, laparoscopy may have complications.[38] In addition, opponents argue that a laparoscopic approach subjects a patient

(with an inguinal testis or nubbin) to an unnecessary laparoscopic procedure in 37–64% of cases.[10,11,15,47] This can be reduced significantly by first performing scrotal exploration when there is any palpable tissue. The finding of hemosiderin or a nubbin with vas and atretic vessels obviates the need for further exploration.[48]

## Advantages to diagnostic and therapeutic laparoscopy

Against this view, advocates of laparoscopy for the nonpalpable testis have noted that it is useful in at least 43–51% of unilateral cases to identify either absence (27%) or an intra-abdominal testicle (16–21%), and for bilateral undescended testicle in 75% of cases, with 17% blind-ending vessels and 58% intra-abdominal testicles,[49] although these numbers vary from study to study. Thereby, an unnecessary inguinal exploration with subsequent extended open abdominal exploration can be avoided in the 'vanishing testis' syndrome and testicular aplasia. Other reports site intra-abdominal viable testicles as high as 52%.[5,50] Thus, surgical planning is improved. Several rare conditions, including absent vasa and vessels with a retroperitoneal testis,[15] persistent müllerian ducts,[51] other intersex states,[52] transverse testicular ectopia, polyorchidism, and gonadal dysjunction from the wolffian ducts, can best be identified and treated simultaneously laparoscopically. Careful intra-abdominal mobilization can be extensive with therapeutic laparoscopy, allowing orchiopexy with or without testicular vessel division. In addition, laparoscopic orchiopexy offers less trauma of access, a rapid recovery, minimal adhesion formation,[45] and potentially less psychological burden from surgery and scarring. In skillful hands, the operating time for laparoscopic orchiopexy becomes equivalent to open abdominal orchiopexy. A time of less than 90 min for bilateral orchiopexy for abdominal testicles is reasonable to expect in most cases.

# Laparoscopic surgery
## Unilateral nonpalpable testes

Preoperatively, the family is counseled concerning the possibilities of an absent testicle, small atrophic testicle, or an intra-abdominal testicle. The possible surgical scenarios are then presented. If a testicle is palpable under anesthesia (18%),[5] an inguinal orchiopexy is performed. If there is palpable tissue in the scrotum, an expeditious scrotal exploration may be performed, looking for a nubbin or deposit of hemosiderin, vas and atretic vessels, all suggesting no need for further exploration.[48] If it remains nonpalpable under anesthesia, then diagnostic laparoscopy is performed. If an atrophic testicular remnant is identified, a laparoscopic orchiectomy might be performed (surgeon's bias). If a subjectively good testicle is found, the laparoscopic options include (1) primary laparoscopic orchiopexy, (2) one-stage Fowler–Stephens orchiopexy, or (3) two-stage Fowler–Stephens orchiopexy (second stage follows 6 months later). The risks of surgery include bleeding, infection, anesthesia risks, injury to intra-abdominal or retroperitoneal organs necessitating emergent laparotomy, loss of a testicle (acute atrophy), mechanical injury to the vas, epididymis, testicular vessels or testis, poor testicular position, or need for a two-stage procedure. An algorithm illustrating the approach to management of the nonpalpable undescended testicle is shown in Figure 14.1.

## Techniques of procedures

### Diagnostic laparoscopy

After adequate anesthesia is attained, the patient is secured to the bed in the supine, frog-leg position with arms tucked. Preparation and draping must be suitable for an open abdominal procedure, be it planned or necessary. A urethral Foley catheter and an orogastric tube are passed. All laparoscopic equipment is assembled and verified. A supra- or infraumbilical skin incision is made and peritoneal access is obtained. Several techniques have been used, including Veress needle, Hasson access, or open access. Given most patients are between 6 and 24 months of age, safety concerns have led most surgeons to abandon blind access techniques (Veress needle) and to use open

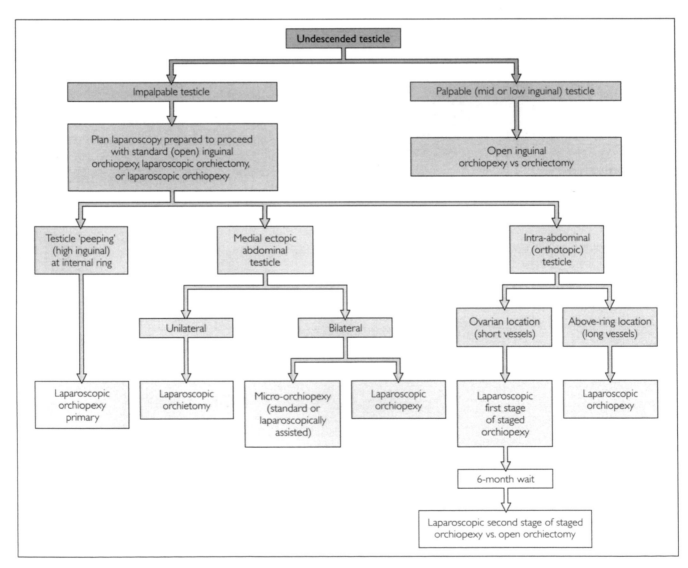

**Figure 14.1**
Algorithm for management of the undescended testicle.

access techniques. Holding sutures are placed in the fascia to help elevate it for the peritonotomy. The authors use the InnerDyne Step introducer system,[53,54] a radially dilating access sheath, to achieve 5 or 10 mm access.[55] Alternatively, exclusively needlescopic 2 mm access (and working ports) can be used, as reported by Gill and colleagues,[53,56,57] but they provide less light and a smaller visual field. After insufflation to 14 cmH$_2$O, a 5 mm 0° camera is used to inspect the abdomen for injury. The patient is then placed in the Trendelenburg position and each internal ring is inspected bilaterally. On the unaffected side, the testicular vessels and vas are easily identified, leaving the closed internal ring (Figure 14.2). Caudal traction on the descended testis can help visualization of its cord structures. On the affected side, the internal ring is noted and the testicle, vas, and testicular vessels are sought.

Several findings are possible on the affected side:

1.  If the ring is closed with a normal vas and normal testicular vessels exiting (see Figure 14.2), the groin is explored for the testis or nubbin by a laparoscopic or open approach. The removal of any remaining testicular nubbin is controversial since 10% of nubbins may contain viable germ cells[58–60] and theoretically could undergo malignant change.
2.  If normal-appearing vas and testicular vessels exit an open internal ring (Figure 14.3), the inguinal canal can be 'milked' retrograde in an attempt to push a canalicular (peeping) testicle or nubbin into the abdomen (Figure 14.4). In any case, if the gonad is not found, the groin must be explored,[61] either by open or laparoscopic techniques.

3.  If blind-ending vessels are clearly identified, ending in a 'horse tail' appearance and often within proximity to a blind-ending vas, the testis is not viable and the procedure is terminated, although some surgeons again would remove any testicular nubbin found (Figure 14.5).
4.  An intra-abdominal testis could be found (Figure 14.6).
5.  A blind-ending vas can be seen without testicular vessels in the vicinity. In this case, the laparoscopic exploration is not complete and must continue rostrally toward the aortic origin of the testicular vessels until the gonad is found. This finding is termed gonadal dysjunction.

Statistically, in nonpalpable cases, an intra-abdominal testis or peeping testicle is identified in 50–60%, an atrophic nubbin in 30%, and an absent testis in 20%. If a testicle is found, it can be seen within 2 cm of the internal ring (30.6%) or peeping (17.4%), typically of normal size with a normal-appearing epididymis, vas, and vessels. Alternatively, the testicle can be found > 2 cm from the internal ring, either along the normal path of descent (44.8%) or in such ectopic sites as beside the bladder, rectum, kidney, liver, spleen, or crossed ectopia (7.1%).[38]

In some cases, the testicle and testicular vessels are not clearly identified with the camera alone. A manipulating instrument is useful to visualize the testicular vessels (if loops of bowel are blocking the view). The Veress needle or other small probes have been used for this purpose and do not require a formal secondary cannula placement. If therapeutic laparoscopy is indicated, the insufflation is

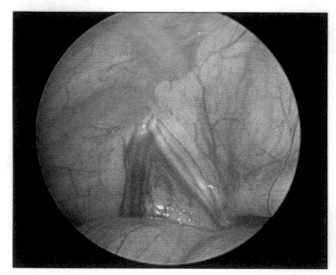

**Figure 14.2**
The laparoscopic appearance of a normal left groin. The spermatic vessel leash can be seen joined by the vas deferens passing through a closed internal ring. Traction is on the testicle, emphasizing the location of the ring.

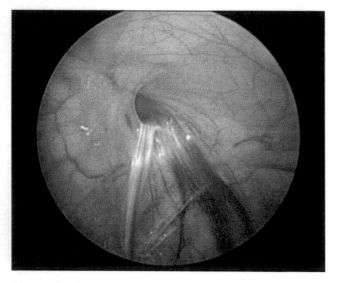

**Figure 14.3**
The laparoscopic appearance of the right groin in which there is a patent processus vaginalis (hernia).

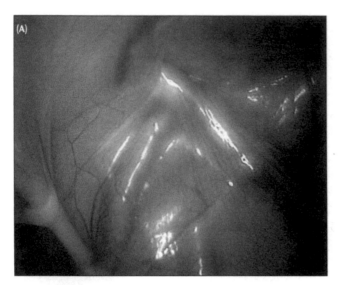

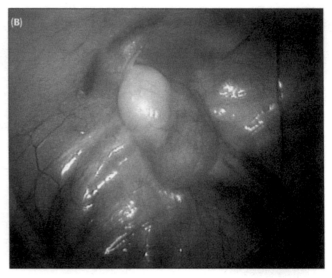

**Figure 14.4**
(A) Laparoscopic appearance of the right groin; the spermatic vessel leash joined by the vas can be seen passing adjacent to the open internal ring (patent processus vaginalis). (B) With gentle pressure on the groin, the testicle can be seen delivered into the abdomen.

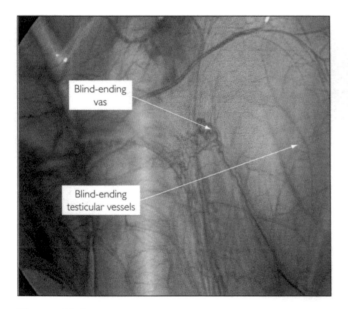

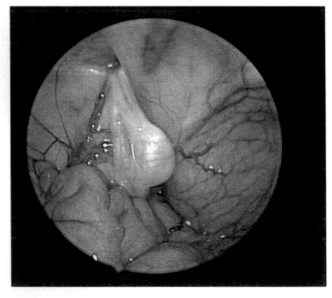

**Figure 14.5**
The laparoscopic appearance of the right groin, with the classic blind-ending vas and blind-ending testicular vessels in proximity to each other.

**Figure 14.6**
The laparoscopic appearance of the low left abdominal testicle.

temporarily increased up to 20 cmH$_2$O while two 2 mm or 5 mm ports are secured at the level of the umbilicus just lateral to the inferior epigastric vessels (Figure 14.7). Using a Maryland grasper and laparoscopic scissors with cautery, the testis is located. Either laparoscopic orchiectomy, single-stage laparoscopic orchiopexy (primary or one-stage Fowler–Stephens), or two-stage laparoscopic orchiopexy is chosen.

## Primary laparoscopic orchiopexy

To perform a primary laparoscopic orchiopexy, the patient is placed in the Trendelenburg position with the ipsilateral side of the bed tilted upward. A peritoneotomy is made just lateral to the testicular vessels. It is carried over the top of the internal ring and continued lateral and superior to the vas, with care to not injure the inferior epigastric vessels or

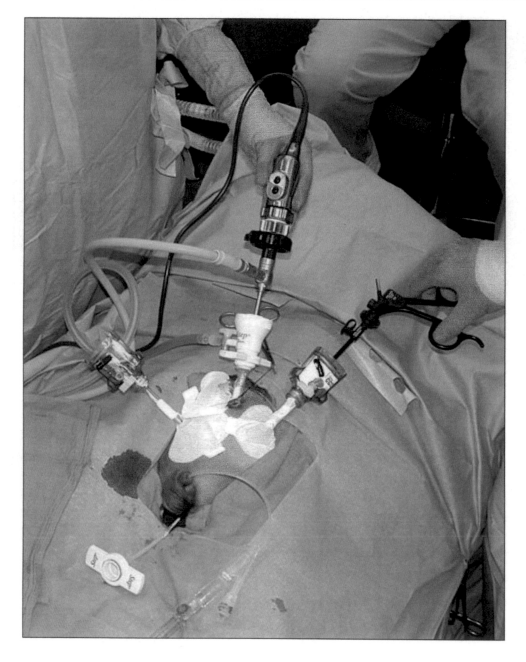

**Figure 14.7**
Typical cannula placement for left laparoscopic orchiopexy.

the bladder. While some urologists make a mirror peritoneotomy medial to the vessels and vas, others (including the authors) intentionally leave the peritoneal triangle between the testicular vessels and the vas undisturbed. Once the peritoneotomy is completed, the testicular vessels, testicle, and vas are elevated on this peritoneal pedicle, thereby dissecting the plane between these structures and the external iliac vessels (Figure 14.8). Care is taken to not harm the external iliac vessels, inferior epigastric vessels, or a long looping vas. The testicle is then retracted rostrally, inverting the processus vaginalis and the gubernaculum. The gubernaculum is thinned and cut across with electrocautery, taking care to watch for a long looping vas. Cautery is used since the gubernacular attach-

ments are vascular, although caution is exercised to avoid thermal damage to peritesticular structures. The testicle is then retracted toward the contralateral internal ring to assess length. In most cases, if the testicle can reach the contralateral internal ring, length is sufficient to place the testicle well in the respective hemiscrotum. While vigorous mobilization of the vas should be avoided for fear of testicular atrophy, the vas must be sufficiently mobilized to prevent ureteral kinking from the paravasal attachments. Any remaining attachments preventing testicular mobility are carefully dissected, and, once adequate length is assured, the testicle can be transferred to the scrotum.

In some instances, length is inadequate. One option is to incise the peritoneum parallel to the testicular vessels as far

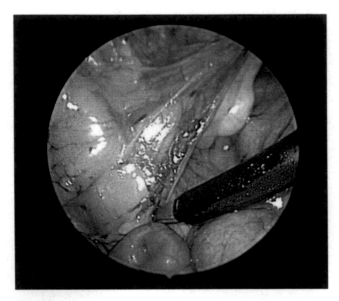

**Figure 14.8**
The peritoneotomies have been completed and the gubernaculum was transected. The testis is retracted medially and ventrally, with the sheet of peritoneum medial to the testicular vessels and vas intact. Tethering attachments on the dorsal side of the peritoneum can be divided as the testis is pulled toward the contralateral internal ring.

proximal as is safe. Then, the peritoneal incision is extended perpendicular over the testicular vessels without their injury. Often this perpendicular incision significantly 'relaxes' the vessels, allowing scrotal positioning. If length still remains an issue and the peritoneum medial to the vas and vessels is intact, the spermatic vessels can be divided (Fowler–Stephens approach – see below).

Several techniques are described to deliver the testis into the scrotum, including retrograde placement of a clamp or port. By placing a port, the pneumoperitoneun can be maintained in the event the testis is 'fumbled'. The authors use the InnerDyne Step 5 or 10 mm for the transfer.[53,54] A 2 mm grasper in the ipsilateral abdominal port is passed medial or lateral to the inferior epigastric vessels, depending on length needs, just over the pubic ramus (Figure 14.9A). A scrotal skin incision is made in the ipsilateral hemiscrotum and a subdartos pouch is generated. The 2 mm grasper is passed through the scrotal incision. The Step introducer sheath is introduced retrograde over the 2 mm grasper (Figure 14.9B). The 5 or 10 mm trocar is introduced through the Step introducer (Figure 14.9C). A locking grasper is introduced through the scrotal port, the gubernaculum of the testis is grasped, and the testis is delivered via the port into the scrotum (Figure 14.10A). The testis is secured intrascrotally in the subdartos pouch by the fixation technique preferred by the surgeon (Figure 14.10B). The intra-abdominal pressure is lowered to 4 mmHg and the surgical field assessed for bleeding (Figure 14.10C).

In children, the fascia of any 5 or 10 mm port site is closed, as hernias have been reported. All $CO_2$ is evacuated and skin wounds are closed and dressed. These children do profit from adjuvant caudal anesthesia and local injection of cannula sites using bupivacaine (Marcaine). The children are awakened, recover from anesthesia, and are discharged. In most cases, the diet is rapidly advanced. With the exception of instructions to keep the child from playing on straddle implements, virtually no physical restrictions are imposed.

## One-stage Fowler–Stephens laparoscopic orchiopexy

If the maneuvers outlined above result in inadequate length of the testicular vessels preventing scrotal positioning, a one-stage Fowler–Stephens procedure can be performed. Via a contralateral 5 mm port, the testicular artery and vein are clipped and transected, preserving the vasal blood supply to the testicle and thus allowing the testicle to be placed in the scrotum with one laparoscopic procedure. However, this technique has a higher risk of testicular atrophy.[38]

## Two-stage Fowler–Stephens laparoscopic orchiopexy

If, at the time of diagnostic laparoscopy, a high testis is found which stands little chance of reaching the scrotum without transection of the testicular vessels, a two-stage Fowler–Stephens laparoscopic orchiopexy may be used.[7] In this case, a contralateral 5 mm port is placed and the only peritoneotomy performed is parallel and immediately medial to the testicular vessels, a safe distance proximal to the iliac vessels. Via this peritoneotomy, the vessels are encircled and a 5 mm vascular clip applier is used to ligate the vessels. The vessels may be transected or left in continuity after clipping, and the procedure is terminated. Six months later, a second laparoscopy is performed following the steps outlined in the primary laparoscopic orchiopexy. The vessels are mobilized to the clips and the mobilized testis is transferred into the scrotum. During the 6-month interval, collateral blood supply via the paravasal arteries is ostensibly enhanced.

Division of the spermatic vessels to 'aid' with orchiopexy was advocated as early as 1903 by Bevan.[62] The staged approach based on collateralization along the long loop of the vas deferens was an extension of the technique described by Fowler and Stephens. Originally a long looping vas was felt to be a prerequisite for the Fowler–Stephens procedure; however, intra-abdominal testicles with non-long looping vas deferens have been successfully addressed. The staged approach has been likened to other forms of delay, a term in the

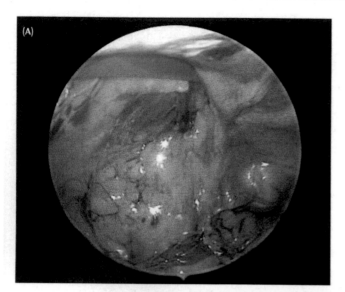

## Figure 14.9

(A) Via the ipsilateral abdominal port, a laparoscopic Maryland grasper is passed medial to the ipsilateral inferior epigastric vessels, over the anterior pubic ramus, and out through the scrotal skin incision. (B) The 10 mm Step introducer is loaded on the Maryland grasper and pushed intraperitoneally as the Maryland grasper is drawn back into the abdomen. Note the Maryland grasper in the ipsilateral port exiting the scrotum. (C) The trocar is advanced into the introducer with visualization via the intra-abdominal camera.

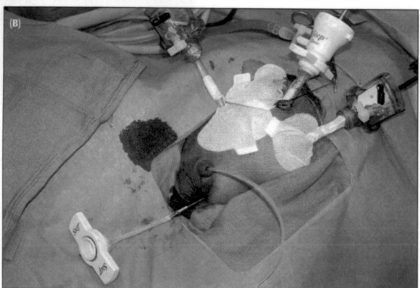

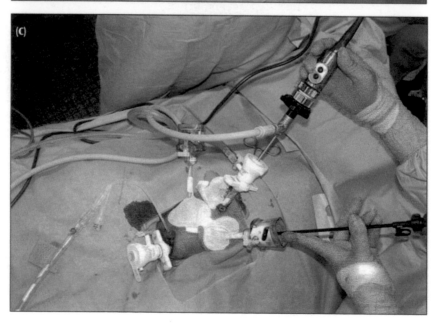

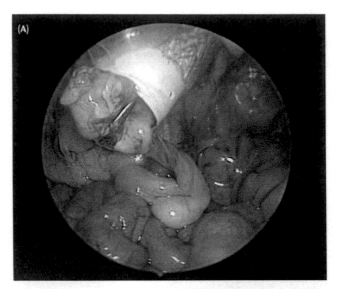

## Figure 14.10

(A) Photograph showing an intra-abdominal testicle being pulled into the 10 mm laparoscopic cannula using testicular grasping forceps. the testicle is then delivered to the right hemiscrotum. (B) Photograph illustrating the outside appearance with the testicle delivered to the level of the scrotum. (C) Intra-abdominal view after the left testicle has been transferred to the scrotum.

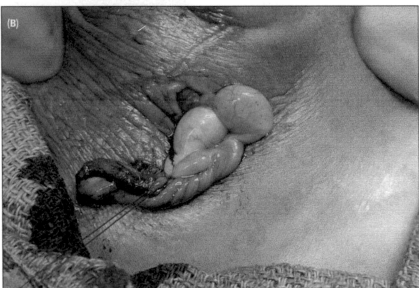

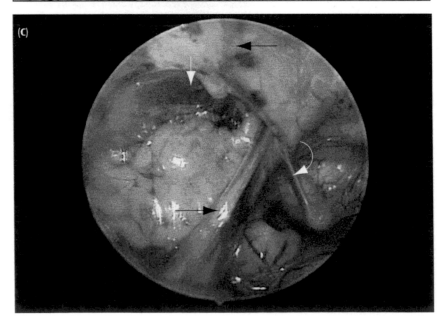

reconstructive literature which implies the transposition of tissue at a first stage, with division of the axial blood supply at a second stage, thus allowing the transfer tissue to survive on random collateralization occurring between the first and second stage. Clearly, the staged orchiopexy does not accomplish this. Instead, the axial blood supply, or at least part of it, is divided at the first stage. There remains a second axial blood supply, but one is led to believe that the second blood supply enhances during the period between first stage and second stage. Whether this enhancement truly occurs has recently been called into question by Koff and Sephic.[63] Clinically, most would agree that the paravasal blood supply, after division of the spermatic vessel leash and a waiting period, does appears to be more prominent. After a 6-month wait following the initial ligation of the spermatic vessels, using either laparoscopic techniques or an open technique, the testicle is brought to the scrotum based on the paravasal vascular supply.

## Intraoperative scenarios

**Common scenarios.**  If normal vessels enter an open or closed ring, an inguinal exploration can be accomplished laparoscopically in virtually all cases. In the case of a high canalicular testis (peeping testis), laparoscopic orchiopexy has been shown to be effective. In the vast majority of low abdominal testes (< 2 cm from the internal ring), primary laparoscopic orchiopexy is most effective. For testes >2 cm from the internal ring, many would consider staged orchiopexy.

**The blind-ending vas and the medially ectopic testis.** It cannot be overemphasized that the undescended testicle is found proximate to the vessels, not necessarily the blind-ending vas. If one finds only a blind-ending vas deferens in the pelvis, one cannot declare the testicle 'vanished' without further exploration and the findings of blind-ending vessels. Occasionally, the gubernacula can appear vascular enough to represent testicular vessels, and give the mistaken impression of vas and vessels exiting the ring when a testis exists proximately.

During descent, the medial ectopic abdominal testicle comes to rest medial to its respective medial umbilical artery. Associated with these testicles are readily apparent vascular gubernacular structures that extend to the respective location of a normal internal ring, usually closed (i.e. no patent processus vaginalis). The vas deferens is quite short; most of these testicles have not been noted to have looping vas or disassociation of the paratesticular tubular structures, and, by definition, the spermatic vessel leash is short. Although these testicles can occasionally be placed in the scrotum using laparoscopic techniques, this is often technically difficult. Also because these testicles are already medial to the obliterated umbilical artery, the advantages

of medial transposition are negated. Because the testicles are not associated with looping of the vas, the advantages of spermatic vessel division, either primary or staged, are likewise negated. These testicles appear to be quite 'ovarian'. The prominent gubernacular vessels are very similar to a round ligament in appearance. There is often a very prominent peritoneal fold, reminiscent of the broad ligament. The testicles, as opposed to having a vertical orientation, appear to have a horizontal orientation. If unilateral, consider orchiectomy or staged laparoscopic orchiopexy. If associated with bilateral maldescensus, aggressive mobilization can be attempted. Another option in the case of bilaterality would be the microvascular reanastomosis of the free transferred testicles.

## Bilateral nonpalpable testes

At birth, approximately 1/600 males have bilateral undescended testes, representing 10–25% of patients with cryptorchidism. Given that normally testicular descent is an event of the third trimester, this may be a common physical finding in premature male neonates. It is estimated that at least 6% of patients with bilateral undescended testes have an endocrine disorder as the etiology.[64,65]

Bilateral undescended testes, when each is palpable, are managed in the same fashion as unilateral palpable undescended testes. However, the finding of bilateral nonpalpable testes represents a special situation that may have life-threatening implications in the neonatal period, especially in association with severe hypospadias. The differential diagnosis of bilateral nonpalpable cryptorchidism includes anorchidism, undescended testicles (bilateral or unilateral with contralateral absence), and ambiguous genitalia due to female pseudohermaphroditism or another intersex condition. It is this last possibility that necessitates an urgent and thorough evaluation to rule out life-threatening congenital adrenal hyperplasia (CAH). A karyotype, endocrine testing, radiographic studies and, if indicated, laparoscopy usually provide the necessary information to make an intersex diagnosis. A normal-appearing masculinized phallus does not eliminate this possibility. Routine neonatal screening for CAH has aided detection of this entity.

In the case where an intersex disorder has been excluded, endocrine studies – human chorionic gonadotropin (hCG) stimulation test, serum müllerian inhibitory substance (MIS) level, or serum inhibin B level – may be useful to differentiate bilateral cryptorchidism from anorchia.[66] hCG administration can be used to stimulate testosterone production by testicular tissue to detect its presence biochemically, and may also cause the gonads to become palpable by physical examination. However, false-negative hCG stimulation testing can occur due to an unresponsive population of Leydig cells. In addition, no consensus has been reached concerning dosing and frequency of hCG. Therefore, hCG stimulation testing is combined with the measurement of gonadotropins to diagnose anorchia. Markedly elevated gonadotropins before puberty are indicative of anorchidism,[66] but all boys with normal serum gonadotropin levels must undergo exploration regardless of the outcome of the hCG stimulation test. Measurement of serum MIS can be used to provide additional evidence that testicular tissue is present and has recently become widely available. Recently, in prepubertal cryptorchid children, the serum inhibin B level has been shown to negatively correlate with serum follicle-stimulating hormone (FSH) levels (basal or hCG stimulated)[67] and positively correlate with the lack of testosterone response to hCG stimulation.[68] However, serum inhibin B levels can also be somewhat low in children with gonadal dysgenesis or the history of testicular trauma. If the clinical experience with this new available serum marker continues to show its reliability, this may supplant the need for the hCG stimulation test.

Thus, with a male genotype, the diagnosis of anorchia can be made with a low serum testosterone, a negative hCG stimulation test, increased serum gonadotropins, a negative serum MIS, a low basal serum inhibin B level, normal levels of adrenal steroid precursors, and radiographic studies demonstrating the absence of müllerian structures. In equivocal cases, diagnostic laparoscopy and/or open surgical exploration with gonadal biopsy may be required to confirm the diagnosis of anorchia. However, some pediatric urologists feel that for the child with bilateral nonpalpable testicles, laparoscopic management is imperative, regardless of the laboratory results after hCG stimulation or serum MIS sampling.

Intraoperative decision making is impacted by the location of the testes with bilateral disease. In patients with high bilateral intra-abdominal testes, most pediatric urologists perform staged reconstructions. Surgery is completed on one side, confirming unilateral testis survival prior to embarking on the contralateral side, since in many of these complex cases a Fowler–Stephens approach must be used.

## Laparoscopic orchiopexy for intersex states

Diagnostic laparoscopy was first described for intersex evaluation in 1973 by Gans and Berci.[69] Advancements in the laboratory diagnosis of intersex states mean the majority of cases have a clear-cut diagnosis prior to surgery. Exceptions include differentiating between true hermaphroditism and the XX male with genital ambiguity and nonpalpable gonads.[52] Nevertheless, therapeutic laparoscopic techniques including laparoscopic gonadal biopsy, gonadectomy (for dysgenetic gonads or when contrary to sex assignment), orchiopexy, and in some cases removal of ductal structures, have a prominent place in the management of intersex children (primarily male pseudohermaphrodites). Minimalization of physical scarring from surgery is paramount in this patient population, who often suffer from poor body and sexual self-esteem.

## Benefits of surgery

By performing an orchiopexy, the often-associated inguinal hernia is repaired and the testicle is fixated in the scrotum, thereby preventing torsion and any psychological issues associated with an empty hemiscrotum.

## Fertility

Clinically, decreased fertility is a well-recognized consequence of cryptorchidism. Even after orchiopexy, fertility is impaired in approximately 50–70% of boys born with one undescended testis and up to 75% of those born with two undescended testes.[70] Since histologic deterioration is thought to be worse with higher testes, fertility has been thought to vary in association with this finding. However, a recent study indicates that paternity (which does not necessarily correlate with histology of the undescended testis in cases of unilateral maldescent) may be similar in both abdominal and extra-abdominal unilateral undescended testes.[71] Since the serum level of inhibin B is considered to reflect Sertoli cell function and seminiferous tubule integrity, the finding of lower levels of circulating inhibin B in boys with a history of cryptorchidism may predict impaired spermatogenesis later in life.[72] Whether or not early orchiopexy ultimately improves fertility remains to be seen. Without treatment, bilateral cryptorchidism ultimately results in infertility. Antisperm antibodies, abnormalities of the epididymis and vas deferens, and surgical injury to the vas deferens during orchiopexy may also contribute to infertility in patients with a history of cryptorchidism.

## Testicular malignancy

Despite the increased risk (9.7×) over the general population, the likelihood of developing testicular cancer in a man with a history of cryptorchidism is no more than 1 in 2000. For this reason, removal of undescended testes is not warranted in the general case. Orchiopexy allows easy examination of the scrotal testis for earlier detection in cases of testicular cancer. Unfortunately, there is no strong evidence that early orchiopexy decreases the risk of testicular cancer.[73]

# Complications of diagnostic and therapeutic laparoscopy for the nonpalpable testis

Diagnostic laparoscopy is regarded as a highly effective and safe procedure to localize and diagnose the nature of the nonpalpable testicle. In most series, a large number of procedures have been performed with >95% accuracy.[5] Many of the complications of laparoscopic orchiopexy have been associated with blind cannula placement Veress needle insufflation, which is discouraged by the authors. Major complications that have been reported with laparoscopic orchiopexy include acute testicular atrophy, bowel perforation,[74] cecal volvulus, bladder perforation,[9] ileus, minor vas laceration, bowel incarceration at the site of the closure of the parietal peritoneum, and spermatic vessel avulsion, which leads to a one-stage Fowler–Stephens orchiopexy.[38]

# Outcomes of laparoscopic orchiopexy

Outcomes analyses always compare to a gold standard. In the case of orchiopexy, open surgical techniques are the gold standard, with the early postoperative outcome variables being testis position (scrotal) and lack of testicular atrophy. In 1995, a meta-analysis of open surgical results[40] found open orchiopexy for the intra-abdominal testicle to yield an overall 76.1% success rate. By procedure, open one-stage Fowler–Stephens orchiopexy yielded a 67% success rate, whereas the two-stage procedure yielded 73%. Transabdominal orchiopexy was successful in 81%, whereas microvascular orchiopexy worked in 84%. In comparison, a 2001 multi-institutional analysis of laparo-

scopic orchiopexy was performed, collating the results from 10 US centers.[38] A total of 310 laparoscopic orchiopexies in 252 patients in a 9-year period were included; 15.2% were lost to follow-up. Primary laparoscopic orchiopexy was successful in 97.2% of 178 testes. One-stage Fowler–Stephens laparoscopic orchiopexy was successful in 74.1% of 27 testes, whereas two-stage Fowler–Stephens laparoscopic orchiopexy was successful in 87.9% of 58 testes. Therefore, if the Docimo 1995 meta-analysis is compared for each type of orchiopexy, the laparoscopic approach yielded higher success rates than the same approach performed open (Table 14.1). In addition, both analyses revealed that one-stage Fowler–Stephens approaches had a significantly higher atrophy rate than the two-stage repair.

In summary, laparoscopic orchiopexy has been found effective, in one modification or another, for the management of all testicles from high canalicular, associated with hernias, to high abdominal. However, the higher the testicle, the more profound the anatomic aberrances. The long-term function of these testes with respect to malignant degenerative potential and fertility will be outcomes analyzed by the next generation of pediatric urologists. The issue then surrounds the advocacy of performing orchiopexy for the severely dysmorphic abdominal testicle. That issue has been extensively argued and will continue to be. However, the development of sperm aspiration techniques associated with various applications of assisted fertilization seems to favor a try at orchiopexy as opposed to reflexive orchiectomy.

# Conclusions

Laparoscopy for the nonpalpable testis has become the standard approach at many US and European centers. Although laparoscopy is invasive and requires general anesthesia, the advantages are felt by most to far outweigh the disadvantages, particularly now that the laparoscopy can be part of the management, as opposed to just the preparation. The experienced surgeon can accomplish identical or even improved surgical results with similar

**Table 14.1** *A comparison of open vs laparoscopic orchiopexy success rates from two large published series. Success was defined as scrotal position and lack of atrophy*

| Study | Primary orchiopexy | | One stage F-S | | Two stage F-S | |
|---|---|---|---|---|---|---|
| | *n* | Percent | *n* | Percent | *n* | Percent |
| Open orchiopexy[40] | 80 | 81.3 | 321 | 66.7 | 56 | 76.8 |
| Laparoscopic orchiopexy[38] | 178 | 97.2 | 27 | 74.1 | 58 | 87.9 |

*n* = number of testes, F-S = Fowler–Stephens.

operative time and diminished surgical morbidity using laparoscopic techniques. It is clear that laparoscopic orchiopexy provides higher retroperitoneal mobilization of the testicular vessels and vas than can be achieved via inguinal open approaches. Given several reports[32,35–39] of testes found laparoscopically after false-negative inguinal explorations, the reports of carcinoma-in-situ in post-pubertal cryptorchid patients,[28,75] and numerous cases of malignancy in retained intra-abdominal testes,[76] a consistent definitive diagnosis by laparoscopy is imperative and outweighs the price of its invasiveness. Laparoscopic orchiopexy is, if not the procedure of choice, an acceptable and successful approach to the nonpalpable testis. Sometimes called a technology seeking an application,[77] it is currently the procedure associated with the highest testicular success rate (scrotal position without testicular atrophy).[38]

# References

1. Berkowitz GS, Lapinski RH, Dolgin SE, et al. Prevalence and natural history of cryptorchidism. Pediatrics 1993; 92(1):44–9.

2. Rajfer J. Congenital anomalies of the testis and scrotum. In: Walsh P, Retick AB, Vaughan ED, et al., eds. Campbell's urology, 7th edn. Philadelphia: WB Saunders, 1998: 2172–92.

3. Levitt SB, Kogan SJ, Engel RM, et al. The impalpable testis: a rational approach to management. J Urol 1978; 120(5): 515–20.

4. Jordan GH, Winslow BH. Laparoscopic single stage and staged orchiopexy. J Urol 1994; 152(4):1249–52.

5. Cisek LJ, Peters CA, Atala A, et al. Current findings in diagnostic laparoscopic evaluation of the nonpalpable testis. J Urol 1998; 160(3 Pt 2):1145–9; discussion 1150.

6. Cortesi N, Ferrari P, Zambarda E, et al. Diagnosis of bilateral abdominal cryptorchidism by laparoscopy. Endoscopy 1976; 8(1):33–4.

7. Bloom DA. Two-step orchiopexy with pelviscopic clip ligation of the spermatic vessels. J Urol 1991; 145(5):1030–3.

8. Jordan GH, Winslow BH, Robey EL. Laparoendoscopic surgical management of the abdominal/transinguinal undescended testicle. J Endourol 1992; 6:157.

9. Bogaert GA, Kogan BA, Mevorach RA. Therapeutic laparoscopy for intra-abdominal testes. Urology 1993; 42(2): 182–8.

10. Duckett JW. Pediatric laparoscopy: prudence, please [editorial]. J Urol 1994; 151(3):742–3.

11. Molenaar JC, Hazebroek FW. Diagnostic laparoscopy should not be routinely done in non-palpable testes. Neder Tijdschr Geneesk 1993; 137:582.

12. Jordan GH. Children's genitourinary laparoscopic surgery: the pro side [editorial] [see comments]. Urology 1994; 44(6): 812–14.

13. Koff SA. Does compensatory testicular enlargement predict monorchism? J Urol 1991; 146(2 Pt 2):632–3.

14. Huff DS, Snyder HM 3rd, Hadziselimovic F, et al. An absent testis is associated with contralateral testicular hypertrophy. J Urol 1992: 148(2 Pt 2):627–8.

15. Moore RG, Peters CA, Bauer SB, et al. Laparoscopic evaluation of the nonpalpable testis: a prospective assessment of accuracy. J Urol 1994; 151(3): 728–31.

16. Tennenbaum SY, Lerner SE, McAlear IM, et al. Preoperative laparoscopic localization of the nonpalpable testis: a critical analysis of a 10-year experience. J Urol 1994; 151(3):732–4.

17. Polascik TJ, Chan-Tack KM, Jeffs RD, Gearhart JP. Reappraisal of the role of human chorionic gonadotropin in the diagnosis and treatment of the nonpalpable testis: a 10-year experience. J Urol 1996; 156(2 Pt 2):804–6.

18. Docimo SG. Re: Is human chorionic gonadotropin useful for identifying and treating nonpalpable testis? J Urol 2001; 166(3):1010–1.

19. Hrebinko RL, Bellinger MF. The limited role of imaging techniques in managing children with undescended testes. J Urol 1993; 150(2 Pt 1):458–60.

20. Wolverson MK, Houttuin E, Heiberg E, et al. Comparison of computed tomography with high-resolution real-time ultrasound in the localization of the impalpable undescended testis. Radiology 1983; 146(1):133–6.

21. Cain MP, Garra B, Gibbons MD. Scrotal-inguinal ultrasonography: a technique for identifying the nonpalpable inguinal testis without laparoscopy. J Urol 1996; 156(2 Pt 2):791–4.

22. Maghnie M, Vanzulli A, Paesano P, et al. The accuracy of magnetic resonance imaging and ultrasonography compared with surgical findings in the localization of the undescended testis. Arch Pediatr Adolesc Med 1994; 148(7):699–703.

23. Yeung CK, Tam YH, Chan YL, et al. A new management algorithm for impalpable undescended testis with gadolinium enhanced magnetic resonance angiography. J Urol 1999; 162: 998–1002.

24. Huff DS, Hadziselimovic F, Duckett JW, et al. Germ cell counts in semithin sections of biopsies of 115 unilaterally cryptorchid testes. The experience from the Children's Hospital of Philadelphia. Eur Journal Pediatr 1987; 146(Suppl 2):S25–7.

25. Huff DS, Hadziselimovic F, Snyder HM 3rd, et al. Histologic maldevelopment of unilaterally cryptorchid testes and their descended partners. Eur J Pediatr 1993; 152(Suppl 2):S11–14.

26. Nagar H, Haddad R. Impact of early orchidopexy on testicular growth. Br J Urol 1997; 80(2):334–5.

27. Lee PA, Coughlin MT. Leydig cell function after cryptorchidism: evidence of the beneficial result of early surgery. J Urol 2002; 167:1824–7.

28. Rogers E, Teahan S, Gallagher H, et al. The role of orchiectomy in the management of postpubertal cryptorchidism. J Urol 1998; 159(3):851–4.

29. Oh J, Landman J, Evers A, et al. Management of the postpubertal patient with cryptorchidism: an updated analysis. J Urol 2002; 167:1329–33.

30. Castilho LN, Ferreira U. Laparoscopy in adults and children with nonpalpable testes. Andrologia 1987; 19(5):539–43.

31. Froeling FM, Sorber MJ, de la Rosette JJ, de Vries JD. The nonpalpable testis and the changing role of laparoscopy. Urology 1994; 43(2):222–7.

32. Perovic S, Janic N. Laparoscopy in the diagnosis of non-palpable testes. Br J Urol 1994; 73(3):310–13.

33. Milad MF, Haddad MJ, Zein TA, et al. Laparoscopy for the impalpable testes. Initial experience of one center. Int Surg 1994; 79(2):163–5.

34. Bell AI. Psychologic implications of scrotal sac and testes for the male child. Clin Pediatr 1974; 13(10):838–43, 846–7.

35. Lakhoo K, Thomas DF, Najmaldin AS. Is inguinal exploration for the impalpable testis an outdated operation? [see comments]. Br J Urol 1996; 77(3):452–4.

36. Boddy SA, Corkery JJ, Gornall P. The place of laparoscopy in the management of the impalpable testis. Br J Surg 1985; 72(11):918–19.

37. Barqawi AZ, Blyth B, Jordan GH, et al. Role of laparoscopy in patients with previous negative exploration for impalpable testis. Urology 2003; 61:1234–7.

38. Baker LA, Docimo SG, Surer I, et al. A multi-institutional analysis of laparoscopic orchidopexy. BJU Int 2001; 87:484–9.

39. Koyle MA, Rajfer J, Ehrlich, RM. The undescended testis. Pediatr Ann 1988; 17(1):39, 42–6.

40. Docimo SG. The results of surgical therapy for cryptorchidism: a literature review and analysis. J Urol 1995; 154(3):1148–52.

41. Gibbons MD, Cromie WJ, Duckett JW Jr. Management of the abdominal undescended testicle. J Urol 1979; 122(1):76–9.

42. Lindgren BW, Darby EC, Faiella L, et al. Laparoscopic orchiopexy: procedure of choice for the nonpalpable testis? J Urol 1998; 159(6):2132–5.

43. Fahlenkamp D, Winfield HN, Schonberger B, et al. Role of laparoscopic surgery in pediatric urology. Eur Urol 1997; 32(1):75–84.

44. Poppas DP, Lemack GE, Mininberg DT. Laparoscopic orchiopexy: clinical experience and description of technique. J Urol 1996; 155(2):708–11.

45. Moore RG, Kavoussi LR, Bloom DA, et al. Postoperative adhesion formation after urological laparoscopy in the pediatric population. J Urol 1995; 153:792–5.

46. Pattaras JG, Moore RG, Landman J, et al. Incidence of postoperative adhesion formation after transperitoneal genitourinary laparoscopic surgery. Urology 2002; 59(1):37–41.

47. Carr MC. The non-palpable testis. AUA Update Series 2001; 20(29):226–31.

48. Belman AB, Rushton HG. Is the vanished testis always a scrotal event? BJU Int 2001; 87(6):480–3.

49. Diamond DA, Caldamone AA. The value of laparoscopy for 106 impalpable testes relative to clinical presentation. J Urol 1992; 148(2 Pt 2):632–4.

50. Guiney EJ, Corbally M, Malone PS. Laparoscopy and the management of the impalpable testis. Br J Urol 1989; 63(3):313–16.

51. Wiener JS, Jordan GH, Gonzales ET Jr. Laparoscopic management of persistent Mullerian duct remnants associated with an abdominal testis. J Endourol 1997; 11(5):357–9.

52. Denes FT, Mendonca BB, Arap S, Laparoscopic management of intersexual states. Urol Clin North Am 2001; 28(1):31–42.

53. Ferrer FA, Cadeddu JA, Schulam P, et al. Orchiopexy using 2 mm. laparoscopic instruments: 2 techniques for delivering the testis into the scrotum. J Urol 2000; 164:160–1.

54. Schulam PG, Hedican SP, Docimo SG. Radially dilating trocar system for open laparoscopic access. Urology 1999; 54(4):727.

55. Cuellar DC, Kavoussi PK, Baker LA, Docimo SG. Open laparoscopic access using a radially dilating trocar: experience and indications in 50 consecutive cases. J Endourol 2000; 14(9):755–6.

56. Gill IS, Ross JH, Kay R. Needlescopic surgery for cryptorchidism – the initial series. Am J Pediatr Surg 2000; 35:1426.

57. Ross JH, Gill IS, Kay R. Needelescopic surgery for cryptorchidism. Dialog Pediatr Urol 1999; 22(9):5–6.

58. Rozanski TA, Wojno KJ, Bloom DA. The remnant orchiectomy. J Urol 1996; 155(2):712–3; discussion 714.

59. Merry C, Sweeney B, Puri P. The vanishing testis: anatomical and histological findings. Eur Urol 1997; 31(1):65–7.

60. Grady RW, Mitchell ME, Carr MC. Laparoscopic and histologic evaluation of the inguinal vanishing testis. Urology 1998; 52(5):866–9.

61. Elder JS. Laparoscopy for impalpable testes: significance of the patent processus vaginalis. J Urol 1994; 152(2 Pt 2):776–8.

62. Bevan A. The surgical treatment of undescended testicle: a further contribution. JAMA 1903; 41:718.

63. Koff SA, Sephic PS. Treatment of high undescended testes by low spermatic vessel ligation. J Urol 1992; 156(2):799–803.

64. Hortling H, Chapelle A, Johansson CJ, et al. An endocrinologic follow-up study of operated cases of cryptorchism. J Clinical Endocrinol Metab 1967; 27(1):120–9.

65. Snyder HM 3rd. Bilateral undescended testes. Eur J Pediatr 1993; 152(Suppl 2):S45–6.

66. Jarow JP, Berkovitz GD, Migeon CJ, et al. Elevation of serum gonadotropins establishes the diagnosis of anorchism in prepubertal boys with bilateral cryptorchidism. J Urol 1986; 136(1 Pt 2):277–9.

67. Raivio T, Dunkel L. Inverse relationship between serum inhibin B and FSH levels in prepubertal boys with cryptorchidism. Pediatr Res 1999; 46: 496–500.

68. Kubini K, Zachmann M, Albers N, et al. Basal inhibin B and the testosterone response to human chorionic gonadotropin correlate in prepubertal boys. J Clin Endocrinol Metab 2000; 85:134–8.

69. Gans SL, Berci G. Peritoneoscopy in infants and children. J Pediatr Surg 1973; 9: 399–405.

70. Cendron M, Keating MA, Huff DS, et al. Cryptorchidism, orchiopexy and infertility: a critical long-term retrospective analysis. J Urol 1989; 142(2 Pt 2):559–62; discussion 572.

71. Lee PA, Coughlin MT, Bellinger MF. Paternity and hormone levels after unilateral cryptorchidism: association with pretreatment testicular location. J Urol 2000; 164(5):1697–701.

72. Schneck FX, Bellinger MF, Fagerli J, et al. Inhibin B: an indicator of seminiferous tubule impairment in children with cryptorchidism. Pediatrics 1999; 104(3):843.

73. Pike MC, Chilvers C, Peckham MJ. Effect of age at orchidopexy on risk of testicular cancer. Lancet 1986: 1(8492):1246–8.

74. Caldamone AA, Amaral JF. Laparoscopic two-stage Fowler–Stephens orchiopexy. J Urol 1994; 152(4):1253–6.

75. Sexton WJ, Assimos DG. Laparoscopy for the adult crypt-orchid testicle. Tech Urol 1999; 5:24–8.

76. Ford TF, Parkinson MC, Pryor JP. The undescended testis in adult life. Br J Urol 1985; 57(2):181–4.

77. Ferro F, Lais A, Bagolan P, et al. Impact of primary surgical approach in the management of the impalpable testis. Eur Urol 1992; 22(2):142–6.

# 15

# Minimally invasive management of pediatric urinary calculus disease

Michael Erhard

## Etiology/Epidemiology

Urinary stone disease in children is relatively rare in developed countries although it is recently observed to be increasing in frequency.[1] Significant renal calculus disease remains endemic in many developing nations, most likely due to dietary and infectious etiologies. In the United States the most common presenting symptoms include abdominal pain (40–75%), gross or microscopic hematuria (25–40%), and symptoms attributable to urinary tract infections (10–30%).[2–6]

Spontaneous passage of a calculus is possible; therefore, conservative management should be undertaken unless there is obstructive uropathy, urosepsis or uncontrolled pain and vomiting. The rate of spontaneous passage will vary according to both the size of the stone and position within the ureter. Adult studies show an overall spontaneous passage of approximately 55% for all stones with those less than 4 mm passing approximately 80% of the time.[7] Other studies have shown that stones within the proximal collecting system pass approximately 22% of the time compared with 46% and 71% for those in the middle and distal third of the ureter.[8] Previous reports in the pediatric literature concluded that calculi less than 3 mm have a greater chance of passing spontaneously while stones larger than 4 mm most likely require surgical management.[9] It has been this author's experience that even small stones which become symptomatic in the proximal ureter are often not likely to advance spontaneously (Figure 15.1). All recommendations are meant to be general guidelines, and every situation needs to be managed individually.

If the clinical symptomatology suggests the presence of a urinary calculus, the most appropriate radiographic evaluation is a nonenhanced helical computed tomography (CT) scan of the abdomen and pelvis [10,11] (Figure 15.2). This will allow complete visualization of the collecting system and we will be able to identify all sizes and types of

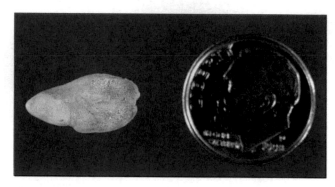

**Figure 15.1**
Even large stones with smooth edges and a tapered leading edge, may pass through the paediatric ureter, therefore conservative management should be the first step unless symptoms warrant urgent intervention.

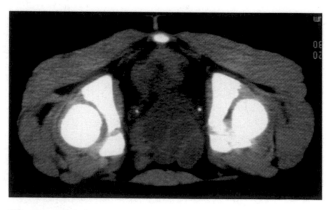

**Figure 15.2**
This young boy had right-sided symptoms and was found on nonenhanced CT scan of the pelvis to have bilateral ureteral calculi.

urinary calculi. If deemed necessary, intravenous contract media can be administered after the noncontrast phase to evaluate for obstruction and focal changes in the kidney, providing more information than a traditional

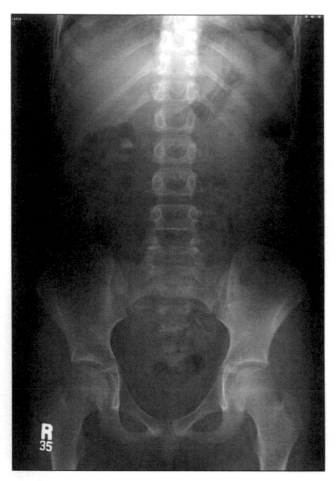

**Figure 15.3**
Many stones can be visualized on plain x-ray of the abdomen, but this should not be a first line x-ray in the evaluation of the symptomatic child due to lack of sensitivity. Also, no anatomic information of the collecting system is obtained making this a less than ideal study.

intravenous pyelogram (IVP). Most pediatric stones are radiopaque and consist of calcium oxalate, which may enable them to be visualized on plain x-ray (Figure 15.3). Although ultrasound is usually still performed to exclude large renal calculi, hydronephrosis or perirenal collections, it has very low sensitivity for detecting ureteral calculi.[12] Total radiation exposure in children is a serious consideration, and CT protocols with minimum dosage need to be devised.[11,13]

Metabolic and genitourinary anomalies which predispose to urolithiasis often coexist in pediatric patients. Metabolic abnormalities have been reported in approximately 48–86% of children with urinary stones.[5,14–16] Common urine abnormalities include hypercalciuria, hypocitraturia and hypomagnesuria. Urinary supersaturation indexes are often elevated and may prove to be a more precise predictor of stone recurrence than traditional metabolic parameters.[17,18] Low urinary volume is also common and treatment should result in urine output of

approximately 35 ml/kg daily.[19] Significant hypercalciuria and hypocitriuria should be aggressively treated in children with recurrent stone disease or signs of the presence of either multiple or bilateral calculi. Serum electrolyte evaluation is necessary in children found to have significant urine metabolic abnormalities.

Conservative management is most appropriate for stones of relatively small size (<4 mm) without signs of obstructive uropathy or urosepsis. It is important to have the child strain all urine so that calculus debris can be obtained and sent for stone analysis. This also gives an end point for conservative management possibly eliminating the need for follow-up radiographic assessment.

Once the child has been cleared of any calculus disease either through conservative management or surgical intervention, it is appropriate to obtain 2 consecutive 24-hour urine samples for metabolic stone risk profiling. These should include an internal creatinine standard to insure completeness of the urine sample. Traditional urinary metabolic parameters include calcium, phosphate, magnesium, citrate, creatinine, uric acid, pH, and voided volume. Pediatric reference ranges should be utilized when available. Serum evaluation should be performed in children with stone recurrence or multiple calculi, and should include calcium, phosphate, uric acid, creatinine, sodium, and potassium. Surgical intervention is appropriate with prolonged hangup of urinary stones or unrelenting symptoms such as pain, nausea, vomiting, and gross hematuria. Proactive treatment of renal stones >5 mm should be considered due to an increased risk of a stone this size causing obstructive symptoms while passing through the urinary system. Treatment strategies should be based upon accomplishing the best stone-free rate for the particular situation with the least morbidity and lowest risk for auxiliary procedures. The most effective treatment plan may include multiple modalities.

## Treatment options
### ESWL

Extracorporeal shock wave lithotripsy (ESWL) in children was first reported in 1988.[20] Initial reports in animal models indicated evidence of significant renal damage following SWL which may have contributed to the delay in its acceptance in children.[21,22] Long-term functional studies on pediatric patients following SWL show no significant change in effective renal plasma flow or mean body height at least 4 years after treatment.[23–25] The safety and efficacy of SWL has also been demonstrated in premature low-birth-weight infants.[26] Morphologic changes such as subcapsular or intrarenal hematomas have been infrequently noted, and usually resolve spontaneously within

1 week. It is not uncommon to experience gross hematuria after SWL, which quickly resolves with resumption of increased fluid intake. Any child with significant abdominal or flank discomfort in the early postoperative period should be evaluated for possible hematoma or obstruction from calculus debris.

Hemoptysis has also been reported postoperatively, particularly in children with significant orthopedic deformities.[27] Small stature and some skeletal deformities increase the risk of the pulmonary field being present within the shockwave path. Prevention of such a complication may be lessened through the use of styrofoam padding, and some symptoms should resolve with conservative management.

Shockwaves are generated and focused by a variety of mechanical systems. The original units are spark gap generated, ellipsoid focused systems which are extremely powerful and have a wide focal point (Figure 15.4). This produces a wider area of shockwave effect, which increases the risk of complications. Subsequent generations of lithotriptors have improved both the scatter of energy and ease with which a child can be placed on the unit. Some units are portable and may be easily transported between operating room suites. In adults it is possible to perform shockwave lithotripsy under light anesthesia, although children may require a deeper general anesthetic for successful completion. Localization of the stone during treatment is determined by fluoroscopy, sonography, or plain x-ray films. Sometimes it is necessary to position a child prone in order to access the stone for effective lithotripsy.

Similar principles are applied to children as in adults, and proper patient selection will help to improve treatment outcomes. Some relative contraindications for SWL include morbid obesity, a large stone burden, increased stone density, congenital skeletal/renal anomalies, and previously failed SWL. The number of shocks, and the maximum energy level should be tailored for each case, and periodic stone visualization during the procedure will demonstrate when adequate lithotripsy has occurred. The primary goal always is to use the least amount of energy necessary to accomplish successful treatment.

## Ureteroscopy

Advances in the design of mini rigid and flexible ureteroscopes have resulted in miniaturization, allowing for use in pediatric patients. Digital imaging as well as enhancements to video technology now allow for clear visualization as well as instantaneous documentation of endourologic procedures (Figure 15.5). The first reported ureteroscopic procedure in an infant was in 1929 by Hugh Hampton Young.[28] He had performed the procedure in a 2-month-old boy with massively dilated ureters secondary to posterior urethral valves. He utilized a 9.5F pediatric cystoscope and was able to visualize the ureter as well as intrarenal collecting system. It wasn't until 1988 that Ritchey and Shepherd independently published articles on the technique of pediatric ureteroscopy for treatment of urinary calculi.[29,30] Since this time, ureteroscopy has gained wide spread acceptance by pediatric urologists.

There exist two distinct types of ureteroscopes: mini rigid fiberoptic and flexible fiberoptic. The mini rigid fiberoptic (i.e. semirigid) ureteroscope has a metal outer casing, which is malleable enough to allow for limited bending without image distortion (Figure 15.6). These endoscopes are particularly useful in the distal ureter, but

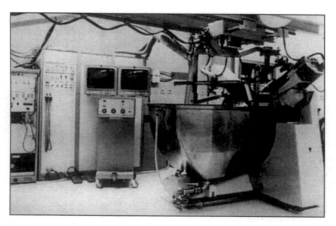

**Figure 15.4**
The original spark gap generated lithotripsy unit was quite effective but cumbersome. Refinements in technology have produced sleeker units capable of being transported between operating room suites.

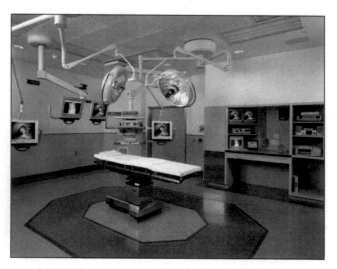

**Figure 15.5**
Modern day surgical rooms can be equipped with state of the art digital video equipment providing improved visualization as well as immediate documentation of endourologic procedures.

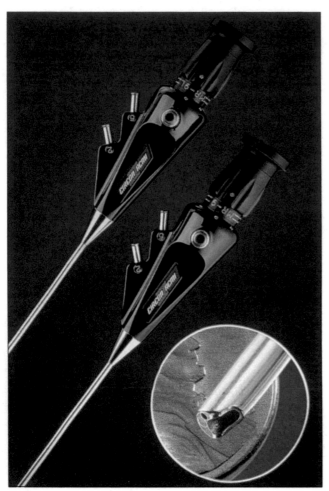

**Figure 15.6**
Semirigid ureteroscopes have an outside metal casing making them more resistant to damage when compared to flexible endoscopes. Fiberoptic image transmission and light delivery provides more room for irrigation and working channels. Many semirigid ureteroscopes can be autoclaved for sterilization.

may be difficult to pass into the proximal collecting system above the bony pelvis. Two working channels allow for simultaneous irrigation as well as placement of working instruments. Varying lengths are necessary, and this author uses both a 15 and 33 cm endoscope tailored to the child's size and location of the stone. These endoscopes are more durable than flexible ureteroscopes and most can be safely autoclaved for sterilization. The distal tip is as small as 4.7F but the malleable metal shaft gradually increases in diameter as you move more proximally towards the eyepiece. Because of this it is necessary to maintain constant vigilance to help limit the risk of meatal injury in the young male infant.

Flexible ureteroscopes are useful within the proximal and intrarenal collecting system due to their active as well as passive tip deflection (Figure 15.7). Some models have the capability of both primary and secondary active deflec-

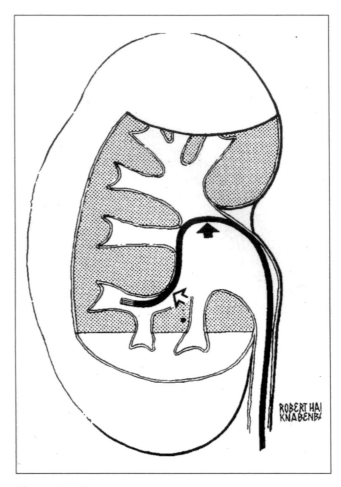

**Figure 15.7**
The open arrow demonstrates distal active deflection while the closed arrow shows passive secondary deflection enabling access into the lower pole calyz. Some models now have the capability of both primary and active secondary deflection.

tion, (our-8 Elite, circon, ACMI) and others have 270° primary deflection in either direction (Flex-ex, Karl Storz). Most flexible ureteroscopes have a working channel of approximately 3.6F, which is adequate for passage of instruments while maintaining space for irrigation. Rarely is secondary passive tip deflection necessary for complete inspection of the intrarenal pediatric collecting system because the arc of deflection is adequate to access the lower pole in most pediatric kidneys (Figure 15.8). Many working instruments will decrease the ability to actively deflect the ureteroscope. It is important to remember to straighten the distal tip of the ureteroscope prior to passage of any working instrument to help prevent damage. Resistance within the working channel may be decreased through the use of a silicone lubricant.

Because of their flexible design, these endoscopes are more prone to damage and need to be handled with care. Recent technologic advancements have improved the durability of both the outside sheath, and deflecting mechanisms, but have resulted in an increased outer diameter.

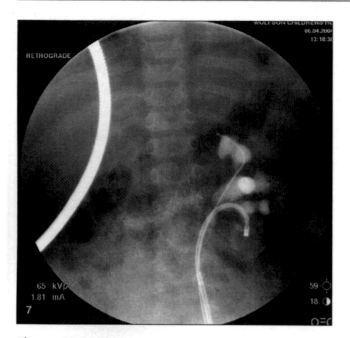

**Figure 15.8**
Most of the time only active deflection is necessary to access the lower pole calyz in the pediatric kidney.

Replacement of the fiberoptic bundles is necessary when the image becomes distorted, and any perforation of the working channel will cause damage to the endoscopes. Flexible endoscopes can be safely soaked in cold sterilization solution or undergo gas sterilization, but cannot be autoclaved. The distal tip is approximately 7.4F but gradually becomes 8.5F or greater at the proximal shaft, which helps to strengthen the sheath and protect the inner bundle fibers. This author prefers the use of three distinct lengths in children (35, 50, and 65 cm) in order to decrease the amount of redundant shaft outside of the body, which helps to prevent damage during use (Figure 15.9).

## Working instruments

A variety of working instruments have been designed for use within miniaturized endoscopes. Guidewires are the most commonly used working instruments in endourology. Not only do they aid in access to the ureter but they also help to prevent intraoperative complications by preventing loss of access to the collecting system. Most have an inner stainless steel core coated by polytetrafluoroethylene (PTFE) to reduce friction. Some have a super-elastic nitinol (nickle–titanium) alloy core which prevents kinking of the wire. There are varying diameters, but a 150 cm 0.035 inch PTFE-coated guidewire with a 3 cm floppy distal tip is the most common type used in the author's practice. The distal tip may be straight or angled and the length of its flexible floppy tip varies. A dual floppy tip wire is the safest choice for passage of a flexible ureteroscope because it minimizes potential damage to the working channel.

A hydrophilic-coated guidewire is helpful for negotiating a tortuous or narrowed ureter and for placement of a working wire proximal to an impacted ureteral calculus. These extremely slippery guidewires need to be kept moist and should not be used as safety wires due to the ease with which they may be dislodged during an endoscopic procedure. Handling of the slippery hydrophilic wires is made easier through the use of a moistened gauze sponge. Extra-stiff guidewires are useful for straightening tortuous or reimplanted ureters (Figure 15.10) and also should be used for percutaneous tract dilatation. These wires should not be used when placing a flexible ureteroscope due to the increased risk of damaging the delicate working channel.

A variety of baskets as well as graspers have been developed to aid in extracting stone debris from the collecting system. They vary in diameter from 1.9–4.5F and most are contained within a hydrophilic sheath (PTFE, Polyimide) to facilitate passage. A variety of designs of baskets exist, but the most significant improvement in basket design has been the tipless nitinol basket. The tipless design makes it particularly safe and useful for extraction of stones within a tight calyx and when deployed allows for near complete active deflection of the ureteroscope due its increased flexibility (Figure 15.11 A,B)[31]. Some of the newer baskets have been designed to allow controlled active angulation of the baskets' wires (Dimension, Bard Urological, Covington, GA) and others enable a canopy to form which may

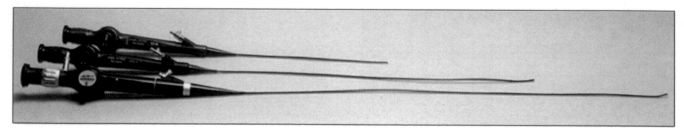

**Figure 15.9**
Varying lengths of flexible endoscopes (35, 50, and 65 cm) are useful in pediatric ureteroscopy to help prevent damage to the endoscope by minimizing the amount of redundant flexible shaft present outside of the body.

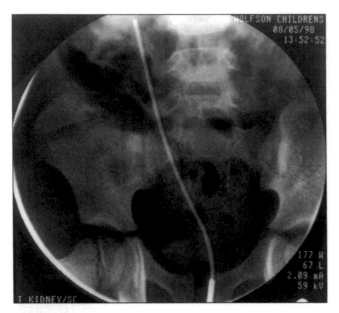

**Figure 15.10**
An extra stiff guidewire helped to straighten this right reimplanted cross-trigonal ureter allowing for easier access during flexible ureteroscopy. Initial access to the reimplanted ureter can usually be obtained with the help of an angled tip guidewire.

engage multiple small calculi. Some baskets have a central channel which allows for the simultaneous placement of electrohydraulic or laser lithotripsy probes once the stone is stabilized.

Grasping forceps are quite helpful during endoscopic stone extraction particularly within the ureter. The most significant advantage is that a grasper will disengage from a stone if it becomes lodged within a relatively narrow ureteral segment. This helps to prevent trauma of the ureteral wall by eliminating entrapment during stone removal. The grasper should be opened only as wide as is needed to engage the stone thus decreasing the risk of ureteral wall perforation (Figure 15.12). It is important to maintain contact with the stone while closing the graspers, therefore slight advancement of the sheath is needed as the forceps are closed.

Proper selection of a stone retrieval device is important for the successful and timely completion of any endoscopic procedure. Several factors impact this decision, particularly the size, position within the collecting system and condition (i.e. impacted vs nonimpacted) of the stone. Ptashnyk et al studied exvivo porcine kidneys and ureters to determine which stone retrieval devices were most effective in certain situations.[32] Their conclusions were that graspers are most efficient at the removal of a single ureteral stone (particularly impacted) with little mucosal damage, and that a helical basket was most effective for Steinstrasse. In another study, nitinol baskets have been shown to be most effective for calyceal stones and those in the lower pole.[33] The flexible mitinol component and the atraumatic tipless basket design allow complete deflection and produce minimal surrounding tissue trauma.

A newer instrument is the Dretler stone cone (Microvasive, Boston Scientific), which is a 0.038 inch

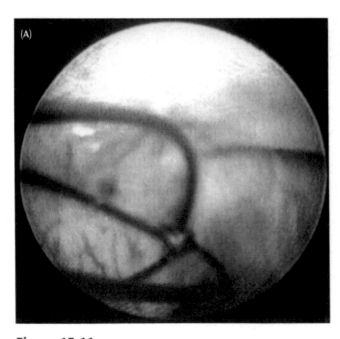

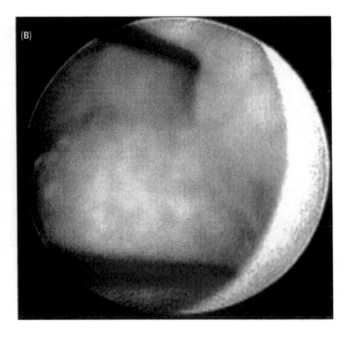

**Figure 15.11**
The strong, flexible, nitinol basket is easily deployed into a tight calyx (A) and produces minimal trauma to the urothelium when used to remove calculi (B). Nitinol baskets also enable near-complete active deflection of all flexible ureteroscopes.

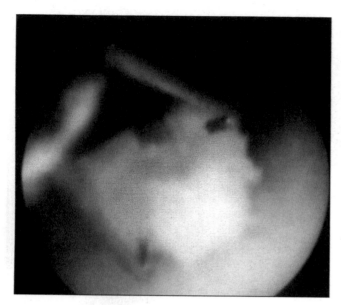

**Figure 15.12**
A three-prong grasper is most effective at removing ureteral calculi. It is important to open the grapser only as wide as needed to engage the stone to decrease the risk of ureteral wall perforation. The main safety feature of the grasper is that it will automatically become disengaged from the calculus if the stone becomes entrapped within a narrowed portion of the ureter.

Nitinol-teflon coated wire which can be coiled proximal to the calculus acting as a backstop to prevent proximal migration. It has been shown to be effective at extracting stone fragments and more successful than flat-wire baskets at preventing stone migration.[34]

Historically there are four modes of intracorporeal lithotripsy: ultrasonic; ballistic (i.e. pneumatic); electrohydraulic (EHL), and laser. Each has been extensively studied and all have unique capabilities and limitations.

Ultrasonic lithotripsy was first described in 1953.[35] The metal probe transmits vibrational energy to the tip, which when in contact with the stone results in disintegration due to cleavage of the crystal matrix. Small solid probes can be utilized through pediatric cystourethroscopes and large probes with a central suction channel are helpful for removal of stones during percutaneous procedures (Figure 15.13). These probes will lose energy transmission with any degree of bending, therefore are most effective when used in endoscopes with a straight working channel. Ultrasonic lithotripsy is safe and results in minimal tissue damage.[36] It is best suited for the percutaneous treatment of large renal stones.

Ballistic lithotripsy involves the pneumatic mechanical impaction of stones by a solid probe. There are no thermal or cavitation effects, therefore risk of tissue injury is minimal. This modality has been effective in fragmenting all types of stones and smaller flexible probes are

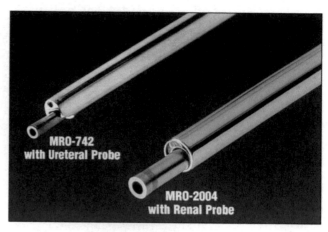

**Figure 15.13**
Ultrasonic lithotripsy probes can have a central channel which is helpful for the removal of stone debris during treatment of calculi. Ultrasonic probes need to be used in an endoscope with a straight working channel to prevent the loss of energy due to bending of the device.

available.[37–40] Retrograde migration due to pneumatic impaction as well as loss of lithotripsy power with significant deflection of the probe are two significant shortcomings.

Electrohydraulic (EHL) lithotripsy was discovered by Yutkin in 1955 and involves the generation of an electrical spark, which produces a cavitation bubble, providing sufficient energy to produce lithotripsy [41] (Figure 15.14). The energy is maximized at a distance of approximately 1 mm from the stone and therefore the tip of the probe should be kept just off the surface of the stone. Electrohydraulic lithotripsy may not fragment all stone compositions but is

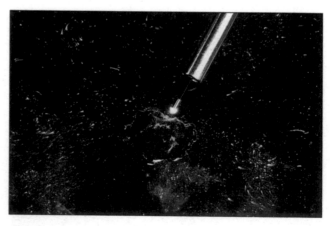

**Figure 15.14**
The generation of an electrical spark producing sufficient energy for lithotripsy is known as the process of electrohydraulic lithotripsy. The risk of tissue damage due to lateral disbursement of this energy is increased when working within the small confines of the pediatric collecting system.

able to be used through both flexible and rigid endoscopes. One significant risk of EHL is lateral disbursement of the energy, which can increase injury to the surrounding soft tissues. Probes are as small as 1.9F which will allow access to lower pole calculi.

Holmium yttrium-aluminum-garnet (HO:YAG) laser lithotripsy is extremely effective at fragmenting all types of urinary calculi.[42] Holmium laser lithotripsy was first reported in 1992[43] and subsequent reports have shown it to be safe in adults and children.[44,45] Holmium lithotripsy involves direct stone absorption of laser energy with subsequent disintegration.[46] Solid quartz fibers as small as 200 μm enable near complete deflection of a flexible ureteroscope allowing access to nearly all parts of the collecting system. Larger fibers are helpful in the disintegration of larger stones contained within the kidney or bladder. Direct visualization of the tip of the probe is necessary to prevent subsequent endoscope or tissue damage during use. The fiber needs to be placed near the stone in order to result in fragmentation. Holmium laser lithotripsy results in dust particles and fragments less than 2 mm which should be able to pass spontaneously (Figure 15.15A,B).

## Ureteroscopy technique

Ureteroscopy in children requires general anesthesia. After the child is placed in the dorsal lithotomy position, he or she is well padded in order to prevent excessive limb abduction or pressure on nerves. The male urethral meatus is carefully inspected and gently dilated if necessary. Cystoscopy is performed and the bladder is inspected and the position of ureteral orifices is visualized. A urine sample is obtained at the time of the cystoscopy and sent for urine culture.

The author first gauges the caliber of the ureteral orifice by using a 0.035 inch guidewire. If the orifice appears 'volcanic' and barely accepts a 0.035 guidewire, then either active dilatation or prestenting of the ureter is performed (Figure 15.16). The ureter has three physiologic areas of narrowing with the narrowest portion being the orifice. These anatomic differences are age dependent and based on work by Cussen in 1971.[47] It is sometimes helpful to perform access to the ureteral orifice using two guidewires one inside the working channel and the other already independently placed in the ureter as a safety wire (Figure 15.17). This helps to control access and to increase the diameter by placing the endoscope directly between the two wires. Reports of balloon dilatation to 15F has been previously reported with no significant complications or reflux, but clearly produces more active dilatation than actually necessary. This author prefers to use a graduated single-shaft dilator, which ranges from 6–10F (Figure 15.18). Dilation to 2F sizes greater than the diameter of the endoscope is usually needed for successful access. Dilatation can be facilitated by performing this over a stiff guidewire or through a 13F cystoscope sheath in order to prevent buckling within the bladder. If these maneuvers do not allow easy dilatation of the ureter, the author believes

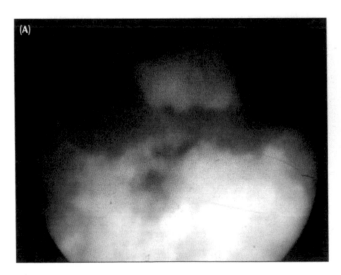

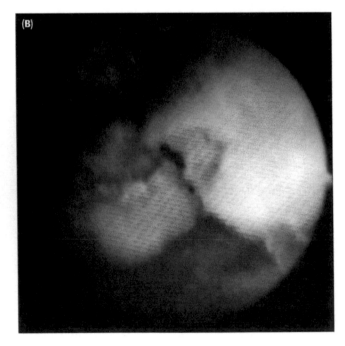

**Figure 15.15**
Holmium laser energy is the most effective way to fragment stones. Dust fragments (A) will pass spontaneously. Larger stones can be precisely cleaved (B) into smaller sizes which facilitates intact removal.

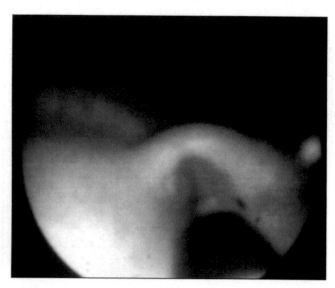

**Figure 15.16**
It is often more prudent to present a ureter which only accepts a 3F catheter.

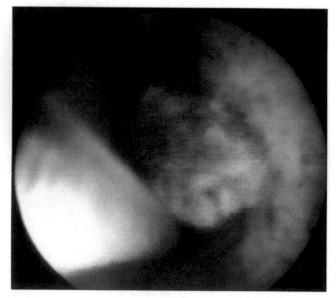

**Figure 15.17**
Dual wire access provides better expansion of the ureteral orifice enabling easier access to the proximal collecting system. One wire is placed through the working channel of the endoscope which helps to safely guide the semirigid ureteroscope.

it is more prudent to place a ureteral stent to passively dilate the ureter rather than performing significant active balloon dilatation. Dilatation of the ureter may be required in approximately 30% of children undergoing ureteroscopy.[48]

When therapeutic maneuvers are anticipated it is important to maintain a safety guidewire within the ureter.

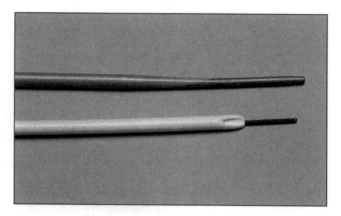

**Figure 15.18**
A 6–10F soft graduated (above) and 10F dual lumen catheter (below) are two helpful tools used for accessing the pediatric ureter.

A hydrophilic guidewire may aid in accessing a tortuous ureter or one with an impacted stone, but should not be used as a routine safety wire due to the ease with which it may become dislodged. A flexible ureteroscope requires either the use of an access sheath or a second working guidewire for placement of the ureteroscope into the proximal collecting system (Figure 15.19A,B) The smallest sheath which accepts flexible ureteroscopes is 9.5F, therefore, in children, prestenting of the ureter is often required in order to dilate the ureter to allow the safe use of an access sheath. Access sheaths should be used with caution and are most helpful when it will be necessary to traverse the ureteral orifice many times when treating large or multiple stones in the proximal collecting system. Fluoroscopic guidance is absolutely necessary during any ureteroscopic procedure.

Previous urologic surgery involving either the bladder neck, ureter, urethra, or ureteropelvic junction is not a contraindication for ureteroscopy. A child who has undergone previous hypospadias surgery may require urethral dilatation prior to placement of the ureteroscope if there is meatal stenosis. It is important to use small diameter endoscopes to avoid disruption of previous bladder neck reconstruction. Oftentimes children who have had bladder neck reconstruction have had ureteral reimplantation at the time of their primary surgery and care must be taken not to over-torque the bladder neck when accessing the previously reimplanted ureter. Access to the ureter after previous reimplantation is clearly dependent upon the type of surgery performed. When either an advancement or extravesical procedure was utilized, access is similar to the unoperated child. When a previous cross-trigonal reimplantation has been performed, access can be more difficult. In this instance, the ureteral orifice is usually laterally located and can be canulated with an angled guidewire. If this is unsuccessful an actively deflecting guidewire can be utilized. Once access has been gained the

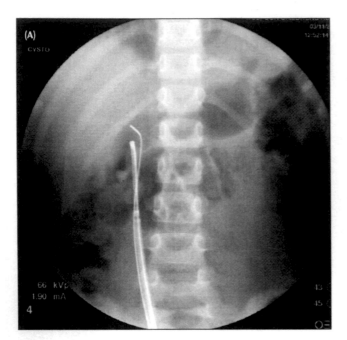 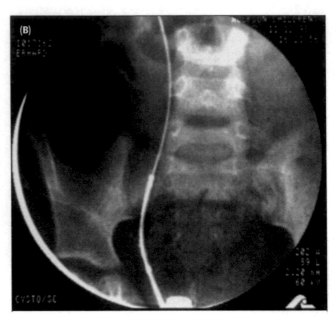

**Figure 15.19**
An access sheath is pictured here with a flexible endoscope exiting the proximal portion of the sheath (A). The safety wire is placed outside of the sheath which provides the largest internal lumen for endoscope placement and stone removal. Access to the proximal collecting system is most often accomplished using a guidewire in a monorail fashion (B). One guidewire is used when a diagnostic procedure is being performed, but two guidewires are necessary when the therapeutic intervention is planned.

initial wire should be replaced with a stiff guidewire which then straightens the intramural portion of the ureter allowing access for ureteroscopy. Dilatation of the tunnel is usually not necessary although it is sometimes necessary to dilate the ureteral orifice. When the procedure is finished the ureter will return to its preoperative cross-trigonal position (Figure 15.20). Recurrent reflux after ureteroscopy in the previously reimplanted ureter has not been demonstrated.

Intrarenal access after previous ureteropelvic junction repair is usually straightforward as long as there has been adequate healing and success of the previous surgery. The ureter remains supple at the site of previous repair and is at no greater risk of injury. Postoperative stenting is not always required, but should be performed after procedures requiring either extensive manipulation or significant active dilatation. If a stent is left in place, the author prefers to leave a dangler string attached to facilitate removal without anesthesia in the office approximately 1 week after the procedure.

A mini rigid ureteroscope should be used for distal and midureteral calculi. It may be used for more proximal stones if it can be successfully passed above the pelvic brim. Flexible ureteroscopy is necessary most of the time for proximal ureteral calculi and should always be used for stones contained within the intrarenal collecting system. Complete access to the intrarenal system is usually accomplished through active deflection alone. Rarely is

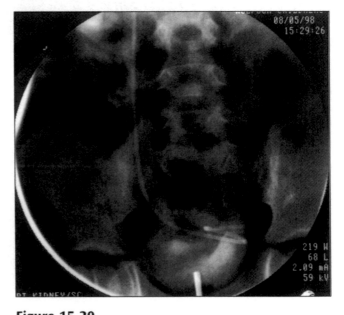

**Figure 15.20**
The cross-trigonal appearance of the right reimplanted ureter is maintained after flexible ureteroscopy. Postoperative reflux has not been an issue in those children who have undergone ureteroscopy after previous ureteral reimplantation.

secondary passive deflection necessary in the smaller pediatric kidney. Instillation of contrast during ureteroscopy will guide you during the complete inspection of the collecting system under fluoroscopy.

Once the stone is encountered it is important to gauge the size of the stone versus the diameter of the ureter. Many ureteral stones can be removed intact through basket or grasper manipulation provided the caliber of the distal ureter is adequate to allow atraumatic retrieval. For stones, which are either impacted or are too large to remove intact, in situ Holmium laser lithotripsy is performed. For an impacted stone, attempts should be made to dislodge the stone into the proximally dilated portion of the ureter. This will allow more room for laser lithotripsy, and decrease the risk of complications. Once the stone is dislodged, the jagged surface is either precisely treated to smooth out rough edges or the entire stone can be cleaved into distinct fragments for subsequent removal. Stones that cannot be dislodged should be treated first on its periphery which should disimpact the stone. It is important to retrieve at least one stone fragment for crystallographic analysis, and once this is achieved it is more efficient to deposit subsequent small fragments within the bladder, which should pass spontaneously. If a stone fragment becomes displaced outside the ureteral wall due to perforation, it is prudent to abandon further attempts at extraction of the migrated calculus.

## Percutaneous endourology

Thomas Hillier in 1865 is credited with the description of the first therapeutic percutaneous renal drainage of what was described as ureteropelvic junction obstruction.[49] Unfortunately, after 4 years of periodic percutaneous drainage the young boy succumbed to septicemia at age 8. It wasn't until 1941 that Rupel described the removal of renal calculus debris through a nephrostomy tract using endoscopic equipment.[50] Percutaneous drainage of hydronephrosis was again reported by Goodwin in 1955, and it wasn't until 1985 that Woodside et al. presented a series of 7 pediatric patients who had undergone a percutaneous procedure.[51]

Early on, percutaneous stone removal was limited to children 8 years of age and older due to fears of significant blood loss and increased renal damage with large (> 24F) tract dilatation.[52] The defect created by a 24F tract in a child's kidney corresponds to a 72F defect in an adult kidney.[53] Increased tract size is directly correlated with increased complication rates, although no significant renal scarring or functional changes can be readily detected after large tract dilatation.[54,55] Subsequent reports have demonstrated that percutaneous procedures are technically feasible for children less than 8 years of age, and that complications can be decreased by utilizing a tract < 22F.

Because of concerns regarding hematologic complications, the technique of a smaller access percutaneous procedure has been developed. Helal et al. presented their experience using a 15F peel away sheath in a 2-year-old child for percutaneous stone removal.[56] A smaller 11F technique using a 'mini perc' approach has also been reported (Figure 15.21). Access to the collecting system is thought to be less traumatic because of the smaller caliber site. There have been no reports of bleeding complications in uncomplicated procedures after mini perc intervention, and the need for postoperative percutaneous nephrostomy drainage is often eliminated. Treatment of large (>3 cm) stones can be tedious, therefore a larger peel-away sheath (15–22F) is recommended to expedite stone fragment removal.

Most pediatric percutaneous procedures are performed for management of renal calculi. It is important that these procedures be performed in an institution where there is an endourologist and interventional radiologist experienced in the treatment of children. Needle access to the kidney is required for tract dilatation and therapeutic intervention, and there is some suggestion that obtaining early access (one day prior to surgery) may decrease bleeding as well as operative time. This is particularly helpful for a 'mini-perc' procedure because the smaller field of view becomes easily obscured by minimal bleeding. Nevertheless, it is possible to obtain access at the time of percutaneous intervention, which does result in safe completion of the procedure.

The proper site chosen for percutaneous access should allow both a direct route to the stone and permit easy access to other areas of the collecting system. The optimal position is usually a posterior calyx with a wide, straight infundibulum. Multiple sites may be necessary, and should be utilized when there is a complete staghorn calculus or any intrarenal anomalies making it difficult to access all stone containing calyces through a single site. Hematologic complications requiring transfusion are not increased when multiple sites are utilized.[57] It is important to obtain the primary access site where it will be possible to maxi-

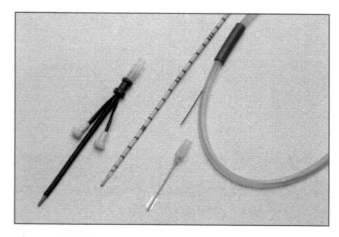

**Figure 15.21**
This prepackaged mini percutaneous access set is available from Cook Urological, Spencer, Indiana.

mally debulk the stone burden, and secondary sites where calyces will be difficult to reach through the primary tract. If the stones are contained within a calyceal diverticulum or a calyx with a narrowed infundibulum, it is necessary to have direct access into that part of the collecting system. Upper pole access sites should be used with caution because of the increased risk of pneumo/hydrothorax. Because of this, a chest x-ray should be obtained at the conclusion of any percutaneous procedure involving upper pole access.

Once needle access has been obtained, a wire is passed down the ureter into the bladder to allow a controlled tract dilatation and to avoid the accidental loss of access to the collecting system. Slippery hydrophilic guidewires should be exchanged for standard teflon coated wires prior to dilatation. The use of a stiff guidewire will facilitate dilatation. If ureteral access is not possible or if access is obtained into an obstructed system or calyceal diverticulum, multiple coils of the wire should be placed within the contained collecting system prior to tract dilatation.

Once safe access has been confirmed, the tract is dilated either using sequential graduated dilators (Amplatz), or active balloon dilatation. Both techniques have proven safe and efficacious, but sequential dilatation of larger tracts may be at increased risk for bleeding due to the potential sheering effect of this technique. Constant vigilance under fluoroscopy is necessary to make certain that dilatation is not carried too far medially, therefore, avoiding disruption of the renal pelvis. The small nondilated pediatric kidney is at greatest risk for this complication and extreme caution must be undertaken to help prevent such occurrences. If there is significant disruption of the renal pelvis or UPJ, it may be necessary to abandon the procedure and to place a temporary nephrostomy or nephroureteral stent.

For balloon dilatation, the distal radiographic marker is placed into the renal pelvis while the proximal portion of the balloon is located externally. The balloon is then inflated to its maximum pressure and then left fully inflated until there is no longer any evidence of fascial constriction (Figure 15.22A,B). The balloon is kept inflated for several minutes to help aid in hemostasis. The access sheath can be placed into the pelvis over the balloon once it has been partially deflated. The balloon size should correlate with the size of the sheath to be used.

If there is any significant bleeding encountered after dilatation, it may be necessary to temporarily place either a large Foley catheter or a tamponade balloon. If these techniques do not result in satisfactory hemostasis, it will be necessary to leave the catheter in place and perform the therapeutic intervention at another time. Uncontrolled hemorrhage requiring transfusion should be evaluated with angiography for possible vascular embolization.

After the working sheath has been placed, the planned procedure is then undertaken. Both rigid as well as flexible instrumentation may be necessary and should be present in the operating room suite in case the need arises. If there is a

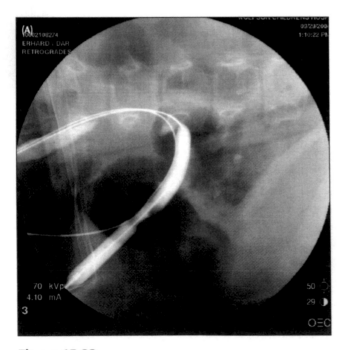
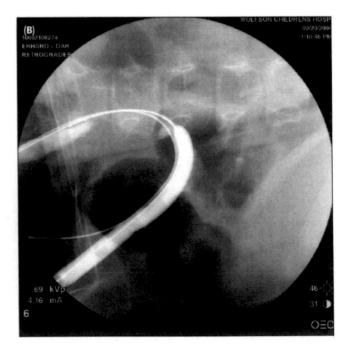

**Figure 15.22**
Percutaneous access is facilitated through the use of balloon dilators. Once you have confirmed proper positioning under fluoroscopy, dilute contrast is used to expand the balloon and is monitored under fluoroscopy. Initial fascial constriction (A) is noted, and the balloon is continued to be inflated to its maximum pressure until all constriction has been eliminated (B). The size of the balloon should be slightly larger than the size of the sheath to be utilized.

large stone burden, then the procedure will be facilitated through placement of a 22F sheath. This allows access with an adult nephroscope enabling the use of larger instrumentation, and giving the capability of removing large intact stone fragments (Figure 15.23). If a 'mini-perc' procedure is performed through an 11F peel-away sheath, then either an offset pediatric cystoscope with a straight working channel or 9.5F modified mini rigid ureteroscope will be necessary to access the kidney. The straight channel offset lens endoscope will allow for the passage of ultrasonic and ballistic lithotripsy probes whereas the in-line mini rigid cystoureteroscope will require the use of the Holmium laser, electrohydraulic, or flexible ballistic lithotripsy devices for stone fragmentation. This author prefers the in-line endoscope because it has two working channels, which allows simultaneous suction irrigation (5.4F), and lithotripsy (2.3F). It also permits 360° rotation of the endoscope for maximum positioning of lithotripsy probes. The endoscope used should be several French sizes less than the internal diameter of the sheath in order to allow continuous flow around the scope, which lessens the risk of significant extravasation. The use of the warmed saline irrigant is encouraged, and this will need to be changed to water or glycine if an electrosurgical procedure is planned. Electrohydraulic lithotripsy is equally effective in saline or water, and thus saline should be used to avoid hyponatremia. Levering of the nephroscope should be limited in order to avoid injury to the infundibulum as well as renal parenchyma during the percutaneous procedure.

Endourologic instrumentation is similar to that used for other procedures. The Holmium laser is particularly useful during small caliber percutaneous access procedures in order to debulk large stone burdens. Extraction of stone fragments is facilitated by using a 4.5F nitinol basket. Ultrasonic lithotripsy is quite safe and can be performed through the straight working channel of either a small-caliber offset cystourethroscope or an adult percutaneous nephroscope. Attempts should be made to remove all stone fragments greater than 2 mm in order to limit a potential nidus for stone regrowth or obstruction with passage of a large fragment. Complete visualization of the intrarenal collecting system as well as ureter should be undertaken. This usually requires the use of a flexible endoscope. Complete inspection is sometimes hampered by limitations of the size of the pediatric kidney and size of the percutaneous access sheath. Significant clots may obscure stone fragments, therefore, every attempt should be made to irrigate them free to allow complete visualization. Most of the time it is necessary to leave a percutaneous nephrostomy tube in place at the completion of the procedure, but it is possible to limit its use. (Figure 15.24) Access to the kidney should be maintained until postoperative x-rays confirm that no second look procedure will be needed.

## Treatment strategies

Many factors need to be considered when deciding the proper treatment modalities for urinary tract calculi in children. Not only do you have to consider the characteristics of the stone (size, shape, location, density, number, etc.), but you also have to look at the characteristics of the child. Body habitus, as well as associated congenital and acquired conditions need to be taken into consideration. Surgeon expertise and available technology may also guide treatment strategy. Each case needs to be individualized in order to choose the best form of treatment in regards to shockwave lithotripsy vs retrograde ureteroscopy vs. an antegrade percutaneous approach.

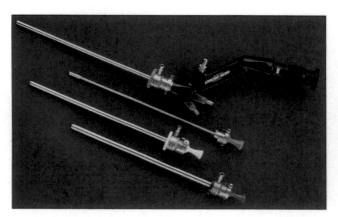

**Figure 15.23**
Fiberoptic offset nephroscopes provide access utilizing a 22F sheath while performing percutaneous stone removal. Fiberoptic technology has resulted in the decreased diameter of the outer sheath while maintaining a large central channel for completion of the procedure.

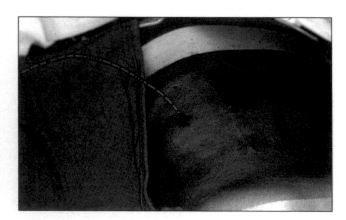

**Figure 15.24**
Placement of a nephrostomy tube is not always necessary after small access percutaneous procedures, but it is important to maintain access to the kidney and ureter until postoperative x-rays confirm that no secondary percutaneous procedure is necessary.

# Renal calculi

Shockwave lithotripsy is the least invasive form of therapy which offers reasonable stone-free rates of greater than 80% with minimal complications.[58–64]

Stones ≤ 1 cm are most efficaciously treated by this modality and often require a single treatment. Higher retreatment rates and the need for ancillary procedures is seen with large stone burdens and in children with renal or collecting system abnormalities.[64,65] Therefore, SWL is not the best therapy when there is evidence of UPJ obstruction, calyceal diverticulum, or infundibular stenosis. SWL is also less effective for ectopic and horseshoe kidneys because of difficulties with precise energy delivery (increased surrounding bony and soft tissue structures) and the presence of an abnormally rotated collecting system which may prevent post-treatment stone clearance. In addition, alternative therapies to SWL should be considered for extremely dense stones (brushite, cystine)[66] and those calculi within an abnormal lower pole (i.e. long, narrowed infundibulum). In these instances the energy may not be sufficient for adequate lithotripsy, and the abnormal intrarenal anatomy may promote fragment retention. Currently, it appears that SWL is best suited for solitary renal stones ≤ 1.5 cm not contained within an abnormal lower pole calyx, and not associated with any congenital or acquired renal abnormalities. Despite this, SWL monotherapy for the treatment of staghorn calculi has been shown to be effective, with stone-free rates of approximately 88% after multiple treatment sessions.

The role of ureteroscopy for the treatment of renal calculi in children remains to be defined. Several reports have demonstrated ureteroscopy to be an effective treatment for stones throughout the entire intrarenal collecting system. It has been successful for the treatment of stone-containing calyceal diverticula of the mid and upper pole.[67] Primary ureteropyeloscopy with stone removal should also be performed when ureteroscopy is being used to treat other ureteral stones. This enables easy access to the kidney for treatment and provides the greatest chance of success with one procedure. Residual fragments after SWL, or failure of SWL as the primary procedure are two other reasons to perform ureteropyeloscopy for stone removal. As mentioned previously, placement of a ureteral access sheath in a presented ureter may facilitate removal of large stones. Concomitant UPJ or intrarenal obstruction can also be treated endoscopically at the time of stone removal.

For intrarenal stones >1 cm, multiple large calculi, staghorn caculi, children with urinary tract malformations or previous reconstruction, a percutaneous approach may be better suited. Stone-free rates after a single percutaneous session range anywhere from 70–100%.[54,68–72] For large stones and staghorn calculi, combined 'sandwich' therapy (percutaneous stone removal followed by shock-wave lithotripsy), provides stone-free rates greater than 90%. A percutaneous procedure does carry risks of excessive bleeding requiring transfusion, but several series have shown that utilization of a tract less than 22F significantly limits this risk. Multiple percutaneous sites may be necessary for complete access to the stone, and have been shown not to increase the risk of transfusion. Long term follow up supports percutaneous procedures as being safe with no significant damage to the pediatric kidney.

Laparoscopy in children has become more widespread and has recently been reported in the management of renal calculi.[73] Patient selection criteria included stones greater than 2.5 cm with failure of percutaneous renal access. Not only does laparoscopy provide a high stone free rate, but also enables the repair of concomitant ureteropelvic junction obstruction. Laparoscopy may also prove helpful in the management of large peripheral calyceal diverticula containing stones by allowing surgical unroofing with ablation of the diverticular neck and lining. Further experience should better define the role of laparoscopy in the treatment of pediatric stone disease.

# Ureteral calculi

Experience with shockwave lithotripsy for stones contained within the ureter has been shown to be effective 54–100% of the time. Retreatment rate for stones within the ureter is necessary up to 23% of the time. Patient positioning may need to be modified for distal ureteral stones by placing the child in the prone position. Stones over the bony pelvis are difficult to treat using SWL because of inadequate visualization and lack of adequate energy delivery.

A review of the literature shows that the stone free rate after pediatric ureteroscopic lithotripsy is 77–100%.[45,48,74–85] Advances in both endoscopic instrumentation as well as Holmium laser lithotripsy have been the major reasons why there has been increased success. One appealing aspect of the ureteroscopic removal of stones is that it offers an immediate stone-free condition at the completion of the procedure. The American Urological Association has issued guidelines to standardize the management of adult patients with stones and Vansavage et al.[82] have published their recommendations for the modification of these guidelines when applying it to the pediatric patient. The ureteroscopic removal of stones contained within the ureter is clearly safe and effective and should be considered the first line treatment for most children.

The percutaneous removal of ureteral stones is rarely indicated. It should be considered the primary form of therapy for children who have impacted stones with significant hydroureteronephrosis and urinary tract infection or urosepsis. The antegrade approach allows for prompt decompression of the obstructed collecting system with antegrade ureteroscopic access for subsequent removal. The technique for antegrade ureteroscopy is exactly the same for the retrograde approach, and has been discussed previously. Flexible rather than minirigid endoscopy should be utilized for antegrade ureteroscopy to limit potential complications.

# References

1. Kroovand RL. Pediatric urolithiasis. Urol Clin North Am 1997; 24:173–84.

2. Choi H, Snyder HM III, Duckett JW. Urolithiasis in childhood: current management. J Ped Surg 1987, 22:158–64.

3. Polinsky MS, Kaiser BA, Baluarte HJ. Urolithiasis in children, Pediatr Clin North Am 1987; 34:683–710.

4. Shepherd P, Thomas R, Haramon EP. Urolithiasis in children: innovations in management. J Urol 1988; 140:790–2.

5. Milliner DS, Murphy ME. Urolithiasis in pediatric patients. Mayo Clin Proc 1993; 68:241–8.

6. Cohen TD, Ehreth J, King LR, Preminger GM. Pediatric urolithiasis: medical and surgical management. Urol 1996; 47:292–303.

7. Ueno A, Kawamura T, Ogawa A, et al. Relation of spontaneous passage of calculi to size, Urol 1977; 19:544–6.

8. Morse R, Resnick M. Ureteral calculi: Natural history and treatment in an era of advanced technology. J Urol 1991; 145:263–5.

9. VanSavage JG, Palanca LG, Anderson RD, et al. Treatment of distal ureteral stones in children: similarities to the American Urological Association guidelines in adults. J Urol 2000; 194 (3 pt 2):1089–93.

10. Heidenreich A, Desgrandschamps F, Terrier F. Modern approach of diagnosis and management of acute flank pain: review of all imaging modalities. Eur Urol 2002; 41:351–62.

11. Strouse PJ, Bates DG, Bloom DA, et al. Non-contrast thin-section helical CT of urinary tract calculi in children. Pediatr Radiol 2002; 32:326–32.

12. Keir A, Fowler B, Locken JA, et al. Ultrasound for detecting renal calculi with nonenhanced CT as a reference standard. radiol 2002; 222:109–13.

13. Spielmann AL, Heneghan JP, Lee LJ, et al. Decreasing the radiation dose for renal stone CT: a feasibility study of single and multidetector CT. Am J Roentgenol 2002; 178:10058–62.

14. Perrone HC, dos Santos DR, Santos MV, et al. Urolithiasis in childhood: Metabolic evaluation. Pediatr Nephrol 1992; 6:54–6.

15. Lim DJ. Walker RD III, Ellsworth PI, et al. Treatment of pediatric urolithiasis between 1984 and 1994. J Urol 1996; 156:702–5.

16. Pietrow PK, Pope JC IV, Adams MC, et al. Clinical outcomes of pediatric stone disease, J Urol 2002; 167:670–3.

17. Parks JH, Coward M, Coe FL. Correspondence between stone composition and urine supersaturation in nephrolithiasis. Kidney Int 1997; 51:894–900.

18. Battino BS, DeFoor W, Coe F, et al. Metabolic evaluation of children with urolithaisis: are adult references for supersaturation appropriate. J Urol 2002; 168:2568–71.

19. Miller LA, Stapleton FB. Urinary volume in children with urolithiasis. J Urol 1989; 141:918–920.

20. Frick J, Kohle R, Kunit G. Padiatr Padol 1988; 23(1):47–52.

21. Kaude JV, Williams CM, Miller MR. Renal morphology and function immediately after extracorporeal shock-wave lithotripsy. Am J Roentgenol 1985; 145:305–313.

22. Fuchs AM, Coulson W, Fuchs GJ. Effect of extra corporeally induced high-energy shock wave on rabbit kidney and ureter: a morphologic and functional study. J Endourol 1988; 4:341–3.

23. Thomas R, Frentz JM, Harmon E. Effect of extracorporeal shock wave lithotripsy on renal function and body height in pediatric patients. J Urol 1992; 148:1064–6.

24. Brinkmann O, Griehl A, Kuwertz-Broking E, et al. Extracorporeal shock wave lithotripsy in children. Eur Urol 2001; 39:591–7.

25. Vlajkovic M, Slavkovic A, Radovanovic M, et al. Long-term functional outcome of kidneys in children after ESWL treatment. Eur J Ped Surg 2002; 12:118–123.

26. Shukla AR, Hoover DL, Homey YL, et al. Urolithiasis in the low birth weight infant: the role and efficacy of extracorporeal shock wave lithotripsy. J Urol 2001; 165:2320–3.

27. Tiede JM, Lumpkin EN, Wass CT, et al. Hemoptysis following extracorporeal shock wave lithotripsy: a case of lithothripsy-induced pulmonary contusion in a pediatric patient. J Clin Anesth 2003; 15:530–3.

28. Young HH, McKay RW. Congenital valvular obstruction of the prostatic urethra. Surg Gynecol and Obstet 1929; 48:509–11.

29. Ritchey M, Patterson DE, Kelalis PP, et al. A case of pediatric ureteroscopic lasertripsy. J Urol 1988; 139:1272.

30. Shepherd P, Thomas R, Harmon EP. Urolithiasis in children: innovations in management. J Urol 1988; 140:790–2.

31. Kourambas J, Delvecchio FC, Munver R, et al. Nitinol stone retrieval-assisted ureteroscopic management of lower pole renal calculi, Urol 2000; 56:935–9.

32. Ptashnyk T, Cueva-Maratinez A, Michel MS, et al. Comparative investigations on the retrieval capabilities of various baskets and graspers in four ex vivo models. Eur Urol 2002; 41:406–10.

33. El-Gabry EA, Bagley DH. Retrieval capabilities of different stone basket designs in vitro. J Endourol 1999; 13:305–7.

34. Dretler SP. The stone cone: a new feneration of basketry. J Urol 2001; 165:1593–6.

35. Mulvaney W. Attempted disintegration of calculi by ultrasonic vibration. J Urol 1953; 70:704–6.

36. Piergiovanni M, Desgrandclamps F, Cochand-Priollet B, et al. Ureteral and bladder lesions after ballistic, ultrasonic, electrohydraulic or laser lithotripsy. J Endourol 1994; 8:293–9.

37. Schulze H, Haupt G, Piergiovanni M, et al. The Swiss lithoclast: a new device for endoscopic stone disintegration. J Urol 1993; 149:15–18.

38. Haupt G, Pannek J, Herde T, et al. The Lithovac: new suction device for the Swiss lithocast. J Endourol 1995; 9:375–7.

39. Ten CL, Fhong P, Preminger GM. Laboratory and clinical assessment of pneumatically driven intracorporeal lithotripsy. J Endourol 1998; 12:163–9.

40. Loisides P, Grasso M, Bagley DW. Mechanical impactor employing nitinol probes to fragment human calculi: fragmentation efficiency with flexible endoscope deflection. J Endourol 1995; 9:371–4.

41. Yutkin L. Electrohydraulic lithotripsy. English translation for US Department of Commerce, Office of Technical Services. 1955; Dic 62–15184 MDL 1207/1–2.

42. Grasso M. Experience with the holmium laser as an endoscope lithotrite. Urol 1996; 48:199–203.

43. Johnson DE, Cromeens DM, Price RE. Use of the holmium:YAG laser in urology. Lasers Surg Med 1992; 12:353–63.

44. Wollin TA, Teichman JM, Rogenes VJ, et al. Holmium:YAG lithotripsy in children. J Urol 1999; 162:1717–20.

45. Reddy PP, Barrieras DJ, Bagli DJ, et al. Initial experience with endoscopic holmium laser lithotripsy for pediatric urolithiasis. J Urol 1999; 162:1714–16.

46. Vassar GJ, Chan KF, Teichman JM, et al. Holmium:YAG lithotripsy: photothermal mechanism. J Endourol 1999; 13:181–90.

47. Cussen LJ. The Morphology of congenital dilatation of the ureter: intrinsic ureteral lesions, Aust NZ J Surg 1971; 41:185–94.

48. Minevich E, DeFoor W, Nishinaka K, et al. Ureteroscopy is safe and effective in prepubertal children. J Urol 2004; 171:551A.

49. Bloom DA, Morgan RJ, Scardino PL. Thomas Hillier and the percutaneous nephrostomy. Urology 1999; 33:346–50.

50. Rupel E, Brown R. Nephrostomy in hydronephrosis. JAMA 1955; 157:891–4.

51. Woodside JR, Stevens GF, Stark GL, et al. Percutaneous stone removal in children. J Urol 1985; 134:1166–7.

52. Hulbert JC, Reddy PK, Gonzalez R, et al. Percutaneous Nephrostolithotomy: An Alternative Approach to the Management of Pediatric Calculus Disease, Pediatrics 1985;76:610–2

53. Jackman SV, Hedkan SP, Peters CA, et al. Percutaneous nephrolithotomy in infant and preschool age children: experience with a new technique. Urology 1998; 52:697–700.

54. Mor Y, Elmasry YE, Kellett MJ, et al. The role of percutaneous nephrolithotomy in the management of pediatric renal calculi. J Urol 1997; 158:1319–21.

55. Gunes A, Yahya Ugras M, Yilmaz U, et al. Percutaneous nephrolithotomy for pediatric stone disease – our experience with adult-sized equipment. Scand J Urol Neph 2003; 37:477–81.

56. Helal M, Bloack T, Lockhart J, et al. The Hickman pee-away sheath: alternative for pediatric percutaneous nephrolithotomy. J Endourol 1997; 11:171–2.

57. Desai MR, Kukreja RA, Patel SH, et al. Percutaneous nephrolithotomy for complex pediatric renal calculus disease. J Endourol 2004; 18:23–17.

58. Kroovand RL. Pediatric urolithiasis. Urol Clin North Am 1997; 12:173–84.

59. Marberger M, Turk C, Steikogler. Piezoelectric extracorporeal shockwave lithotripsy in children. J Urol 1989; 142:349–52.

60. Thornhill JA, Moran K, Moomey EE, et al. Extracorporeal shockwave lithotripsy monotherapy for paediatric urinary tract calculi, BJU Int 1990; 65:348–50.

61. Picramenos D, Deliveliotis C, Alexopoulou K, et al. Extracorporeal shockwave lithotripsy for renal stones in children. Urol Int 1966; 56:86–9.

62. Van Horn AC, Hollander JB, Kass EJ. First and second generation lithotripsy in children: results, comparison and followup. J Urol 1969–1971.633.

63. Rizvi S, Naqvi SA, Hussain Z, et al. Management of pediatric urolithiasis in Pakistan: experience with 1440 children,. J Urol 2003; 169:634–7.

64. Tan AH, Al-Omar M, Watterson JD, et al. Results of shockwave lithotripsy for pediatric urolithiasis. J Endourol 2004; 18:527–30.

65. Al-Busaildy S, Prem A, Medhat M. Pediatric staghorn calculi: the role of extracorporeal shockwave lithotripsy monotherapy with special reference to ureteral stenting, J Urol 2003, 169:629–33.

66. Chuong CJ, Zhong P, Preminger GM. Acoustic and mechanical properties of renal calculi: implications in shockwave lithotripsy. J Endourol 1993; 7:437–44.

67. Erhard MJ. Pediatric endourology. Clinical Pediatric Urology, Fourth Edition 2002: 253–5.

68. Jayanthi VR, Arnold PM, Koff SA. Strategies for managing upper tract calculi in young children. J Urol 1999; 162:1234–7.

69. Badawy H, Salama A, Eissa M, et al. Percutaneous management of renal calculi: experience with percutaneous nephrolithotomy in 60 children, J Urol 1999; 162:1710–13.

70. Al-Shammari AM, Al-Otaibi K, Leonard MP, et al. Percutaneous nephrolithotomy in the pediataric population. J Urol 1999; 162:1721–4.

71. Zeren S, Satar N, Bayazit Y, et al. Percutaneous nephrolithotomy in the management of pediataric renal calculi. J Endourol 2002; 16:75–8.

72. Desai MR, Kukreja RA, Patel SH, et al. Percutaneous nephrolithotomy for complex pediatric renal calculus disease. J Endourol 2004; 18:23–7.

73. Casale P, Grady RW, Joyner BW, et al. Transperitoneal laparoscopic pyelolithotomy after failed percutaneous access in the pediatric patient. J Urol 2004; 172:680–3.

74. Caione P, DeGennaro M, Capozza N, et al. Endoscopic manipulation of ureteral calculi in children by rigid operative ureteroendoscopy. J Urol 1990; 144:492–3.

75. Thomas R, Ortenberg J, Lee BR, et al. Safety and efficacy of pediatric ureteroscopy for management of calculous disease. J Urol 1993; 149:1082–4.

76. Shroff S, Watson GM. Experience with ureteroscopy in children. Br J Urol 1995; 75:395–400.

77. Scarpa RM, DeLisa A, Porru D, et al. Ureterolithotripsy in children. Urology 1995; 46:859–62.

78. Smith DP, Jerkins GR, Noe HN. Urethroscopy in small neonates with posterior urethral valves and ureteroscopy in children with ureteral calculi. Urology 1996; 47:908–10.

79. Kurzrock EA, Huffman JL, Hardy BE, et al. Endoscopic treatment of pediatric urolithiasis. J Ped Surg 1996; 31:1413–16.

80. Minevich E, Rousseau MB, Wacksman J, et al. Pediatric ureteroscopy: technique and preliminary results. J Ped Surg 1977; 32:571–4.

81. Wollin TA, Teichman JM, Rogenes VJ, et al. Holmium: YAG lithotripsy in children. J Urol 1999; 162:1717–20.

82. Van Savage JG, Palanca LG, Anderson RD, et al. Treatment of distal ureteral stones in children: similarities to the American Urological Association guidelines in adults. J Urol 2000; 164:1089–93.

83. Schuster TG, Russell KY, Bloom DA, et al. Ureteroscopy for the treatment of urolithiasis in children. J Urol 2002; 167:1813–15.

84. Bassiri A. Ahmadnia H, Darabi MR, et al. Tranureteral lithotripsy in pediatric practice. J Endourol 2002; 16:297–260.

85. Satar N, Zeren S, Bayazit, et al. Rigid ureteroscopy for the treatment of ureteral calculi in children. J Urol 2004; 172:298–300.

# Index

Page numbers in *italics* indicate figures or tables

Printed and bound by CPI Group (UK) Ltd, Croydon, CR0 4YY

26/10/2024

01779571-0001